Best Marathons

Jog, Run, Train or Walk &
Race Fast Marathons
or your First Marathon

By

David Holt

Also by David Holt
5K Fitness Run;
Running Dialogue;
Best Half-Marathons;
10K & 5K Running, Training & Racing

And e-books:
301 Balanced Eating & Nutrition Tips
401 Injury Prevention & Treatment Tips

NOTICE

The information in this book is not intended to be a substitute for professional fitness or medical advice. As with all exercise programs, seek medical approval before you begin running and if discomfort occurs during or after exercise.

Contents   page

Holt's other Books Include.

Running Dialogue, 5K to the Marathon, 280 pages ISBN # 0965889742...An excellent first running book for beginners at short distances such as the 5K and 10K, through to the marathon.

Holt gently eases you into regular exercise and gives tips for your first race day, plus numerous programs based on the amount of time that you can spend exercising, or on the number of miles you wish to train. Includes nutrition, cross training, cartoons and essays.

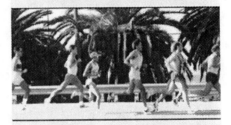

RUNNING DIALOGUE

A humorous look at HOW TO TRAIN...

FROM 5 k TO THE MARATHON

BEGINNER TO EXPERT

By English 31:16 10 K runner DAVID HOLT

Registered Nurse

5K Fitness Run, Walk, Jog & Train for Fun, Health & to Race the 5K. 232 pages, ISBN 0965889750. Jog and run programs, health tips, motivation, cross training and finding the time to run 12 to 30 miles per week.

Both books have numerous training programs to set you up for:

The program which starts at page 75 of this marathon book.

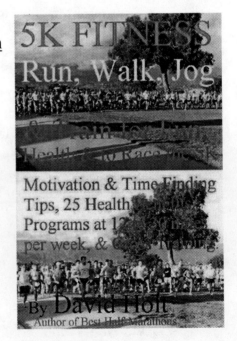

5K FITNESS Run, Walk, Jog

Motivation & Time Finding Tips, 25 Health Programs at 1 per week, &

By David Holt
Author of Best Holt Marathons

Introduction

Sir Isaac Newton's cousin said that "It takes strength to overcome inertia. The first movement can be the hardest." What she meant of course was that you had to get off your butt to get fit or to run a marathon.

Develop the resolve or strength of mind to maintain a steady diet of exercise, with most of that exercise consisting of running at the appropriate intensities and for a reasonable duration, and you'll be successful at the marathon.

These are exciting times for marathon running with Khalid Khannouchi, 5 times World x-country champion Paul Tergat, and Paula Radcliffe setting new world records by running their second half faster than the first half of the marathon. They all did so after years of racing at shorter distances. In September 2,003, the 34 year old Tergat and Sammy Korir became the first members of the sub 2:05 club; Tergat won by one second, so the record is his.

"The will to complete a marathon or the will to set a new personal record in the marathon is not as important as the will to prepare for that marathon," is this authors paraphrasing of New York City Marathon record holder Juma Ikangaa, who said "The will to win..." Winning the race is not an option for most of us, no matter how many miles we're willing to run or how fast we're willing to run some of those miles. Marathon completion or personal records are our victories.

Marathon training is not hard work; in fact, it's not work at all. You just put one foot in front of the other, alternating the lead foot for a few steps while _not_ getting short of breath. That is, you run at easy pace. Don't be afraid of the marathon. It is not a buffalo bearing down at you on a narrow, wooded trail. But like the shortsighted bison, the marathon can be a beast if you approach it from too short a distance. For the most part, keep your distance from the marathon.

However, by adding a small amount of mileage n weeks and a little bit of modest paced speed running, you gradually get used to more exercise, and of course, shift more rapidly during that exercise. You still won't out-run a buffalo, but you'll be able to run a marathon.

Fear of failure is given as an excuse not to run the marathon, yet if you train for the 10K and then the Half-Marathon, you'll easily move up to a whole marathon. You can squelch race day anxiety by having raced many times at the shorter distances, and by talking to people who have already done marathons.

You don't have to run the whole 26.2 miles for your finishers medal. One minute of walking every mile relaxes your running muscles, makes staying hydrated easier and is highly recommended for people who run slower than 9 minutes per mile. Eight minute mile runners should probably walk for 10 to 15 seconds through the liquid stations for fluid replacement too, but don't over-drink. Most of you will have more enjoyable marathon experiences by including walks in the race and during long training runs.

If you can tolerate 8 hours of work per day 5 days per week, you have the tenacity to run a marathon. If you've got the endurance to work 47 weeks per year, you can develop the endurance to complete a marathon. Endurance after all is:
*   The ability to hang in there;
*   To go the distance;
*   Sustain continuous activity for several hours;
*   The determination to keep going...based on having done something very much like it before;
*   Not quit due to laziness.
These are things that you achieve with every workday. You are a winner in life, and will successfully complete a marathon if you get up for work, or go out running on five days of most weeks, while doing the variety of running as shown in the first seven chapters of this book.

Problem with motivation or got a problem which you think will prevent you from doing a certain run? Get over it and get on with the run. Sometimes life is harsh. No matter. You still have things to do, including running. Cruise 30 miles per week while racing 10Ks if you have lots of stress. When your life is more stable, you can start a marathon program. Your short races and running will still be a positive achievement in your extended time of stress, and they will help you to cope with your stress.

Completing a marathon program is a major achievement. Adopt the right attitude about running and you'll achieve one mile farther every two or three weeks, and you'll achieve half a mile more of modest paced speed running compared to last month. Be a pessimist and you'll miss training days and you should commit yourself to the 5K or 10K instead.

Marathon training is not about giving your best effort every day. You need to exercise below the maximum that you could train at in order to conserve something for tomorrow's run. You achieve endurance for running by building up over several years (I hope) or many months.

You don't need a huge amount of time to train for a marathon. One hour on 3 or 4 days a week gives you most of your base training. On two of those days you'll train at modest intensity for the middle 30 to 40 minutes as shown in Chapters Three to Seven.

Once a week, you'll eventually need to devote 2 to 5 hours to the art of covering up to 20 miles at a time. You don't have to go beyond 2 hours until 6 months before your marathon, so even this does not dominate your life. You don't do this long run every weekend either. In fact, one week in four, you'll run half your of your usual mileage:
*   To rest up while your muscles adapt,
*   And to race for fun at the end of your easy week.

Best Half Marathons contains numerous tips on finding time for your short runs including: There's always enough time for the important things in life, but you have to decide what ˙ important to you. Walk a quarter mile to warm up w/

taking a few deep breaths to switch off from the rest of your life; organize nutritious snacks for just before and straight after exercise; always keep a set of running togs in your vehicle, and at work, and at your most frequently visited place; keep a set of cleaning items such as periwash or handi-wipes, a small towel plus deodorant; run before other people get up or before distractions have a chance to take over your day; it's OK to appear selfish at times, so block out a set time of the day and make your run the only priority for that time; run to or at the same time that your kids are doing their organized sports; adopt a dog; train to or from work, or park before you get home and do your run. Put a hammer to your TV and most people will find 14 to 21 hours per week for physical activity! Yet it's only during the last three months of marathon training that you need 10 of those 14-21 hours.

Don't run far in the early days; enjoy part or most of every run by moving at the right speed for that day. Relax at conversational pace and most runs are not hard or exhausting.

Run in pleasant low-stress surroundings such as parks and forests. While you will time most of your runs to work out your mileage, (total time divided by your approximate running pace per mile equals the distance you ran), on some familiar routes you can leave the watch at home and base the speed entirely on how you feel.

Marathon training will strengthen your mind, and give you greater confidence to finish a long task. Never run farther than 2 miles in your life? Don't worry. Add just 100 yards every day and you'll be adding 2 miles every five weeks. You'll move from 2 to 12 miles in 26 weeks.

Meantime, you're burning calories, getting stronger and fitter and more productive at work. Here's a surprise: Over time, active people gain less fat than inactive people.

Feed yourself properly and hydrate (Chapters 8 & 9), run slowly for the most part, and with people some of the time, do it 5 times a week, and a marathon is in your future.

In the second period of 26 weeks you can move from 12 miles to 22 miles in training, and be ready for a marathon. 2

times 26 weeks is a full year, which is less than half of the time you should allocate if you're not currently running at all. Yes people, take at least 2 years before you run a marathon.

There are 15 week programs in this book for the runner who is already doing an 18 mile run twice a month, and two speed sessions per week. But for newer runners the first rule of marathon training applies: Take it one step and one race distance at a time.

Inspired to get off the sofa after watching 20,000 people run a marathon? Running too much, too soon, can lead to injuries and burnout, so use *Running Dialogue* for a year of base training and to get fit for life while experiencing the 5K; then use *Best Half Marathons* to double or quadruple your race distance and perfect your running form.

Marathon racing is even friendlier and less intense than 5K racing. You will be running slowly enough to talk and be sociable during the entire race. The only challenge to the marathon is that you have to commit yourself to regular running, sensible eating and sufficient rest to be able to do it comfortably. Yet you should not need to run any more mileage than you would for competent 5K racing: you'll just run those miles in a slightly different combination. Marathon running will give you health, fitness, plus stress relief while achieving a modest challenge which half a million Americans accomplish each year.

Marathon training requires that you stress your muscles, then rest them to improve your running potential…the so-called hard training alternating with easy training method. A hard session is a run which is done for longer or is faster than your average run at your current level. Easy days are the relatively short and steady paced sessions, or cross training or complete rest from exercise.

Best Marathons and *Best Half Marathons* use the same running philosophy: Build up mileage and speed running in a sensible and graduated fashion using training phases to increase your chance of successful racing.

Best Marathons contains the extensive muscle and joints injury advice and over 60 pages on food and nutrition.

Best Half Marathons includes a detailed stretching chapter, 40 pages on cross-training, and health benefits of running.

The remainder of this introduction is adapted from *Best Half Marathons*. This author recommends that you <u>run</u> at least three half marathons, and <u>race</u> at least two more before embarking on a marathon training program. Then check runnersworld.com (Race Calendar) to find your marathon.

A Harvard study showed that 24 minutes of intense aerobic activity gives you most of your cardiovascular fitness gains:
* You need to get into shape to do 24 minutes intensely.
* Warm up, stretch and cooldown after your 24 minutes.
* So, 40 minutes per "session" will keep you fit.
In 2,002, the Institute of Medicine recommended 60 minutes of moderate activity every day to decrease risk of heart disease, high blood pressure, diabetes and cancer, and to burn enough calories to keep your weight stable. Moderate activity includes "brisk" walking at 4 miles per hour, and you can get most of the benefits from splitting your 60 minutes throughout the day.

The goal of this book is to take you well beyond healthy: The goal is to run the marathon or to run the marathon faster.

Currently overweight? Bill Bowerman, Dr. Kenneth Cooper and the late Arthur Lydiard were overweight and out of shape before they each discovered running for fitness and they influenced millions with their "Jogging and Aerobic" books and coaching advice.

The marathon is not a survival test...unless you enter it with insufficient training or start off too fast. The first mountain you climb should not be Everest. Your first race should not be a marathon or a half marathon.

The best way to train for a marathon is to actually train for a 10K, while also doing a 15 to 20 mile run most weeks; then train to race the half-marathon, while including a 20 mile run every 3 weeks; then go back to training for the 5K, while also including 15 and 18 mile runs; then commence a 15 to 40 week marathon program. Do each distance for one year, and you'll get 4 years of fun before your first marathon.

Or to paraphrase 1972 Olympic Gold Medalist Frank Shorter, "Train well and (occasionally) hard over a period of years, while avoiding major injuries, and you'll be successful at the marathon."

This book gives you the tools with which you can get into shape, or get into better shape! Some caveats:

* Start slowly if you're overweight.
* Start just as slowly if you're not overweight!
* Start even slower if you have cardiac disease. You are 10 times less likely to suffer a cardiac event during exercise if you're heart healthy. Got a history of cardiac disease? Start slowly and only after medical clearance. Your risk will go down as you lose weight and get fitter.
* Add only 15 minutes of exercise each week to your current exercise level.
* This will give you 10 to 15 miles per week or about three hours of exercise per week by the end of the third month if you're coming from sofa dweller.
* Set modest goals for this week and this month, while also looking forward to how you will feel next year. This way your goals will be achievable and sustainable.
* Review your goals every month or two.

Do this exercise for you, for how you will feel. Plan to see a healthier you in the mirror, and exercise often enough to make it happen. Then exercise for the rest of your life.

Make fitness fun and you'll exercise often. Be patient, enjoy every exercise session by moving slowly, without getting short of breath, for sustainable healthy exercise.

Enjoy the achievement of finishing your first mile OR your first 40 minute run. Do most exercise at 60 percent of your maximum heartrate...at about 110 to 130 per minute.

After a few weeks, do some exercise at modest tempo as shown in Chapters 3-7 and cross-train every week.

Run a variety of routes and distances, while wearing running shoes and running shorts. Then run longer or faster...as part of a graduated training program for a race, and enter more races in preparation for your marathon.

Make your children proud of you. Be their role model.

Train with other people sometimes, but run by yourself on some days. Both have their merit.

Push yourself moderately hard for a few minutes on some days while working on running form. Do not hammer your workouts. Instead of working out...exercise.

Eat healthfully without going to extremes. Review Chapters 2, 8 and 9. Train wisely by adapting any program in this book to your needs and abilities.

These marathon training programs will show you how to run often enough and far enough to build strength and endurance for the marathon. You will also run gently at speed to stimulate and educate all of your energy metabolism systems to cope with the marathon.

You'll take easy days after harsh runs. An 80 mile per week, 2 hour 30 minute marathon runner may run 7 miles at 7 minute pace on her easy days; a 40 mile per week 3:00 hour marathon runner may cruise 3 miles at 8 minute miles on his rest days. Either runner could add 30 minutes of cross training and still consider it a restive day.

Treat injuries by decreasing the type of training that caused them. Became injured two days after a track session? It was probably too intense or too long for you. Cruise steadily through this marathon training to keep injury risk low.

David Holt
Santa Barbara, January 4, 2005

CHAPTER ONE

BASE BUILDING

With LONG RUNS & MILEAGE

Chapters One and Three will take you from 30 or so miles per week with a long run of 10 miles each week, to 40 or 50 miles each week with a long run of 18 miles every other week. This phase will take you from one week to six months. Not currently running an average of 30 miles per week? Please put down this book, and go back to 10K training and racing until you can handle 30 miles per week.

Actually, the beginners program starting at page 74 starts at 20 miles per week, and builds to 45 miles over 25 weeks to reach your first half marathon. If you currently race 10K on 30 miles per week, you can get through this first phase of marathon training, and to your first half marathon in only 10 weeks.

Feel and act confident and optimistic about a successful outcome, and provided you restrain your bravado or pace, you'll complete the marathon.

However, the marathon has no mercy. Fail to run mileage and build aerobic muscle endurance and you will suffer.

Marathon training requires runners to be committed...err, that is, to be committed to mileage and endurance training. Once you've built a solid base or foundation to your training, you can move onto formal speed training.

Keep your hard earned and efficient running form from years of 5K, 10K and half-marathon training during your mileage phase. Run efficiently and you'll be ready to embark on a marathon training program with minimal injury risk. Run striders and fartlek, but restrict other speed running to low key intervals if you're increasing your total mileage.

Every type of run has a purpose. You will improve your running biomechanics and your aerobic ability during base training. As you know from half-marathon preparation, mileage training increases muscle size and strength; it strengthens tendons, ligaments and bones.

Continue to use cross training and weight training for additional strength, but don't bulk up; use many reps at modest resistance in weight training. Choose exercise which closely mimic running for your aerobic cross-training.

Marathon Training: Mileage Base for Strength Endurance.

To run a marathon, you have to run far and often. Aerobic endurance comes from long runs. Long runs strengthen your heart and other running muscles. Run long:

* Often: which means most weekends;
* Slowly: at 60 to 70 % of maximum heartrate;
* Slowly: 60 seconds per mile slower than marathon day;
* Sometimes with company: They'll remind you to hydrate;
* Relaxed: find some scenery and run with good form;
* Build up gradually: add no more than one mile per week to your longest runs;
* The long run you did two weeks ago will give you the confidence and endurance for this weeks run.

Your average weekly mileage means little unless you've also run far enough during your long runs. This continuous work bout is the most important run each week.

10K & 5K Running, and *Best Half-Marathons* strongly suggested that you race the shorter distances off of the same mileage as marathon training. However, for the marathon you <u>will</u> allocate your miles in a different way. Your long runs and your main speed session will be lengthened to add the endurance required to run a marathon in comfort.

Fairly new runners who are opting for the marathon at:
* *40 miles per week;*
* *For a 40 to 46 week training schedule;*
* *With little prior racing experience:*

will stay in Phase One of marathon training to build stamina, aerobic pathways, mitochondria, red blood cells and Myoglobin. Patience here will prepare you for the hill running, anaerobic threshold pace training and VO2 max enhancing intervals, which you will do in the next three phases. Better yet, spend at least a year training for the 10K, then another at the half-marathon to decrease your grief.

As you will see in Chapter Three, you fairly new runners will not ignore speed running during base training. You should run <u>fairly</u> fast every week of your life, but you should rarely run at maximum speed. Eight times 100 meters on the grass at 5K race pace is very relaxing 5 days after any long race; 8 relaxed striders are also superb the day after an 18 mile training run. Avoid running really fast let alone at close to maximum speed. Practice fast leg turnover at 5K pace with your striders, fartlek and hill sessions of Chapter Three and Four, while simultaneously getting used to longer runs.

To run well at the marathon, you need to put in long runs, and decent mileage. How long should your long run be?

Top British coach, and frequent contributor to the British Athletic magazines, Frank Horwill, says that "Physiologists believe steady runs should be at least 35 minutes to get a training effect.

"Exercise physiologist David Costill reports the volume of steady running alone at 80 percent VO2 max improves fitness by as much as 12 percent to 80 miles per week. After that, there is very little return for the mileage expended. A good way of building to this volume is to add 5 minutes per day per week to the running. A 35 minute per day runner will reach 70 minutes in seven weeks."

Not all of your runs will be 70 minutes. Some days you will cruise for 50 minutes or cross train as a rest day. Stress your muscles too often and you will injure yourself or get chronically fatigued resulting in a decrease in performance instead of improving performance. You need rest to improve, so the basic schedules of Chapter Three and beyond are based on 4 key runs per week, and three easy days.

Sadly, while we can measure VO2 max, it's a poor predictor of marathon performance. However, while you are improving your VO2 max, you're also improving your running economy, which can vary by 30 percent, and can give you more than twice the 12 percent improvement that the improved VO2 max offers your marathon.

Lets get back to that crucial longest run of the week.

In *10K & 5K Running*, this author recommended that no more than one third of your weekly mileage be done in one run. However, low mileage marathon runners may need to run half of their weekly miles in one run on alternate weeks. The 40 mile per week person will run several 20s leading into the marathon race. The schedule in Chapter Eleven shows that these people also run a 14 to 16 miler in their easy weeks. To get through these long runs in comfort, start out at the pace that you can maintain for the entire run, or perhaps 15 seconds per mile slower than that for the first 5 miles and then gradually speed up to goal pace for the day.

Just like in the marathon itself, you need to have interim goals. The knowledge that you will run the first 6 miles in 62 minutes, and the next 6 miles in 60 minutes sets you up to run at the right speed, to hydrate and fuel during the first two hours, and to enjoy the third 6 mile segment in 58 minutes. Keep the running fun by being at the right pace for your legs.

If you're feeling bad after what should have been an easy 6 miles at the start of your run, try to assess what is wrong. It could just be a bad patch; most of us have them. It could be that the temperature is 15 degrees higher than usual and so you'll need to slow down by 10 to 15 seconds per mile.

Note: The 60 miles per week runners' long run will only be one third of their weekly training.

True beginners to this game will now be training for a 5K while edging mileage up toward 20 miles per week. Some of you will need to alternate substantial periods of walking into your runs in order to stay upright instead of uptight for 40 minutes at a time. *5K Fitness Run* is probably the book for you, or you could use Chapter Sixteen of this book if you have some kind of disease which requires that you do mainly walking for a marathon, or which precludes you from ever going above 25 miles per week while preparing to complete 26.2 miles in one day.

For the rest of you, remember that the action of running 5 miles sets the physical ability and the motivation to run for 6 miles. Running a six reinforces that you'll reach 10 miles in another 6 to 8 weeks. Find the right groove and relax your way through gradually increasing long runs.

Run at the right intensity, especially in your early days. The muscles adapt quite fast to increasing demands but your bones, ligaments, tendons and joints take much longer to get stronger. Keep your cardiovascular system under minimal stress by running at 60 percent of your maximum heartrate until your entire running frame is used to regular physical activity. Talk a lot while you run because it will decrease the tendency to run too fast. When you've raced a 5K you'll be ready for the gentle speed running of Chapter Three.

Visualize success while following Chapter Three's build-up and enjoy these longer runs. Feeling tired? Get on with the run at the right speed, with good running form, and picture your perfect run in ideal conditions. Swap positive thoughts for your negative thoughts. You still have muscle fibers in reserve, just waiting to help out, so change pace by 10 or 15 seconds per mile for variety. After 200 meters a bit slower, and 200 a bit faster, settle back to even speed and do form checks for arm movement, head position and stride length.

Pace changes on long runs with friends are best done by easing off for a hundred yards or more to drop back 10 or 15 yards behind, then cruise back up to the group. You can also practice pushing off with the entire foot to use the calves properly, but take shorter strides and land softly.

You'll discover your running boundaries by gradually increasing mileage and the intensity of some of that mileage. Most of you have enormous possibilities for improvement.

Many of you are currently doing a long run of 8 to 10 miles each week. Add one mile each week until you reach 17, then add one mile every other week while doing a 16 on your easy weekend. You'll cruise up from a 10 mile run to alternating 16s and 20s after 13 weeks or 3 months.

Long runs are a chance to daydream and get the stresses out of your life by taking a break from them or find the resolution to a problem. You can also daydream about running 400 meter repeats 2 seconds faster per repeat next month as you get fitter, or imagine yourself in races for Gold medals, or running down opponents. Do these while running at appropriate pace and they'll do you good.

Visualization is another useful trick to help you maintain good running from in the last few miles of long runs, or the last third of speed sessions. Visualize success, prepare for it mentally and physically and your outcome is more likely to be what you want, especially if you run with good form.

Every 4 to 6 weeks take a lower intensity week to:
* Consolidate your fitness gains;
* Allow your muscles and connective tissues to adapt;
* As you rest up for a race at the 10K.

You will also end your marathon program with one or two runs which keep you on your feet for the same length of time that your marathon does. Because you'll be running one minute per mile slower than marathon pace, these runs will be about 22 miles.

If you take longer than two and a half hours for your long runs, it is prudent to insert walk breaks of one to two minutes every 15 to 30 minutes, usually in the shade and in conjunction with your hydration breaks.

If you take longer than three and a half hours for your long runs, it is prudent to do part of the run later in the day, that is, split your 20 miles for the day into a three hour morning run with the balance of your mileage in the evening. The long run is the key to marathon success, so once a month, cruise with walk breaks for up to four hours in one session.

The American College of Sports Medicine recommends taking in 5 to 12 ounces of liquid every 15 to 20 minutes. At 15 to 48 ounces, this is a huge range. Do page 53s sweat loss test to find out how much *you* need to replace every hour, and then train your stomach to absorb higher amounts of liquid during long runs. Make allowances for the 4 pints you'll be getting from metabolism of glycogen etc.

Marathon runners have a 70 percent less risk of dieing from a heart attack than unfit people, especially if you heed Chapter Two's hydration advice and don't make sudden changes to your training.

What about Fast Running?

Your commitment to mileage and the long run for endurance training should not neglect striders, fartlek or your current interval training. Your current speed running should sustain and improve your running form while you get used to longer runs. Don't give up your legspeed and efficient running form during this strength phase.

If you've been running marathons without any speed running, ease into the fartlek training of Chapter Three.

For newer runners, your increased mileage may take you close to your injury threshold...the point where you are close to injury; the decisive mileage ceiling could also be the amount you can handle mentally. It may be 40 miles or it could be 60 or more miles per week.

Increase mileage by about 10 percent per week on average, until you reach your unique limit, or if you are lucky, your goal. Your muscles improve if stimulated by the right amount of exercise and if given sufficient rest. The training effect is best achieved with a structured training program in which you gradually increase duration and intensity of training, with copious rest days for your muscles and enzyme systems to make their improvements.

The schedule on pages 75 to 76 takes 20 weeks to double your mileage toward your first half marathon race. Any time you feel twinges in your muscles, consolidate for a week or two before increasing again. Sick with a cold during week 14? Enjoy a couple of short easy runs, then repeat weeks 12 and 13 before resting up for your 10K race. Don't worry if you need 30 weeks for this first stage.

If you ran 60 miles per week last year, but you've been enjoying a low-key 35 miles for several months, jumping back to 55 miles over two weeks may not strain your already sound physique. But why rush? Adding 10 percent per week requires only six weeks to reach 60 miles.

While building up your training you can add a few minutes to each run, or you can add half a mile at a time: the net result is increased mileage.

Taking short, yet rapid strides during all running reduces your injury risk. By landing with a slightly flexed knee, between the outer heel and the midfoot and then rolling rapidly through the ankles for quick cadence, and pushing forward instead of upwards from the end of your toes, you can stay low to the ground, decreasing landing shock. Run over the ground with a light step, as if onto eggshells, instead of through the ground. Practice short strides at 90 to 95 steps per minute for each foot during easy runs *and* speed running, and you'll run more economically.

Seek Variety.

The runner who was on low mileage while racing short distances, or the newer runner may have problems coping with boredom during high mileage and long runs.

Unless you have a death wish, avoid headsets for entertainment. Instead, use your brain to plan out different routes, then use it again while running, and you'll rarely be bored. You're rarely stuck on a motorized belt to nowhere. Even if you do run on a treadmill occasionally, other athletes in the room will amuse you. Practice the art of observation and their antics can entertain for hours. Don't get involved with the silliness of people competing for exercise equipment.

Most of your running will be outside. The sheer volume of running makes treadmills a poor choice to prepare for a marathon. According to a study by exercise physiologist Sarah Hooper, people enjoy outdoor running more than they do indoors and get a better workout, running faster for the same heartrate when outside, which is amazing when you consider there is no wind resistance on a treadmill. However, treadmills can help you to run at constant pace while you practice economical running form. Most runners take shorter strides on a treadmill, so this will decrease your overstriding.

Make your higher mileage even more fun by using parks, trails, quiet streets and bike paths. Give way to horse riders and cyclists as appropriate, soak up the scenery, and think about your running form. Exercising outside is a mood enhancer, especially in the winter, and in daylight.

Those of you with a long history of marathon training can still run high mileage in Phase One, but restrict your longest run to 15 miles half of the time. Leave your muscles fresh to practice fast running the rest of the week.

Keep "economy enhancing speedwork" in your weekly schedule if you're increasing mileage, but keep most of the new mileage at 70 percent of your maximum heartrate. Maintain the higher mileage for at least eight weeks before working through phases two to five of marathon training.

No matter how much you like the person, don't follow someone else's training program. Don't even follow the programs in this book. Instead, develop a training mix that is appropriate for you. Running more than fifteen miles twice or three times per month is not for every runner. You may function better at the marathon with one twenty mile run per month and a fifteen three times per month.

Basic Marathon Training Program:
This is one way to allocate your miles: For details on gradually reaching this level see page 75.

Day One *(Saturday)* Some form of speedy running at no faster than your 5K race pace or 95 percent of your maximum heartrate (max HR); Afterwards or later, cross-train.

Day Two *(Sunday)* Longest run of the week at 60 to 70 % of max HR.

Day Three *(Monday)* Short easy run, including 4 to 20 gentle striders of 100 meters but not sprints.

Day Four *(Tuesday)* Cross train and an easy run.

Day Five *(Wednesday)* Your second speed day, usually at 85 to 92 percent of max HR, or half marathon to 10K pace.

Day Six *(Thursday)* The second longest run of the week.

Day Seven is for a rest.

Detailed schedules are in Chapters 3, 11, and 13 to 15.

Beginners, Intermediate and Experienced Runners, or, Serious, Moderate and High Intensity Marathon Runners.
There are many levels of training intensity. For convenience, coaches concentrate on three main intensities of training. All three types are represented at all weekly mileage levels.

Some high intensity trainers race the marathon on 40 miles per week; some lower intensity runners enjoy 60 miles per week. Intensity is partly dependent upon how many total miles you put in each week, but also depends on how many quality miles you run, or how many miles you run faster than marathon target pace.

High intensity runners will run faster than marathon pace about three times per week, and amass 25 to 30 percent of their mileage at 5K to half marathon intensity or speed. Most high intensity trainers will run a quality fast session on Saturday, then run off the effects during the long run the following day. They've probably been running for several years and will rotate many familiar speed sessions on Saturdays. All training will improve your running form, speed and strength provided you either learn to relax at speed, or to relax while doing a long run.

Day One might be five miles of 400 meter repeats or quarter miles at 5K pace, or 800 meter reps at 10K pace, or it could be five times one mile at 15K pace, or hill repeats. If you've been used to running these sessions while training for 10Ks and half-marathons, you can still run VO2 max, anaerobic threshold, or hill sessions during base build-up, but do keep the emphasis on increasing your base by increasing the length of your long run.

The **moderate intensity runner** may have just as much running experience as the high intensity person, but choose to run fast twice a week, getting 15 to 20 percent of her mileage at 5K to half marathon effort. Fast running is only hard on your body if you jump into it suddenly. Add a quarter mile at modest speed each week to avoid the harshness of faster than marathon pace running. For many runners, two speed-running sessions per week is the perfect scheme to achieve fast and satisfying marathons.

The <u>serious runner</u> may train at speed once per week, for about 10 percent of his mileage. In the early days, your long run may feel quite harsh...it can feel like a hard run. In the early days of marathon training it is crucial for you to start your runs slowly. Run too fast and your muscles will get tired and fill up with lactic acid, the waste products of anaerobic running. Your running action becomes labored. You'll be forced to slow down...which is demoralizing. Start all your runs at 60 percent of max HR.

Keep the pace to 60 percent of your max HR until it begins to feel easy to you. Then increase toward 70 percent for the second half of long runs. Pace should be one to 1.5 minutes per mile slower than marathon goal pace.

Most writers would call this the novice or beginner group, and shun speed running. This authors' philosophy is that the people who benefit most from speedwork ARE the novices. Speedy running improves your running form and efficiency. One fartlek session per week can bring the same benefit as half of your other mileage. There are no recreational runners in marathon running. When you're running one speed session each week, you are at least serious runners; many runners in this group have been training for years.

The training levels then are:

High intensity;

Moderate intensity; and,

Serious runners.

At all three levels, the long run is crucial. At all three intensity levels, you should be able to run just as fast tomorrow as you do today. Don't run so hard or fast or long on any day that it prevents you from doing a similar session tomorrow. Of course, during Chapter Three and Four's hill training you will not run hill repeats every day for 10 weeks. Instead, you'll do them once a week but be able to cruise 10 miles effortlessly the next day. Don't completely exhaust your muscles with any one session. It's the accumulation of four balanced runs per week which gives you "marathon training" instead of huge sessions that you detest and an injury. You should not run 20 miles on back to back days, but the pace of training runs must be slow enough that you could.

Several studies show that you can complete a marathon on 4 runs per week provided you include many long runs during your build-up. Don't skimp on or wimp out of your long runs. Include at least one speed training day each week at the right pace and you'll increase the enzyme activity in your muscles, giving you more energy: you'll also be off of the marathon course quicker than most people.

Your Mileage Base Will:

* Add muscle: 3 to 5 percent more muscle mass, giving you strength or endurance, which is the foundation for additional strength training with hills in Chapter Four.
* Develop strength endurance in your diaphragm and intercostal muscles, allowing you to breathe in deeper, more often, more forcefully. Ventilatory muscle movement or breathing can use 10 percent of your oxygen, so make them deep enough: no panting.
* Enlarge the chamber size and stroke volume of your heart, increasing the quantity of blood pumped out with each heart contraction, improving you cardiac output by 35 to 40 percent. Note: Elite athletes will still have almost twice as high cardiac output than you, but only a 50 percent higher VO2 max than you.
* Expand your capillary network, to bring in nutrients and excrete waste products.
* Increase your blood volume, which takes most of the carbon dioxide to your lungs for excretion. Your red blood cells (RBCs) get diluted by your blood volume, so you may appear anemic on blood tests.
* Increase the size and total number of (RBCs) in your system, which brings oxygen to your muscle cells. The hemoglobin in RBCs has a high affinity for oxygen, which allows it to pick up oxygen through the lungs alveoli.

* Increase Myoglobin within the cell, which delivers oxygen to the mitochondria.
* Increase the size and number of your mitochondria, which are the engines of oxygen use in your muscle cells.
* Build bigger muscle fibers...in your heart and in your other running muscles.
* Net result: you take in and distribute more oxygen.
* Improve your fat burning ability. Forget about the fat burning zone because we burn fat all day. Long runs teach your muscles to burn fuel efficiently. The muscle cells burn fat and sugar (glycogen) but you'll learn to conserve the sugar if you do many long runs during your training.

Expect a reduction in your body fat by 10 percent and a reduction in your body fat percentage too.

The more of the above factors which you improve with training, the more you will enlarge your aerobic ability, or your maximum oxygen uptake capacity. You'll gain resistance to fatigue or increased fitness as a high percentage of your muscle fibers are able to contract for long periods. You also train your Type II muscle fibers to work for long periods at modest capacity instead of only for sprinting.

You will also do some quality running to educate your muscle fibers and nerves to improve your biomechanics to work efficiently at faster than marathon pace.

Marathon Running Ability is determined by:

* Mechanical efficiency or physical economy, including how much of your energy you retrieve through your elasticity to pass onto the next stride.
* The efficiency inside your muscle cells. Getting ATP from glycogen and glucose, plus muscle fibers contracting on minimal recovery.
* Contractility: Your force or power.
* Resistance to fatigue of muscle and of your mind.

Fortunately, running is very simple: You train moderately hard, and then take a rest. This is the stress / rest or hard then easy approach. Stress your muscles a bit, let them rest and they'll gradually get better at doing what you ask of them. Rest regularly each week and take an easy week once a month (to rest up for a race at 5K to 10K on fresh legs).

Rest is different for each runner. High mileage runners may run 10 miles at 70 percent max HR on a rest day; Serious or beginner marathon runners may get insufficient rest from an easy 3 mile run. They may need a complete rest from impact with the ground exercise. The rest week every three to five weeks should be 25 to 40 percent fewer miles than your normal training week. You will normally celebrate the end of your rest week with a race of about 10K.

The Right Speed.

The higher mileage build-up for racing a good marathon should not be a slow mileage build-up. Run your long slow distance at or just above 60 percent of maximum heartrate. Stay close to 60 percent in the early runs; once you've run several long ones, further stimulate your cardiopulmonary or cardiorespiratory system by running at 70 percent.

For most runners, 60 to 70 percent of max HR is about one minute per mile slower than marathon pace. In your early marathon training, your pace will be slower because you lack aerobic fitness and you lack running efficiency. You get tired easily.

When you've done many long runs your maximum oxygen uptake or VO2 max will increase, so you'll be able to, indeed you'll have to run faster to reach 60 to 70 percent of max HR. The long runs will also teach you to run economically, so you'll use less oxygen per mile, and you'll therefore run faster still at 70 percent of your max HR.

Economical running will make up for a low inherited VO2 max. If your VO2 max is 60 but you're able to run a 10K at 95 percent of your VO2 max, you'll be faster than the uneconomic runner with a VO2 max of 70 who despite a sensible training program can only maintain 80 percent of his VO2 max for a 10K.

Note: 80 to 82 percent of VO2 max would be an average athletes marathon pace. 95 percent is an average athletes 5K pace, so maintaining 10K at 95 percent of VO2 max requires truly efficient running.

There is little point in getting your VO2 max tested because it does not predict how economically you're able to run. Your races give a better predictor of performances at other distances.

How fast should you set your marathon goal time?

Multiply current 10K race time by 4.66 and you'll have a rough target. Run a 34 minute 10K? 34 x 4.66 = 2:38:27.

Noakes (*Lore of Running*) page 80 uses 5.48 x 10K time minus 28 minutes. Thus (5.48 x 34) − 28 = 2:38:19

See Chapter Ten for other prediction options, then work out your pace per mile for the marathon and add 60 to 75 seconds per mile for those long runs. Not raced a 10K yet? Spend a year at that distance as an apprentice runner before contemplating races at longer distances.

The 10K is a great predictor of marathon performance because it factors out natural strength / speed demons who fade at longer than the 5K, and factors in much of your fatigue resistance from mental and physical resources. The mileage which develops your coronary arteries and your muscle capillaries to run a great 10K will also be key ingredients for maintaining close to 10K pace for the entire 42K and 195 meters of the marathon.

The 10K time to slot into the prediction equation is your best time after spending a year at constant mileage, preferably the same mileage that you will use to prepare for your marathon. You should also have done the types of training espoused in this book's Chapters Four to Seven, namely 15K to 3K pace, including hill training.

44

Sixty to 70 percent of your max HR is also your easy running pace for rest days, allows you talk easily in 8 to 10 word sentences and is slower than marathon goal pace.

These short runs:

* Satisfy your need to exercise through running, and
* Improve your marathon fitness. Provided you:
* Keep the easy runs short enough. Probably 30 minutes for low mileage and newer runners and up to 60 minutes for experienced guys.
* Keep your muscles fresh enough to run your quality sessions well, and
* Complete your quantity sessions (long sessions of speedy running) in reasonable comfort.

Maximum Heartrate Calculation.

Long runs at 60 to 70 percent of maximum heartrate teach your muscles to burn fat for fuel. Burning fat takes 10 percent more oxygen per mile than burning glycogen or sugar; fat burning predominates only at modest speeds.

So, start your runs at 60 percent of max HR, and you'll burn more fatty acids early in the run. Speed up to 70 percent of max HR for the second half of the run, and you'll be able to burn the glycogen supply which you had conserved. This practice is still more effective if you are on high mileage.

Run eighteen miles once every three weeks for 6 to 12 months during your marathon preparation, and you will be well on the way to educating your muscle cells in the skill of fat use and glycogen conservation.

Untrained people store about 280 grams of carbohydrate in their muscles, but well trained runners store up to 720 grams after just one or two rest days, and 880 grams with carbo-loading before a marathon. Your liver also increases its glycogen store by 30 percent, which helps to maintain blood glucose levels to your brain during exercise, which will keep you more alert to cope with your fatigue. You're better able to motivate yourself to maintain pace in the last quarter of long runs and races. Your long runs also teach your muscles to store more glycogen for use during future long runs. It takes a series of long runs to completely train your marathon muscles to store energy and to run economically. You also need to consume a moderate amount of carbohydrates!

You can't completely exhaust your glycogen supply or ATP: some of it is never available for you to run. It stays in reserve to keep you alive after you've collapsed!

How do you know what your maximum heartrate is?
Newer runners can subtract their whole age from 220.
Veteran runners can subtract half of their age from 205.

Been running several months? You're ready for a max heartrate test. Two weeks and one week before your max HR test, warm-up, and run 6 to 8 x 100 meters fast so that you're less likely to strain a muscle during the actual max HR test.

For your test, warm-up with about two miles at gentle pace. After stretching, run three or four striders of about 100 meters. Then, run all-out for 60 to 90 seconds. Veterans can do this up a hill. After a rest, run all-out again, but pace yourself to reach total exhaustion at 60 seconds. If you reach exhaustion midway, you'll be running slower at the end and the lower reading from the heartrate test will mislead you into a slower pace (at which) to do your steady runs.

At the point of maximum exhaustion, check your pulse for ten seconds and then multiply by six. Or read your heartrate monitor. The number will either be your maximum heartrate (HR), or the maximum level at which your body or pain threshold allows you to exercise.

Steady mileage trains all of your Muscle Fiber Units.

Sarcomere: The Muscle Contraction Unit.

The sarcomere is the contractile unit of muscle: It's an all or nothing situation. The sarcolemma (the nerve), either fire the sarcomere to contract or it doesn't. It's just like an electric switch, either on or off. The total amount of a muscle's contractile power is dependent upon how many of your sarcomere contract at one time, how strong the sarcomere or fiber is, and how long it takes before they can contract again.

Your Mileage & gentle Speed Training will:
* Boost the number of sarcomere which can contract at any one time,
* Make each sarcomere stronger,
* Increase the frequency at which they can contract.

Improve all of these factors and you will be able to run fast for a longer distance. You'll be able to run a marathon closer to your half-marathon race pace.

Muscle efficiency is stimulated and improved by long runs, but also by quality running such as fartlek and hill training. Weight training and other cross training also play a role in making muscle cells more efficient, provided your extra muscle bulk does not adversely effect your running form.

Twice a week weight training can reduce injury risk by 44 percent. Strength training improves agility, flexibility, speed and balance, especially if you include exercises such as lunges while holding dumbbells. Cross training gives your cardiovascular system a good workout, strengthens running muscles, plus exercises the muscles which don't usually work much during running, and reduces injury risk.

Weight and resistance training increases the number of myofilaments in each sarcomere. When letting the weight down in the leg press it's an eccentric contraction, which fatigues and damages the quadriceps just like downhill running or overstriding does. The muscle fibers get stretched while the muscle acts as a brake. So do regular weight training to build up your muscles and run perpendicular to the slope with short strides to improve your elasticity and resistance to fatigue and see page 97.

Muscles work in groups. Some are <u>synergistic</u>; they help each other to do one main function. For example: the rectus femoris, one of the quadriceps, lifts the thigh and makes the knee go straight. In lifting the thigh, it is assisted by its synergists the iliosoas muscle group and the sartorius. Its knee extension role is assisted by the other three quadriceps.

For most muscles, there's also a muscle or group of muscles which relaxes as the first group does its work. When the quadriceps fires and shortens in its work phase, the hamstrings at the back of the leg lengthens simply by resting or not contracting. The hamstrings are the <u>antagonist</u> for the quads, although this author prefers <u>complementary muscle</u>.

A run only program can make some muscle groups too strong and they strain their complementary muscle due to imbalances. Weight train twice a week and cross train and you'll be balanced for running, and also decrease injury risk.

Running when injured can strain all of a synergistic group. Strained the middle of your rectus femoris with hill training? Take some rest time or you risk straining the now overworking sartorius and iliosoas muscles. Train through an injury and you also risk straining the muscles in your other leg as they compensate for your weaker leg. Use these tips:

* Don't make sudden changes to your training schedule;
* Add a mile or two to your long run every two weeks;
* Add half a mile to your speed session every two weeks;
* Work within the limits of YOUR body;
* Don't add more than 10 percent per week, and only for three weeks at a time. Consolidate, then move up again.

If something hurts, stop running. However, if it is just mild fatigue from yesterdays fairly long session, and you feel relaxed after an easy first mile, keep going.

First time marathoners may take 26 weeks to reach their mileage goal. During these 26 weeks you should also bring in the fartlek running which is discussed in Chapter Three.

Running is easier after Stretching.

Stretch regularly and slowly because flexibility or long muscles will reduce your injury risk. Stretch before and after running to maintain your full range of movement.

Newton said "that for every action there is an equal and opposite reaction." Runners convert much of the forces (action) on landing instead of wasting it. Up to 30 percent of your propulsive power comes from the stored energy of your springs and shock absorbers on landing. Keep your muscles and tendons strong and flexible with weight training and stretching, and feed your collagen fibers well to maintain their elasticity, or their ability to stretch on the run.

Be pedestrian with these exercises: do them slowly, with no bouncing. Stretching slowly avoids the myotatic reflex...which shortens your muscles and can lead to micro muscle tears. Hold each stretch for 15 to 30 seconds and repeat each stretch two or three times. Breathe rhythmically. Warm up with a little walking before your stretches.

Here's a set of stretches for the major muscle groups.

<u>Calf Muscles:</u> Stand 3-4 feet from a wall, put your outstretched hands on the wall, shoulder width apart. Keep the knee straight and the heels flat on the ground. Lean in toward the wall slowly, keeping the body and knee straight: Stop when you think the calf is at its limit; when it and the Achilles tendons feel stretched.

Next: as above but 2-3 feet away. Bend the knees until you feel the stretch. For both stretches keep your heels on the ground. Try to press your heel into the ground

<u>Quadriceps and Psoas & Iliacus</u>: (the last 2 are also called the iliosoas group). The front of the thigh. Stand upright, hold one foot and pull it up toward your bottom while keeping the knee pointed downwards. Get the bent knee even with your weight bearing knee if possible; keep your hips tucked inward. You can do this stretch in the prone position too, or lying on your side. Knees should be next to each other.

Or, Kneel on a comfy surface, and bring your left foot forward to rest between your hands, then push your right knee back slightly but keep it on the floor. Push your hips forward and feel the stretch in muscles of the right thigh. You'll also stretch the left legs gluteals. Push your chest up for a deeper stretch. Switch legs.

Hamstrings: Back of the thigh: Sit on a soft surface, keep the knees straight and bend forward at the waist. Move your head down toward the knees or beyond.

Or: Place your foot on a support at knee height or a little higher. Some people say that your weight bearing leg should be straight. You're stretching the muscles of the leg which is up, so the choice is yours. With hips facing forward, a slightly bent knee if you wish to reduce the strain, and a straight spine, ease your chest toward your knee.

Inner thigh: Sit on the floor with the soles of your feet together. Push your knees slowly toward the floor.

Or lie next to a wall on your back. Keeping your butt close to the wall, swing through 90 degrees to place your feet up the wall with straight legs. Gradually split your legs to a 90 degree angle at the groin.

Hip muscles, which include the gluteals: Stand upright, or lie on your back on a comfortable surface. Grasp one leg at the shin; pull your knee up toward your chest.

Ileotibial or I-T band: As above, but bring the left knee across the chest toward your right armpit; then re-stretch it toward the right side of your pelvis. Do the right knee to your left side.

Trunk: Stand with your feet apart; keep your hips facing the front. Bend over to one side as far as possible, hold, and then repeat to the other side.

Next, keeping the hips facing forward, rotate the top of the trunk to look behind...hold, swing slowly around to the front and then to the other side.

Lower Back: Feet together or apart, knees bent or straight. Bend over and ease your hands toward your feet. Just hang loose; let the tension go, but don't force it.

Fatigue takes longer to affect a strong trunk or core and reduces your injury risk, so do resistance training too.

The all-purpose leg stretch (below left) does most of your running muscles if you do it with alternate legs on a support. Elliptical training (right), pool running and cycling encourage gentle eccentric or elastic stretching while you exercise, and also reduces the cumulative damage from ground impact.

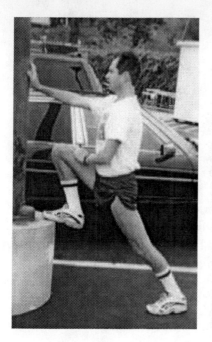 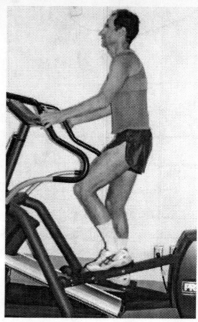

Find a training buddy for some of your runs. You don't need the same goals, though a similar pace makes life easier. The long run at the weekend and the key speed sessions are easier in a group. Friends make catching temperature related dangers and injuries easier.

Safety is vital when you're running solo. Take a self-defense class for its tips on avoiding trouble spots, see page 44s tips, including to carry mace or halt in your hand, and never try to out-run a dog.

Unless you're on a treadmill, never use a musical device.

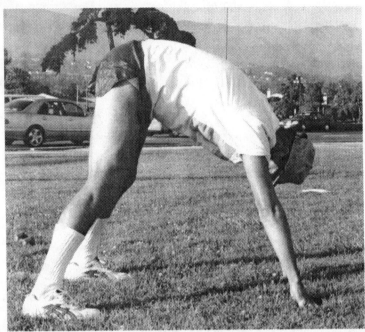

Yoga's downward facing dog (above) is a great way to stretch the hammies, calves, Achilles tendons, shoulders and lower back. You, of course, will be in an inverted V.

Stretch or myotatic reflex.

Near the junction of tendon and muscle lie muscle spindles and Golgi tendon organs (also called proprioceptors) which initiate the tendon-muscle reflex to prevent a muscle from lengthening too far. If the muscle tension is too high, the muscle will not be allowed beyond a certain length. Hold a stretch for 20 or so seconds, and this deep myotatic reflex eases...your muscle is allowed to go a percent or two longer...which is why you should hold a stretch, then seek a little extra pain free elongation after 20-30 seconds.

Mental or physical fatigue?

Dehydration, lack of carbohydrate, starting too fast and many other mistakes can make us feel running fatigue earlier than usual. Correcting the mistake and relaxing running muscles can reduce the amount of energy needed for X-pace. When you add repeats in later chapters, you'll need all of your resources to get through some sessions. So, begin to practice associating with your little aches. Use all of your running muscles to propel yourself forward, and picture yourself achieving your first 12 mile run or whatever run it is today.

You can also use progressive relaxation of muscle groups once a day. Lie down in a peaceful setting and tense, and then relax each muscle group in turn. Breathe slowly.

Using association, progressive relaxation, plus keeping a running diary or journal will decrease your injury risk.

Don't get worked up before any workout or you'll stimulate your sympathetic system, which wastes energy by increasing heartrate, oxygen consumption and lose of fluid. Stay relaxed for track sessions and races too. Got 12 times 400 meters at 5K pace planned today? No problem, because you did 10 repeats at the same speed three weeks ago. By staying relaxed with good running form you'll feel just a bit more fatigue than last time. If you get too excited, you'll waste energy with the sympathetic nervous systems overkill, run 4 seconds too fast for your first repeat, and do only 8 repeats.

Control is even more important on race day. If you let your adrenaline surge take you through the first mile 20 seconds too fast, your day will be hilarious for its discomforts instead of for your achievements. Practice pace control with a race at 5K to 10 miles every 4 to 5 weeks.

Long Runs in the remaining Four Phases. The best way to run fast and comfortable marathon races is with negative splits, which means running the second half faster than the first. Starting off too fast due to poor pace judgment dooms you to discomfort and a slower second half. Years of practice races at the shorter distances and preparation with over 50 runs at 15 miles or more will teach you how to pace your marathon.

Most runners only need to run too fast in the first 5 miles of a 20 mile run on one occasion to learn their lesson. Also:

* Set a realistic target based on performances at 10K to the half-marathon. 4.66 times your 10K time is realistic if you run 50 miles per week, with 10 runs of 20 miles during the 26 weeks leading into the marathon, and with an average of 10 miles per week (split between two sessions) at faster than marathon pace. Longer races are more reliable, so multiply your half marathon time by 2.15. Practice negative splits by picking up the pace by 10 to 15 seconds per mile for the second half of your long runs.
* Run negative splits in short races. Practice with mile repeats in which the last half mile is 5 seconds faster than the first half a mile. Start fartlek sessions at 15K pace and run your last few efforts at 5K pace.
* Hydrate and feed your muscles.

Getting ready for your first half marathon? The race predictor by Pete Riegel predicts your half marathon to be about 2.223 times your 10K, or 1:14:40 for a 33.35 10K runner who will slow by 17 seconds per mile from 5:25 per mile to 5:42. A 46:11 10K runner should slow from 7:27 miles to 7:50s or by 23 seconds per mile. On race day, you should run 10 seconds per mile slower for the first 6 miles, then speed up to dream pace to come in one minute slower than Riegel's prediction. Next time aim for even pace at 2.223 x your 10K. Page 75 to 76 has a program to run your first half-marathon.

Speed up on long runs.

Average pace for your long run 8 minutes? Run the first ten miles at 8:10 pace and the second ten at 7.50 pace. This will teach your muscles to conserve glycogen because you'll be running slowly enough to burn more fat in the first half. Make the last mile an 8.10 as your cooldown, and you'll feel greater motivation next time because you ended the session in comfort. You'll also decrease stiffness with a cooldown. Cool downs after speed running also leave you feeling pleasant.

In your marathon, be more positive. Run the first ten miles two percent per mile slower than average pace. The eight minute marathon runner will start out at 8.10 pace. Note: Our 8 minute per mile marathon <u>trainer</u> of the previous paragraph should be racing at 7 minutes per mile average. Two percent gives you a 7.08 per mile start and 6.52s for the second half.

On courses with early downhills such as the California International, you would need to run at 7.08 mile effort, which would give you about 7 minute mile running pace for the first 10 miles. The second half is flat, so 6.52 effort should give you 6.52 miles. Your finish time ought to be faster than for a flat course because the elevation loss gives you up to two minutes for nothing. Run any faster in the first half and you'll have dead legs from the downhill impacts, and a shortage of glycogen because you worked instead of cruising the first 13 miles. The downhill affect is even more significant at the Boston and St. George Marathons.

After a few of these negative split training runs, add two miles at close to tempo intensity during some of your long runs. At mile 15, speed up to marathon pace for a mile, then return to training pace. Three weeks later do the same thing, but add a second mile at speed from mile 17 to 18. You will still have two miles to cool off.

Fartlek Pace for Novices:

Do a couple of 5K races to find the maximum speed at which to run during fartlek training. Run half of your fartlek efforts at 30 seconds per mile slower than that 5K intensity, and then run half of your fartlek efforts at 5K intensity (enlightenment comes in Chapters 5 and 6). Or run one whole session at 30 seconds per mile slower than 5K pace, with a separate session each week at 5K intensity. Either way will give you nicely balanced yet enjoyable speed sessions. Run them on grass and trails and your muscles and joints will adore you.

Now, a sidebar on the joys and perils of heat and cold.

Chapter Two

Safety First.

Long runs have the potential to increase your "exposure" to the risks of hypothermia, dehydration, hyperthermia, heat exhaustion and heat stroke.

If you feel warm at the start of a run or race, you're probably overdressed, and will soon overheat. You can overheat due to too much clothing on chilly days, and you can get hypothermia on quite mild days due to under dressing and the wind chill.

Cold causes three times more injuries than heat, so lets start with:

Hypothermia:
Coping with Training or Race Day Cold. In a
design fault of its maker, the human body is more efficient when its temperature has risen to just over 100 degrees Fahrenheit. This is one of the reasons you need to warm up before speed sessions and races.

On cold days, you must stay at this temperature, so dress to keep it in. You may require tights or lightweight track bottoms for the legs; you may need a long sleeve running shirt with running vest on top and possibly a T-shirt between. Make sure two of these tuck into the shorts...many shirts shrink over a period of months.

Synthetics are better than wool. The layer next to your skin must wick moisture away so that your body heat evaporates it through your top layer while your skin remains essentially dry. Wear lightweight gloves. To avoid over-heating, these can be dropped off at a friend's feet if the race has circuits; you can also arrange for someone to be at for example, the three mile point in a long road race. Or drop them off at the one mile point, and pick them up in the warmdown.

Except in long races, avoid the cold drinks on offer. Dehydration is rarely a problem in winter...unless you were drinking alcohol the previous evening, or forgot your fluids in the morning. A warm drink one hour before and half an hour before the start may be required if the race is more than 10K.

Avoid standing for long periods before the start. It will make you tired and allow you to cool. Go to the start area at the last practical moment after your warmup. Wear a throwaway top layer and stay out of the wind.

Provided you start at realistic pace and wear the right amount of clothing, chilly days should not be a problem. Even pace is vital: if you slow during the second half, the cold soon gets to you. If you have any doubts about your fitness, give cold race days a miss. The onset of a cold or throat infection must be treated seriously: give the medics a break and stay at home.

During training runs, you're more likely to need a hat and a waterproof, breathable jacket. However, this form of jacket can cause over-sweating, and lead to dehydration or chills. The hat is the best temperature regulator; take it off to lose 25 percent of your heat.

Wearing several layers of clothing will insulate you from a certain amount of cold, but you need to keep moving or despite that inner layer wicking the moisture out, you'll get cold because you're not dressed for slow walking or standing.

Take care of your appendages in cold weather. Keep the ears, nose and hands covered if it's below freezing. Vaseline works nicely, and cover the vaseline with clothing when appropriate. Some days you'll be dressed like a bank robber in ski mask; other days, you'll look less menacing.

If you get your feet or hands wet on training runs, be prepared to change course to get dry stuff on sooner. You can always do your last 5 miles in different shoes and dry socks if you went through icy puddles. No dry cloths available? Keep moving or get inside a warm building and exercise until you either warm up enough to get home safely, or your ride arrives to rescue you. Swallow your hubris and make that phone call to get you home.

If it's raining, poor planning is the number one cause of cold injuries. After all, if the temperature is below 32 F the precipitation will not usually be rain. Metal manhole covers are slippery when wet, so ease across them with a light step. Jumping them can lead to falls or strained hamstrings.

Running on fresh snow is a thrill. Running on iced snow is more dangerous and slippery. When the snow is too deep for running shoes, you can do what 1983 World Champ Grete Waitz and the late Emil Zatopek did...wear boots. You could also run in the newer design and narrow snowshoes. Only got a small section of road that is runable? Waitz would run back and forth over the same quarter mile when she needed to.

Hypothermia is technically, a body temp below 94 degrees Fahrenheit. However, some people exhibit the following signs at higher temps:

* Fatigue: extremely tired, more so than usual;
* Cold: the whole body may feel chilled, sweating ceases;
* Shivering; Slow pulse;
* Lightheaded: not high, just silly...leading to
* Slurred speech, as if drunk and less alert;
* Loss of body actions: the running becomes a stagger or shuffle and you'll wander across the course;
* Unreasonable behavior: loss of temper, perhaps violence, and of course, the runner insists he or she can finish the race or training run; Can lead to complete collapse.

Treatment:

Get yourself or the person you have spotted with this problem out of the cold and wind.

Remove wet clothing. Wet skin can lose 25 times more heat than dry skin. Replace with layers of warm, dry clothes.

A shower or bath can restore warmth to the body, but a cold, drafty shower room is of little use. Gradually increase the temperature of the water toward 105 Fahrenheit. No heat pads because there's a high propensity for burns.

Do not rub the body to warm it up; gentle massage may be of use. Putting feet or hands into warm water will help; blood flow to the extremity increases, takes in the heat and takes it back into the central core. Tingling on re-circulation is good. No tingling, or skin numb when warm? See an MD.

Give warm drinks, plus a simple energy source such as chocolate. Then give warmer, nourishing drinks once the body can handle them. Keep soup on hand for emergencies.

If you're able to do so, keep the person moving and they will generate their own heat. Otherwise, use warm blankets or the heat retaining foils such as Mylar.

No alcohol. Alcohol doesn't warm you, but it can kill you by further dilating skin blood vessels, which results in losing still more of your precious body heat.

Exposed skin can freeze: On the other hand, running in the cold air cannot hurt the lungs because your air passages and bronchial system warms the air.

Respect the cold but don't be frightened by it. Heed the wind chill factor. While 40 to 60 degree windless days may seem ideal for setting fast times, many personal records have been set by people wearing three shirts.

As the temperature is usually lower at night, lets consider additional night running safety.

* Wear reflective clothing and something white to be seen.
* Carry a small flashlight to help you see and to be seen.
* Know your terrain from daylight runs.

* Yet vary your actual route and time of running to avoid predictability from potential assailants.
* Know the neighborhood; know what types of people are in this area at the time of day that you run.
* Seek out lighted running or biking trails and bike lanes, or run toward the on-coming traffic, or the left side of the road in the United States.
* The sidewalks at cross streets are high: don't fall, trip, or run into vehicles. Obey foot traffic rules.
* Don't use a musical device or look well dressed. Leave the Rolex at home and wear long sleeves covering your $20 stopwatch.
* Find a couple of busy running tracks to run gentle striders even if you don't socialize with anyone.
* Carry halt or mace and keep your senses alert to the potential to use it. Stretch only in a safe area.
* Don't run to exhaustion. When training through Chapter Five's anaerobic threshold sessions, focus on mile or so efforts with a 2 minute mental and physical breather instead of 30 minute efforts.
* Run with someone, especially if you are female.
* If you've come to your senses and realized that life is not better for having a cell phone, cancel the service, but keep the phone charged because you can still use it for 911 calls. Carry it on your runs.

Wind Chill.
How wet you are, the speed you're moving at, the temperature, and the wind, all play a factor in heat loss.
* Wind chill index is below -25 Fahrenheit? Avoid biking.
* Warm up before stepping out of the door.
* Layer your clothing.
* Wear a HAT which covers your ears; 25-40 percent of heat loss is from the head.

* Exercise at the warmest time of day, or when the wind is at its slowest and run into the wind on the way out and get pushed back on the return.
* Exercise in sheltered areas when possible. Houses perpendicular to the winds direction and woods offer protection from the wind.
* Change into dry clothes immediately after exercising.
* Don't hang around getting cold while talking afterwards.

	Wind speed (mph)								
	Zero	5	10	15	20	25	30	35	40
	50	48	40	36	32	30	28	27	26
T	*40*	37	28	22	18	16	13	11	10
e	*30*	27	16	9	4	0	-2	-4	-6
m	*20*	16	4	-5	-10	-15	-18	-20	-21
p	*10*	6	-9	-18	-25	-29	-33	-35	-37
	0	-5	-24	-32	-39	-44	-48	-51	-53
	-10	-15	-33	-45	-53	-59	-63	-67	-69
F	*-20*	-26	-46	-58	-67	*-74*	*-79*	*-82*	*-85*
	-30	-36	-58	*-72*	*-82*	*-88*	*-94*	*-98*	*-100*
	-40	-47	*-70*	*-85*	*-96*	*-104*	*-109*	*-113*	*-115*

Note the relatively large increase in the chill factor at modest wind speed. There is a much greater increase from 5 to 15 mph than there is from 25 to 35. Mild winds can kill.

Running in the Heat.

Just like the internal combustion engine, you waste prodigious amounts of your energy as heat. You only use 25 percent of your energy to make yourself move. Most of the rest is wasted as heat. Fine in winter, but getting rid of internal heat can be a problem in summer.

Losing this excess heat works best when:

1/ The air temperature is below your body's, so that you don't absorb more heat from the atmosphere.

2/ There is air movement, the body moving or the wind.

3/ The air is able to take up more water, or to evaporate the sweat. Very little sweat will evaporate at 100 % humidity.

The worst situation is a high temperature, high humidity day with a slight wind from behind. Think **danger.**

What is the effective (or wet bulb) temperature experienced by your body during your typical 8 mile run at 95 degrees and mere 70 percent humidity? The table below shows 124 Fahrenheit. However, do your run early in the day or later at 85 F, and despite the fact that the humidity will have risen to about 90 percent, your effective running temperature is a mere 102 F. You'll still need to take liquids with you, but 102 is much more tolerable than 124.

If there is a 10 mile per hour breeze this day, have someone drive you 8 miles out so that you can run into the wind for the entire run. This technique can take the effective temperature down another 10 degrees. Stay hydrated with minimal clothing on and most people can run effectively during the summer.

Got a threshold pace session on a high temperature and high humidity day? Slow down and run it based on heartrate instead of speed, or do it later. Stay out of the sun when possible. If it's 90 degrees out, and there has just been a short shower, the humidity can go up 20 to 30 points as that moisture quickly evaporates. Unless you're running while it's actually raining, and running into the slight breeze which often accompanies these showers, the equivalent temperature can go up 25 degrees or more.

		80	85	90	95	100...real temperature
		Equivalent Temperature (Fahrenheit)				
Rela-	40	79	86	93	101	*110*
tive	50	81	88	96	*107*	*120*
	60	82	90	100	*114*	*132*
humi-	70	85	93	*106*	*124*	*144*
dity	80	86	97	*113*	*136*	Death Valley
(%)	90	88	102	*122*	Death Valley	

More heat index info at crh.noaa.gov/arx/heatindex.html

When the index is above 105, curtail your pace and include modest amounts of salt and potassium in your liquids.

The smog factor is often a concurrent problem on hot days. Most people know the smoggy areas and time of day that it peaks at home. Check air quality at weather.com for more guidance. Example: the ozone peak for Los Angeles is late afternoon…but ozone is a greater danger in the mountains around Arrowhead downwind from the smog source.

The general rules are to:
* Exercise up-wind from smog sources,
* Early in the day, and
* Stay at least 50 feet from congested streets at all times.

Slow moving vehicles pump out huge amounts of carbon monoxide and nitrous oxide. Run in the central part of parks and avoid the trails which are often 20 feet from a road.

Dehydration.

According to one study, almost half of the exercisers at a major fitness chain *started* their exercise session dehydrated. Drink before you get out of bed and while driving to the gym.

When training in even modest temperatures, humans sweat, and blood vessels near the skin dilate to allow heat to escape. This takes up to 20 percent of your blood to the skin and away from your muscles and takes fluid out of your circulatory system. The end result is dehydration. Your heart has less volume to pump out and eventually you'll sweat less and your body temperature rises.

Exercise and sweat for long enough periods without replacing liquid and your performance decreases. You may also become dizzy, creating many dangers for you.

Once you're dehydrated, your heartrate would have to increase to maintain the same volume per minute through your muscles, enabling you to maintain the same exercise intensity. If you're already at the maximum that you can sustain for your current run, you'll be forced to slow down.

Alternatively, if you stay at the same pace, and force your heartrate up, you will not be able to keep running at the same pace for as long as you had planned. Your body does try to acclimatize when you first go to a hotter environment.

* Urine output decreases; blood volume increases;
* Sweating becomes more efficient;
* But it takes two to three weeks to adapt to the heat;
* Avoid the harshest workouts for the first few days of a heat wave or vacation.

To Reduce Dehydration Risk,

do your anaerobic threshold running as long repeats on dirt trails and with two minutes rest in the shade instead of as a tempo run on asphalt. Run them based on heartrate, not pace; you'll be closer to half-marathon pace than 15K pace on hotter days. When you do VO2 maximum training as intervals of one to two minutes, take recoveries in the shade.

Running longer repeats at 5K pace with short rests gets you out of the heat faster. Example: Excluding warm-up and cooldown, 20 x 400 meters in 90 seconds with 90 second rests takes 58.5 minutes. Running 4 x 2K with a 3 minute rest only takes 39 minutes, plus you'll get a far greater percentage of the 5 miles of speed running at your goal heartrate.

Plan your racing to decrease heat problems. Atlanta doesn't seem like the ideal place to race a 10K in July, yet thousands of runners do so without problems.

Preparation for hot race day conditions is easy to

plan, but can feel harsh while you're doing it, so make your changes gradually. To prepare for hot and humid conditions:

* Run close to the hottest time of day, which for many places is 2 to 5 pm, whereas the suns worst damage to your skin occurs between 10 am and 2 pm.
* Wear a synthetic shirt that provides some SPF protection, because these usually let you get rid of heat very quickly; an additional teashirt on top gives you heat training.

* If you live in a cooler part of the country, a lightweight tracksuit or tights will stimulate the body's response to racing in the heat. Don't overdress though.
* Put your sunscreen on and run in the sun to get used to the heat, and for the delight of feeling it on your SPF 30 protected skin. Wearing sunscreen also helps you to dissipate heat faster. Lotions, sprays and zinc oxide all have their uses for skin protection.
* Make a point to avoid the shade while wearing a dark cap to keep the heat in. On race day, a white mesh cap with a bill could be your choice. Poor water on it too.
* Run on asphalt for some of your mileage for its refracted heat instead of dirt and grass which would keep you cool.

Run two quality sessions per week in the cool, or using heat avoiding techniques so that you can run fast enough to maintain your legspeed.

Hot weather running is a form of resistance training. Just like you do at altitude, you can train at a slower speed for the same heartrate on high humidity / high temp days. At slower speeds, you're less likely to get a muscle injury. But stay well hydrated and consume plenty of fruit for their electrolytes.

In the early stages of a long run at modest pace, say 70 percent max HR, you will be able to maintain pace. However, as the run proceeds, as you become more dehydrated, you'll be working at and then beyond 80 percent of max heartrate. Yet the damage to your legs will be at 70 percent of maximum speed. You would have an altitude training effect from the dehydration, but it is something you should avoid because of its potential to harm. Stay hydrated and your heartrate can remain at 70 percent of maximum!

Racing on Hot Days.

Most races start before 9 a.m. On the big day, wearing your lightweight running vest which the breeze goes through, you can concentrate on the race. Clothing should be loose and light in color. Avoid standing in direct sunlight for prolonged periods pre-race. Find a breezy, shaded spot. Better yet, stay in an air conditioned area until the last moment to decrease glycogen use, to slow lactate build-up, and most importantly, to delay your gradual temperature increase. Gentle stretching will suffice for the warmup; do a few gentle strides without a tracksuit and you'll be ready to go.

Drink sufficient fluids before the race. Some peoples' stomach cannot handle citrus fruits just before a race due to their acidity: Try actual melon, cantaloupe and grapes, plus apple or cranberry juice to provide liquid, electrolytes, simple calories and rapid liquid and sugar absorption. The fructose will be converted to glucose in your liver and come online in hour two of your race or training run. During the race you'll need glucose, maltose, glucose polymer, maltodextrins or high glycemic foods for more rapid uptake and to preserve your liver and muscle glycogen. Fructose is absorbed slowly, though it is useful if combined with other sugars.

Get used to drinking on the move. This is best done by taking half a cup of liquid, cover most of the top with your hand, and pour a mouthful at a time. You can tuck a straw in your shorts to make it easier to drink. Sponges can be used to cool the head, neck and the main muscle groups (thighs). Cooling your head can persuade your brain that you are not too hot, but liquid inside of you will actually keep you below 104 F longer. Don't get all your running stuff wet; wet socks increase your blister risk; shoes get heavy.

Even pace is the aim. When the temperature or heat index is really high, start off slower than normal. If you misjudge the pace, you must consider dropping out. Although you will feel bad at the time, you'll feel better than if you'd ended up in the first aid or medic vehicle with heat exhaustion.

You can have your good run another day. The other reason to drop out is to avoid the plodding and suffering for the last three quarters of the race. This will leave a mental scare of greater magnitude than dropping out.

The damage from starting off too fast is usually done in the first two miles or the first 10 percent of the race. The damage from failing to rehydrate is done in the next 10 miles or 40 percent of your race. Sadly, the USA Track & Field recently changed its fluid guidelines to "drink only when you are thirsty." The Marathon Medical Directors Association recommends a mere 8 ounces every 20 minutes.

Please ignore both ideas and drink based on your sweat loss rate of page 53. Rehydrate early, before you feel the need. Like the inactive bulk of the population, your thirst center is a laggard. You will not get the message to drink until you're already 2 to 3 percent dehydrated, and at race pace, you'll never catch up the fluid deficit. Most of us can run 10 miles without feeling the need to drink, but we are definitely dehydrated by then, and your last 16.2 miles is ruined because you never catch up the deficit. If you only run fast enough to sweat out 24 ounces per hour, that is the right intake for you.

Most of the above is relevant when training. Organize your long runs around drink sources. Wear a fanny pack to hold your liquid bottle because hand held bottles effect running form. You also have to carry the weight twice if it's in your hand, and move it too. Diluted fruit juice (one-quarter strength) or sports drink (add a little sodium to both) decreases your risk from dehydration. The pleasant taste will encourage you to drink more of it, and the electrolytes will replace the minimal amount that you lose in sweat.

Part of your hot or humid day training course should be shaded. There should be several cut-off points so that you can shorten runs. Listen to your body. Is it over tired from the previous day's training, or are you at the beginning of a slight illness? In the former case, a long run at a sensible pace will be ideal; in the latter, a shorter run or rest is required.

Eating smaller, more frequent cold meals can help during a hot spell, preferably, with cold drinks. Stay in a cool place before and after exercise to help prepare for exercise and to recover from your session.

Avoid chronic dehydration by checking the color of your urine. This should be nearly clear before you start running. To conserve liquid, your kidneys virtually shut down on commencement of exercise. Your urine will usually be dark or orange after a session; it should return to its normal pale yellow within a few hours if you drink during and after the run. If you consume B vitamins, your urine will remain dark for several hours, so use the volume of your voids to estimate hydration status. Daily weight is also a guide. If you suddenly drop 4 pounds in two days like on crash Hollywood or high protein diets, it's obviously a shortage of liquid.

Use a good mix of several fruit drinks and vegetable juices, decaffeinated tea or coffee, non-fat milk and water after your runs; if you want to avoid most nutrients, use sports drinks.

Use caffeine in moderation. While caffeine does not dehydrate over the course of the week, it's a diuretic in the short-term. Caffeine an hour before running is a stimulant to your bowels and your running, and encourages you to consume liquid. One to two caffeine servings will not dehydrate you if you start exercise soon after its consumption, but drink caffeine free stuff to flush out the caffeine and to make sure your liquid intake is high enough. Caffeine constricts blood vessels, which can be fine if you want to clear a headache, but is not good for running muscles.

For hydration, it doesn't matter what you drink, according to a University of Nebraska Medical Center study. During a three day period one group took half its fluid from plain water while the other group had only juice, coffee, and coke. At the end of the trial there was no difference in hydration. The caffeine may keep you awake, and excessive empty calories will make you fat, but at least you will not be dehydrated!

If you take a 9 day winter trip in the south, starting with a race on the first day, remember to do your other 8 high mileage and high quality days at *modest* pace. Days 2 and 3, recover from the race with steady runs at 60 to 70 percent of max HR. You could do anaerobic threshold intensity on the

4th and 6th day, but leave your VO2 max session for day 8 or 9. If you've had months of steady running, do it at 5K pace; don't push for 2 mile pace. Then you can finish with the longest run of the vacation the day before you go home, and feel pleasantly wasted for a day or two afterward. After all, you'll appreciate a couple of very easy days on return to colder climes. It will take at least a week of gentle training to recover from the 9 days of heavy training, and for your body to adapt fully to the vacation's effort.

Attempting a track session when free of encumbering track suits at 3K pace early in the week invites a frustrating vacation via an injury. You don't go south to lounge around by the pool with an injured hamstring because you assaulted your body with 3K speedwork just 2 days after a 15K race.

Sweat Rate or Sweat Loss Test.

The standard sweat test is to weigh yourself, run for 30 minutes under normal conditions, then re-weigh yourself. Your naked weight (before and after running), on an electronic scale will allow you to work out your weight loss via sweat. Multiply by two to get your hourly loss. Here's a more accurate system for real endurance athletes.

Start off well hydrated and run for 30 minutes. By now you've warmed up your muscles and your sweat rate has reached a high level to dissipate the extra heat. You lose minimal sweat until your muscles are warmed. Any weight loss in the first 30 minutes gives an ineffective number to use for your marathon training, let alone your racing.

Void, drink one pint of low sugar and electrolyte liquid, strip off and weigh yourself. Because you've warmed up, your kidneys will now conserve water; you should not need to void in the next hour. Put your damp clothing back on. You lose heat by evaporating your sweat, so don't start with another set of dry clothing or the test is lame. Your wet clothing allows you to lose muscle heat by conduction; your clothing may get a bit wetter during the test hour, but sweat loss will show a closer correlation to the middle miles of your marathon than the first 30 minutes of exercise would.

Put 24 ounces of liquid in your bottle holder to keep you psychologically comfortable during your <u>one hour</u> test run. Run out for 30 minutes, then run back to your scale. Drink about 6 ounces every 12 minutes and your last drink will be 12 minutes before the end of the test.

Because you need to know how much you'll sweat on race day, an anaerobic threshold session from Chapter Five is the logical choice for this sweat test. Three minutes at half-marathon pace alternating with 3 minutes at 30 to 45 seconds per mile slower than marathon pace as recovery works well. If you're doing this test after working through Chapter Five, you could do a marathon pace tempo run for most of the 60 minutes, or 5 times 10 minutes with a 2 minute rest.

Do the test under harsh conditions. Race day expected to be 90 degrees? Test yourself in these conditions.

Finished your hour run? Strip and re-weigh yourself. Original weight plus the 1.5 pounds of fluid taken in, minus finishing weight gives an accurate weight loss per hour.

The number of ounces you lose per hour is the number of fluid ounces you need to replace each hour. When running, liquids should be replaced with an ounce for every ounce of weight loss. Divide your hourly loss rate by 6 if you rehydrate every 10 minutes; divide the loss rate by 4 if you drink every 15 minutes. You do have some wiggle room though.

* Because you can hyperhydrate, you can start off with a couple of bonus pints inside you.
* Carbo-loaded? Glycogen stores water too and should provide 3 pints (1280 grams according to one study – because three-quarters of glycogens weight is water).
* Give yourself a one percent body weight buffer.

Performance drops off significantly at more than a two percent of body weight loss due to liquid shortage. A 150 pound runner therefore has 3 pounds to play with before slowing down. Use half of this liquid buffer only if you must, such as during the last six miles or 40 minutes of your marathon. Hardly drink at all in the last section as it will not be in your circulation in time to benefit you, unless of course you've already bonked due to poor hydration status.

Lose a net 4 pounds in your sweat test and you'll need to consume 4 pints per hour during long runs and races. Take four hours for the marathon? That's 16 pints. However, the three stared items on page 54 give about six pints of liquid, leaving you only 10 pints to drink during the race. That's still 8 ounces every 10 minutes, or one pint every 20 minutes!

The three hour marathon runner gets a bigger bonus. Her 12-pint sweat loss, minus the 6 pounds from the stared items means she has essentially only 6 pints to replace. She needs a mere 8 ounces every 15 minutes. The 6 pint intake is <u>essential</u> to prevent her losing more than two percent of body weight.

Calculate weight loss based on your weight three days pre-race. Your extra drinking and carbo-loading adds liquid to your system. Avoid losing more than two percent of your normal weight during the marathon and your speed will not be decreasing due to dehydration. However, speed in the last 10 miles may be decreasing due to lack of training, increased or decreased body temperature, or from starting off too fast.

It takes less than a 2 percent fluid loss for your thermoregulatory system to begin failing. At 2 to 4 percent body weight loss, muscular endurance decreases. At 4 to 6 percent loss your muscles are significantly weaker and cramps occur...leading at greater than a 6 percent loss to heat exhaustion, heatstroke, coma and death.

Sipping and perspiring is for girlies. Runners drink and sweat. While wacky Aberdeen researchers did show that gulping fluids down after a workout leads to more urine production, which is actually a good thing, if you only sip your liquids it's awfully difficult to replace the 4 pints that you lost in the last hour of running. In the first 10 minutes post run, zap a goodly amount of liquids into your belly my fellow runners, then continue to press that liquid out of your stomach by topping it up every few minutes. Include tomato juice, V8 and fruit for their electrolytes, gradually get back to your pre-start body weight, and stay there until your voids are of sufficient quantity and frequency.

Shower with a deodorant soap before a marathon and you will not need to decrease your sweating with an anti-perspirant. Don't block the sweating process or you'll lose less body heat. Use deodorant if you must, but it will be hours before bacteria working on your sweat could give you BO. Some runners do have smelly sweat, but it's usually due to the food they eat, burning protein or fatty acids secondary to low carbohydrate intake.

So, dehydration and raised body temperature lead to a decrease in performance. Heat injury risk increases. Drink water or a 5 percent sugar solution before, during and after exercise. Drinking fluids has a more profound effect on your cooling system than pouring it over your head. If copious supplies are available though, a dunking can help. The first cup always goes inside.

Beer has many things in its favor as a source of electrolytes and energy, but most of the energy is not from sugar. Alcohol dehydrates, and increases the sensation of fatigue on any day, so decrease consumption prior to racing in hot spells. You can decrease alcohol dehydration by matching each pint of beer consumed with a pint of water. However, don't use it as an excuse to do the reverse.

Don't drink more than 2 alcohol servings any evening before a key training session because your muscles will hurt more and fatigue earlier. Practice alcohol moderation after hard runs too. Other factors that decrease the liquid in your muscles' circulatory system include:
* A fever, diarrhea or diabetes;
* A high protein diet such as the zone or Adkins;
* Taking in too much sugar and electrolytes: Liquid will rush to your intestines to dilute and absorb the sugar.

While it's busy doing that, it will not be bringing oxygen to your muscle fibers. (see hyponatremia on page 58)

Chronic dehydration occurs from daily exercise or saunas and jacuzzi time without catching up on the lost liquid.

Heatstroke & Heat Exhaustion:

For most people, the first is a nasty exacerbation of the second. However, you don't actually need to exercise to get heatstroke. Sitting in direct sunlight on a hot day can give you heatstroke. Fatiguing your muscles in relatively modest temperatures can give you heat exhaustion. Official temperatures are 105 Fahrenheit for heatstroke and 102 for heat exhaustion. You may get heat exhaustion at 101 or 103.

Some sources say that heat exhaustion is when our muscles can no longer perform due to fatigue or dehydration; they add that heatstroke may not involve fatigue, but is mainly a very high body temperature. Don't worry about the nuances because most of the treatments are the same.

The body will feel hot with pale, clammy skin. Thirst, headache and dizziness are typical. Reduction of the brains blood flow causes confusion, and poor or complete loss of coordination. Other signs are similar to hypothermia concerning how the body feels and reacts. The result is loss of coordination and confusion. If the high pulse rate does not decrease on cessation of exercise, and if sweating has ceased, total collapse can follow.

Got heatstroke or heat exhaustion?

* Get out of the sun and stop exercising;
* Cool the body by getting more air contact;
* Face the breeze or a fan, or have someone fan you;
* Removing the shirt is optional. A wet shirt can cool you if the shirt is refreshed with cold liquid;
* Sponging or pouring cool water over yourself helps too.
* Drink cool liquids with electrolytes and sugar (see below);

* A cold body of water such as a lake, ocean, river or shower is invaluable. Supervise the person. Keeping the clothing on is fine. You do not have to strip off.
* Get those water and sports drink bottles out of the ice container and ease your friend in to his shoulders while having him sip a cool salty drink. Ice packs help too.

Low blood sugar (hypoglycemia) may be a concurrent problem; simple sugars may be required to get the brain back into action. A small amount of salt may also be needed to replace what's been lost in sweating. As a general rule, extra salt is not required once the body is used to warm weather running: minimal salt (half a teaspoon, about 2,000 milligrams, in 2 pints of sugared solution) can be given for the initial muscle cramps.

Cool fluid and cooling the body is the important thing. Get them to drink as much as they can tolerate without becoming nauseous. Don't overhydrate. Reach pre-race or pre-run weight. Don't exercise to the point of nausea in the first place. If the pulse rate doesn't decrease, the runner should be taken for medical attention.

An overstated problem: Sweating too much, combined with low sodium intake, and if further exacerbated by drinking too much liquid, can lead to hyponatremia, a blood-sodium level which is below normal. The man who died at the 2,002 Boston marathon was drinking excessive amounts of sports drink, and diluted his blood to its low sodium level despite the presence of some electrolytes in his liquid. At a sodium osmolarity of 20 mmol per liter, most sports drinks contain only one-third the amount of salt that is in our blood (60 mmol). If you drink water or sports drink, sodium rushes into your intestines before you're able to absorb the liquid. You therefore decrease your blood sodium if you drink too much of almost any drink while exercising.

A solution at 50 to 60 mmol does not deprive your circulation of sodium, and gets absorbed faster to help you to lose heat. It actually increases your blood volume and decreases urine loss compared to sports drinks.

Add juices too for the sodium and potassium content. An 11.5 ounce can of V8 contains 880 mg of sodium and 780 mgs of potassium and counts as two vegetable servings! Other good potassium sources include citrus fruits, bananas, apricots and raisins, all of which provide a nice carbo boost. Salted pretzels allow you to eat your sodium after a run, while also giving you fat free carbohydrate.

Don't over-hydrate during an event. Drink enough to maintain your weight, or lose the two to three pounds of liquid you stored up with your carbo-loading. Generally, you only need minimal amounts of electrolytes during and after exercise because your body conserves its electrolytes. However, eating a few salty foods is wise on hot and humid days because the salt encourages your body to conserve its water while also encouraging you to drink more liquid.

Sweating out too much salt or drinking excessive amounts of water are traits of under trained exercisers. Build up the length of your long sessions, and your body will learn to conserve water and electrolytes while dissipating heat efficiently. You also learn to consume the minimal amount of electrolytes which you need with your liquid replenishment.

In your early sweating days you may lose one to two grams of sodium per liter of sweat. As you get fitter, you'll lose less. Novice and also drank too much water? Drink 16 ounces of V8 or tomato juice, and shortly afterwards a pint of non-fat milk, and you'll be well on the way to homeostasis.

Unless you exercise for greater than 5 hours and or take in excessive amounts of plain water, hyponatremia is like a rattlesnake on a 70 degree F. day. Be aware of its potential to show and know what to do if it does show. Include sodium with your liquids, and don't overhydrate.

Start your long training sessions in equilibrium and take in a few calories and electrolytes during the session. While resting and cooling a heatstroke person makes them feel better, rest and cooling a person with hyponatremia has little impact. They may also vomit forcefully, exacerbating the exit of body electrolytes.

Don't let the above problems put you off running and racing in extreme climates. Unless you have a weak heart, you should cope well with all but the very worst days. Most runners have a slight decrease in their performance. Running within 10 minutes of your best marathon time on a hot day could be the equivalent of a personal best in ideal conditions.

As mentioned before, you can get decent heat or humidity acclimatization in about 14 days. Training in high humidity will prepare you for hot but dry areas and vise versa. Do short exercise sessions early on, and gradually increase the duration and intensity of sessions. Include plenty of fresh vegetables and fruit for your electrolytes, and once your resting heartrate has got back to normal, you're ready for serious training.

You retain most of your hot whether running ability for over two weeks if you continue to exercise. You can also train faster in low temps due to your acclimatization.

Other sun and heat issues.

Wearing a cap with a bill shades your eyes, reduces the squinting which tenses the face muscles and which can spread lower. It also improves your running form.

A cap will make you look up, encouraging you to run tall. It can help you to run better. Toward the end of a marathon, the people who slow down have a tendency to look down. Keep your eyes focused about 75 yards ahead and your head will stay up, your lungs will be able to fully expand and keep taking in tons of oxygen to fuel your weary muscles.

Training in sunlight is mood enhancing due to stimulating the release serotonin, dopamine and beta-endorphins. It is also an efficient way to produce vitamin D for your bone health. To make vitamin D you'll have to expose some skin without sunscreen.

<u>Treadmills</u> help you to avoid heat or cold. See page 89.

* Dress appropriately to avoid overheating.
* Practice taking in liquids while treadmill running.
* Don't cheat the machine by bouncing up higher on each stride or jumping up and down. Jumping and bounding are great strength exercises, but don't spoil your form with excessive vertical lift during the rest of your training. Push off with the calves to go forward, not upwards.
* Unless your goal is the Pikes Peak Marathon, it's unlikely that going above a 6 percent grade will help you. You're likely to mess up your running form and strain a calf muscle or Achilles tendon.
* Running feels easier outside. You actually run faster for the same effort, so don't do too much on the treadmill.
* Keep your eyes focused about 12 feet away at eye level to avoid looking down at the controls all the time, which will spoil your running form.

<u>The well trained athlete</u> derives minimal benefit from the energy in drinks, provided his glycogen stores are adequate before he commences the run. The under trained athlete lacks endurance because his muscles have not been educated (trained) to exercise for long periods.

If you're under trained, 16 ounces of a sugared solution before the start, then 8 ounces of sports drink taken every 15 minutes during a run can increase the distance you're able to run at a set speed...by 12 percent. Half of the increase will occur with water alone, that is, by staying hydrated.

Muscles cannot work hour after hour unless they are trained to work at modest effort for hour after hour. Energy is a secondary problem for under-trained muscles. Under-trained muscles are not experienced at storing glycogen because they have not been stimulated with numerous long runs (that is...trained) to store huge amounts of glycogen. Bombarding under-trained muscles with sugar during a run is no substitute for your weekly long run. Train your muscles to conserve energy by only consuming water on most long runs, but practice with 5 to 8 ounces of sports drink every 15 minutes once a month to be ready for race day.

Beware of the research on this subject. Until you see a group of international class <u>runners</u> being tested for improved endurance while drinking sugared liquid, take the research with a grain of salt, err, electrolytes. The test should also be based on their ability to run 5 miles at 30 seconds per mile slower than anaerobic threshold (preceded by say 20 miles at 45 seconds per mile slower than threshold). Many studies are done with bikers who can consume all the liquid they wish. (Tour de France cyclists have "clocked" 44 ounces per hour.) Your training is the best way to get faster. If you have no interest in going beyond 40 miles a week, sugar drinks can help to delay one aspect of the wall during a marathon.

Most of the sports drink research is also based on sprinting ability at the end of say a 20K effort. However, you're running 42.195K at a constant pace. If you're able to sprint the last 195 meters, you obviously did not run hard enough from 20K to 42K. A bit of carbohydrate in your fluid intake does help you in the marathon by:

* Giving your muscles fuel, saving your liver's fuel, thus delaying the wall; and
* Giving your brain fuel, which decreases your perception of fatigue.
* To take advantage of the fact that fructose is absorbed slowly, include juices and fruit with your first three pints of liquid after runs.

Blood Donation.

This author is amused to read "experts" advising people not to run on the same day that they donate blood.

True, giving blood will take about one tenth of your Red Blood Cells (RBCs) and one tenth of your blood volume, so you'd think it would decrease your performance by 10 percent: Alas, it will decrease your performance by less than 2 percent. Other factors, including:

* The amount of air and oxygen taken in by the lungs;
* Your muscle power, including the number of muscle fibers which are eager to contract at a moments notice;
* The number of mitochondria in your muscles;
* The quantity of Myoglobin in your muscle cells;
* Your inherent ability and your background training;

Are all still completely intact.

Provided you consume an extra pint of liquid compared to your usual intake, the blood *volume* is replenished within a few hours. And your blood is less viscous, so it flows more easily, reducing the workload on your huge heart.

This is clearly not the week to increase your training, but you don't need to decrease it either. It's not the day to run your first ever track session either. But:

If your usual 400 meter repeats take 100 seconds, you should be able to run 102s at the same effort level 6 hours after giving blood...provided you hydrate properly. If you usually run at 3K pace, you'll be running at 5K pace on a donation day, yet your heart and lungs will still be at 3K intensity. The cardiovascular system at 3K effort while your lucky legs rest at 5K pace is a win-win situation.

Over 75 % of Carbon Dioxide waste is excreted via the plasma, or the fluid portion of blood. Thankfully, most is in a buffered form as bicarbonate. So, donating a tenth of your RBCs has minimal effect on CO_2 excretion or CO_2 levels.

After the donation, RBCs production - just like when you're at altitude - will increase. The extras will come on line at 2 weeks and get you back to normal levels in 4 weeks. Make sure you consume vitamin C with your iron sources and you'll soon regain your normal hemoglobin level.

Giving blood twice a year gives you a reason to back off from racing for a few weeks, and helps save a life.

CHAPTER THREE

BASE BUILDING Part Two

FARTLEK RUNNING

Speedplay or fartlek is a controlled OR uncontrolled system to accomplish quality running and speedwork. It can be a "run fast when you feel like it" session, or you can have a set plan such as 20 efforts of 200 to 300 meters. Another day, you might run roughly half miles. A true fartlek session uses a combination of distances. Use sections with the safest footing, or least traffic, or most mud, or enjoyable slope; after each fast section, run easy at pace to recover.

Marathon training requires that you stress your body a little bit, give it some rest to get stronger, then stress it again. You'll do this stress and rest for many months as you increase the length of your long run followed by easy days; you'll also increase the duration and the speed of the fast sections during speed training. This hard / easy approach has been perfected over the last century, but sadly, it's different for every person. Some runners can do 3 speed sessions per week, plus long runs; others can handle one speed session per week. Give yourself a realistic chance of finding your level by controlling your speed in all running. Don't run yourself into the ground in an individual session and there's a good chance that you can train moderately hard twice or three times each week.

According to Olympian and author Jeff Galloway, "The long run is the most important component in your training program, and bestows more conditioning benefit than any other." Galloway adds that, "Fartlek is the best form of speed training, because it conditions the mind for racing, as it gears up the body for top performance."

Although they have separate chapters, you'll be increasing your long run <u>and</u> incorporating speed running with fartlek over the same time period. Each element feeds on the other element. The ability to relax at speed makes your long runs easier and they eventually take less time because you run them at a faster pace for the same heartrate. The speed training becomes easier as you develop an economical running form plus the endurance from your long runs.

Short speed sessions at modest pace sharpen your legspeed or cadence, and give you an excellent heart/lung stimulus while you're still on modest mileage. You can sharpen your speed <u>and</u> aerobic ability and develop your cardiorespiratory system to get huge quantities of oxygen into your muscle cells. You also stimulate the mitochondria inside the cells to use the oxygen to power yourself to marathon success.

You can accentuate the training stimulus by taking short rests during fartlek running. After a 30 to 60 second strider, take a mere 15 second breather before setting off again at 5K pace. Do this a several times during each fartlek session but keep most of the session a bit more casual.

Some runners like to time the amount of fast running, but don't concern themselves with the actual distances they run; they will cruise back to base once they have achieved the allotted goal. Others count the number of short or long efforts as the schedule on pages 75-76 suggests.

When you're feeling fatigued it may take 50 minutes to amass 20 minutes of fast running and take 25 fast efforts because you're inclined to run for 45 instead of 90 seconds;

on inspired days, on straight, smooth trails it could take only 35 minutes to get the fartlek finished because you're inclined to take shorter rests and run longer efforts. You'll still need a mile or two of easy running before and after your speedplay. However long the fartlek session takes, don't ever run faster than 5K effort, and in your early days, run most efforts about 30 seconds per mile slower than 5K effort.

Your actual speed will be different depending on factors such as the softness of the terrain, the weather conditions and your level of fatigue. Aim for 85 percent of your maximum heartrate for the early efforts; as suggested in Chapter One, ease the pace toward 95 percent later in your sessions. Your running pace changes by about 35 seconds per mile.

Fartlek during Base Training.

If you're new to fast running, you can start with 6 to 8 gentle striders. As we English say, "Any twerp can sprint 50 meters to catch a bus." If the twerp doesn't have a heart attack, said person could sprint again in a month or two! A 100 meter strider or build-up is much slower than an all out sprint. This is supposed to be gentle training...not a straining of muscles.

You're going to progressively increase the amount of your fast running, so add a quarter of a mile each week and build to two miles of easy speedplay at one minute per mile faster than your steady run pace; gradually increase the speed to half-marathon race pace. This fast running will improve your running form; it will make your running more efficient.

When you've got used to your increased mileage, you can bring the last few strides down to 10K speed. Over the course of several months, by changing one stride a week to the faster pace, most of the speedplay can become 10K race pace or at about 92 percent of your maximum heartrate. As you will see in Chapters Five and Six, the preferred paces to train at are 15K and 5K speed. During this first phase though, you can be generic, 10K pace is a safe goal.

After a few more weeks, move up to three miles at speed, or if you've been here before, take it up to 10 percent of your weekly mileage in one or two sessions per week.

As you will be alternating moderately long runs such as a fifteen with long runs of 18 to 20 miles at the weekends, you can also do a race every other weekend. Note the term "do a race". Your goal should not be personal records at 5K or 10K. Instead, aim for a pleasant and painless experience while running 15 seconds per mile slower than PR pace for each distance. You'll get plenty of pace judgment practice with these races, and you'll be running on the roads with company.

Limit yourself to the 10K so that you're fresh for the 15 miler the next day, and to recover for a good fartlek session 2 or 3 days after the 15. You need to recover quickly from training races while also benefiting from the speed training.

Midweek and on the Saturday before your longer runs, do your fartlek session on soft terrain to save your legs for Sunday. Plot your routes to include some soft surface running for your long runs too. If you have tons of trails available, do all but 2 to 3 miles on soft surfaces. Run a couple of miles on the road each week to practice the steadier and economic style that you will need in a long race.

In later phases you will rest up to race at 10K to the half-marathon, then take an easy week before moving your training up a notch. During this phase stay with short races.

Fartlek Running is:

* Quality aerobic conditioning speedwork;
* A great way to recover after long runs;
* An ideal extra session during your high mileage build-up;
* A great anti-aging device for masters' running:
* Fartlek is a great play tool.

Most distance running for the marathon needs to be fun. When playing, that is running, use fartlek training for:

Quality Aerobic Conditioning.

All distance running helps your aerobic conditioning. However, fartlek's speedplay brings in those reluctant fast twitch muscle fibers and gets all your muscle cells into action.

Most marathon runners own predominantly slow twitch muscle fibers. The 10 to 30 percent of your fibers which are fast twitch need to be trained. Once your slow twitch fibers are fatigued during long runs, the fast twitch fibers are forced to work: you educate them to work like slow twitch fibers to keep a steady pace going.

You need to maintain their fast contractile abilities by running quite fast. Put your muscles through a full range of motion at least twice a week to maintain good running form.

Runners with over 30 percent fast twitch fibers find speed training easy because they're naturally fast. You should still run fartlek, but the striders must not be sprints. Your goal is to teach these short acting, yet fast acting fibers to work at low capacity for a significant time, namely, the hours it takes to run a marathon. Fartlek sessions at modest pace, and long runs will improve the endurance of these fast twitch fibers. You'll improve their ability to work sub-maximally for hours at a time just like your slow twitch fibers do.

Post Long Distance Run Recovery.

A soft surface is best for fartlek. Long runs at modest pace can make your leg muscles feel dead. Fartlek running on soft grass or trails brings pep back to your legs…but gently. Two days after a long run, try some 100 to 400 meter striders over varying terrain, at different speeds or paces.

When to do Fartlek Running?

High mileage runners can do these gentle fartlek sessions the evening after a long run, (unless it was longer, or faster than you've been used to) or the morning of the day on which you plan to run miles of track repeats. Fartlek at the right pace for you will make you feel looser in both situations.

Most of you will be training once a day. You will run a short fartlek session the day before your long run, and a longer fartlek session three days after your long run.

Leg Strength and Masters Anti-aging.

Fartlek keeps your legs strong as you train through the masters' age groups. All quality running helps to keep or increase your natural leg strength. Use fartlek to gain or maintain leg strength at all ages.

Speedplay also stimulates endorphin production inside your body for healing and health. The endorphins make us feel good too; the endorphin produced by our body is more potent than morphine. The endorphin or runners high may never happen to you, or you may get it during and after most runs (especially the good ones).

Officially, endorphins don't cross the blood-brain barrier. Anandamide does though, our bodies make it in abundance at 10K to half marathon intensity, it tickles a happy brain receptor and also dilates your blood vessels and bronchioles, which can make your running feel effortless, and you feel high. However, most of us will still call it an endorphin high.

Feeling exhausted from a tough day. You'll feel better after running provided you don't run too far in total, or run the speedplay too fast for your situation. These runs make you feel more positive about your life and about your prospects of completing a marathon because you'll run 20 to 40 seconds per mile faster than marathon pace for your fartlek efforts.

Fartlek running is your chance to experiment at speed. See how much easier, (or harder) it is to run at a certain pace with higher knees, or short rapid strides, or a ground hugging running style. Find the running form which suits you best.

Former 5,000 meter specialist?

Maintain legspeed or cadence with 30 to 90 second efforts. Play around with your knee lift and stride length. Push off from the toes and enjoy your 5K speed. Run some longer efforts too. Run at a nice relaxed tempo for 3 to 7 minutes while feeling the power in your legs from your new mileage base. However, don't run all-out.

Are you an Experienced Marathon runner who rarely ran speedwork in prior marathon preparations? Be gentle with your first few fartlek sessions. Run fartlek once a week for four weeks, then twice a week for at least four more weeks before moving onto Chapter Four.

Runners who did regular speed running in their earlier marathon preparation will have no problems with fartlek. Just run a variety of distances and paces.

Low mileage recreational runners and joggers will find fartlek the most humane way to incorporate speedwork into their 40 to 50 miles per week marathon training.

Maintain Running Economy and Efficiency

Feeling tired toward the end of a long run, or the last few efforts during a fartlek session? Don't develop poor running technique. Keep your shoulders loose; keep your arms down; don't lean forward too much.

* Keep your stride length short and your legspeed high to avoid overstriding. Aim for 180 strides per minute. Overstriding stresses the joints and muscles. Land with your foot directly underneath you and knee slightly flexed.
* Feet should be moving backwards when they land on the ground so that they do not act as brakes. They are then ready to propel you forward.
* Land with the knee flexed at about 15 degrees to reduce ground impact from slamming into your planets surface.
* Land on the outer edge of the heel or mid-foot, then roll inwards to a neutral position as you move toward push-off. Push off from the end of your toes in a straight line forward, not upward.
* Make your ankles roll as you glide along.

* Push yourself forward powerfully with the calf muscles: Extend the trail leg to its full length, and
* Run upright; run tall. Some say a one percent forward lean helps, but only if you keep your body straight! Practice a slight lean when standing still and tall with your abs tensed, back straight, knees slightly flexed and pelvis perfectly under your shoulders. Lean forward with the only movement coming from the ankle joint. When you practice this while running, extend your legs back on each stride to maintain balance, and keep your leg-speed high.
* If in doubt, bring your hips forward.
* Make your feet hug the buttocks as they swing through on each stride. Whip those feet through.
* Then do some striders of 50 to 100 meters. Think legspeed when you do this drill. Don't land daintily on the toes, or with a locked knee, or copy sprinters.
* Keep your arms quite low; move them in rhythm with your legs: move them just enough to stop your shoulders from rolling. This should stop your head from rolling too and keep you running rhythmically. Don't swing your arms across your body; swing them back and forth.
* Keep your hands loose and relaxed. A clenched fist transfers its tension to the shoulders. Save the energy for your leg muscles by keeping the fingers lightly curled.
* Look well ahead of you to keep your head up, but scan from side to side to avoid locking up.

Use the above pointers as a guide to help you run smoothly: avoid wasteful motions because efficient use of your meager oxygen supply is 90 percent dependent on running form.

Jack Daniels, Ph.D. recommends 180 strides per minute as the most economical rate (90 stride cycles – count the left foot landing for 60 seconds). Take short, rapid strides to achieve this rate, but include speed running, hill repeats, other strength training plus flexibility work to allow your stride length to eventually increase while you're at 180 per minute.

Speed comes from being strong and by relaxing. Then practice relaxing at speed at every level of your strength gaining process. You'll be stronger or slimmer next month, so just like during that growth spurt of adolescence, your coordination at speed needs to be practiced…every week.

Get the tension out of your body as you cruise gently at speed to teach your muscles and the nerves to move you rapidly over the ground. Over the ground that is, not through the ground. Land lightly as if onto eggshells. Fartlek should not hurt you. You cannot relax at speed if you're hurting in the early sessions. Mild discomfort can come later, but you'll learn to relax with that too, as you think about good running form during longer and longer repeats at 5K pace.

Keep your shoulders low and relax your hands, drop your lower lip a little to relax your face, and to enhance air intake. Arms forward and back with no lateral motion. You're running forward, not sideways. Keep your muscles ready for speed with daily stretching, especially the hamstrings, butt and calf muscles.

More on Fartlek Pace.

If you're a very experienced runner, use appropriate running pace and distances for a more formal fartlek session. Use long reps at 15K pace for anaerobic threshold training, mixed with long reps at 5K pace for VO2 Max training.

For a harder training session, run the same amount of time at fast pace which you'd run in an interval or tempo session. Use a different section of the forest or park for each effort. Let perceived intensity and breathing guide your speed.

Should you call 6 x 800 meters a fartlek session? Not really. Six efforts of 2 to 4 minutes would qualify though, especially if you ran some efforts at 5K pace and some at 15K race pace. A purist might say that you ran 2 x 2 minutes; 2 x 3 minutes; and 2 x 4 minutes, instead of a fartlek session.

True fartlek means a variety of distances. If you want to time yourself between two landmarks close to the beginning of the session, and again toward the end of the session, go ahead. Or run two times a set distance for pace judgment in the middle part. Try to keep most of your fartlek free flowing.

Working predominantly the aerobic or the anaerobic system depends on which intensity you concentrate your fartlek efforts upon. You can do all fartlek at anaerobic threshold or all at VO2 max by running at 15K or 5K pace respectively. However, whichever pace you train at, you also stimulate the other system.

Fartlek improves your "fuel economy" as European 5,000 meter champion Bruce Tulloh calls it, or running efficiency, taking you farther on each 1,000 calories.

Alternative Resistance Training. Moving through the airs resistance takes effort. Running just behind someone in a marathon can save you 3 to 5 minutes depending on whether you're a 2:20 or a 4 hour marathon runner. More if the course is predominantly into head winds and you run in the middle of a pack. The worst spot is next to the leader of a pack because you both have to break the wind: your combined volume takes more effort than if you were on your own.

When training however, running into the wind can make a session of two hundred meter striders, or fartlek harder: you'll gain more heart and lung fitness at modest speeds. So, run fartlek 200 to 600 meter efforts into the wind.

Run a few striders with the wind for relaxation, and to focus on running form. Don't bounce, but do maintain fast cadence to protect your knees.

The advantage of doing speed running into the wind is that it will slow you down, thus decreasing the tendency to overstride. You'll incur lower ground impact forces and save your leg muscles for your next run, and your joints, tendons and ligaments for the next few decades.

As mentioned in Chapter One, new runners may take more than 26 weeks to reach their weekly mileage goal, and another 10 to 16 weeks to reach the long run of 18 to 20 miles every other week. According to a survey in the August 2,002 *Runner's World*, 63 percent of marathon runners do a longest run of 19 to 22 miles. Get used to these distances on a regular basis to improve your running economy.

During this extended period of building up your long run, you should be bringing in the fartlek running at the rate of an extra quarter mile to half a mile each week. Run another eight weeks at high mileage with your full fartlek session and you'll be ready for a race at the half-marathon.

You can do two fartlek sessions each week or gradually add hills on Saturdays while running your fartlek mid-week. Your hill training tips are in Chapter Four. Runners in their fourth year of training will only need 2 to 10 weeks in the fartlek and mileage base phase before bounding over to hill training for the third or 10th time.

Still a recreational runner? Here is your 25 to 29 week schedule to prepare for your first half-marathon. This schedule incorporates hills starting from Week One.

Currently doing a 12 mile run most weeks plus quality running? Join the party at week 10 of this schedule by racing at 8K or 10K. You'll be ready for a 10 mile race in weeks. If you've got more running experience join at your level.

Coming from a low mileage background?

The aim is for a gradual increase in training quantity, while also adding small amounts of quality running. The overall training load needs to rise progressively over several months. Apply a modest stress to your muscles, give them time and some rest and they'll get stronger.

If you add just five miles per week each month to your training, you'll be running 30 miles per week more than your start level by month six. Your half-marathon and 10K race times will improve for another six months at this increased training level. Your marathon can wait a few months while you reap the running endurance and leg strength gains at your new mileage level.

If you start this program as a 20 miles per week recreational runner, cross train for 30 to 60 minutes on Monday and Wednesday, and the rest of your weekly training will progress something like this:

		Day One	Two	Four	Six	
		Probably Saturday	Sunday	Tuesday	Thursday	
		Hill reps	Long	Fartlek	Medium	Total
		(in meters)	run	*	run	miles
Wk	One	4 x 400	5 miles	12 / 1.5	4	19.5
	Two	3 x 600	6	3 / 2.0	5	22.5
	Three	6 x 200	7	16 / 2.0	6	24
	Four	3 x 300	7	3 / 2.0	5	22

* 12/1.5 means about 12 efforts to total 1.5 miles at speed. 3/2.0 means about 3 efforts to total 2 miles at speed. As mentioned before, your long efforts should be about 35 seconds per mile slower than 5K pace; short efforts should be at 5K pace intensity.

Every fourth or fifth week should be an easy week to rest up for a race. Instead of hills on Day One, (7 days pre-race) run the 300 meter reps on flat grass

The 15 to 20 mile per week recreational runner increases mileage to an average of only 22, but:

* Learns to run hills slowly enough to avoid exhaustion.
* Learns the ideal pace of speedplay to improve running form at 30 seconds per mile faster than marathon pace.
* Increases the long run by 40 percent to 7 miles.
* Incorporates 3 to 5 miles at 75 to 80 percent of maximum heartrate during the Thursday run. You will be running at close to marathon pace for these middle miles.

Note: Had you increased mileage by the maximum recommended 10 percent per week, you could be at 29 miles...which is close to the average for weeks five to eight. Don't rush to higher mileage. Instead, learn to run fast and efficiently while gradually increasing mileage.

The goals over the next 20 to 30 weeks are to increase the distance which you run, while also increasing your speed running at sensible paces so that you run efficiently. 5K pace is fast enough and helps you avoid injury. If you did all of your running slowly, you'd only train yourself to run slowly. Changing your muscle structure requires rest, and most of you have 3 restive days per week for body adaptation.

This schedule is similar to step one for the half marathon, and you'll race a half marathon at around week 30 or 35 or 40, depending on how many sections of 4 to 5 weeks you need to repeat.

Week #	Hills	Long run miles	Fartlek	Medium Long	Total
Five	Race 5K	7	20 / 2.5	6	26.5
Six	6 x 400	8	5 / 3.0	7	27.5
Seven	4 x 600	9	24 / 3.0	7	28.5
8	10 x 200	10	6 / 3.5	8	31
9	5 x 300	8	20 / 2.5	7	26
10	Race 8K	9	28 / 3.5	8	35.5
11	8 x 400	11	6 / 4.0	9	34
12	6 x 600	12	32 / 4.0	9	35
13	16 x 200	13	6 / 4.0	9	36
14	8 x 300	10	20 / 2.5	7	29
15	Race 10K	11	7 / 4.5	10	39
16	10 x 400	14	32 / 4.0	11	39.5
17	8 x 600	15	8 / 5.0	12	42.5
18	20 x 200	16	32 / 4.0	10	40.5
19	10 x 300	12	4 / 2.5	7	31.5
20	Race 12K	12	32 / 4.0	10	41

Most runners should then consolidate by repeating weeks 15 to 20. When you feel ready, move to week:

21	12 x 400	17	8 / 5.0	12	45
22	8 x 600	18	32 / 4.0	12	45
23	20 x 200	18	8 / 5.0	10	44
24	12 x 300	14	24 / 3.0	8	35.5
25	Race 10 miles:				

Because you've just done a long run in the form of the 10 mile race, it's probably best to run only 5 miles the day after or bicycle for an hour. It takes about one day to recover from each mile of racing, so don't plan on running hard until the middle of the following week. Two very gentle fartlek sessions with 3 miles at speed on Tuesday and Thursday will give you a 33 mile recovery week. It will set you up nicely to repeat weeks 21 to 24 prior to a half-marathon race.

Week 21s first session 7 days after a 10 mile race is hills. Run the 400 meter hill reps slower than usual as part of your race recovery. If your next half-marathon course is flat, consider replacing one hill session with a 5K race.

Note that the week before each race you're doing less mileage than the previous 3 or 4 weeks. This is resting up or a mini peak for a race. Accentuate the resting up by:

A. Running relaxed 300 meter striders on flat grass at 5K pace 7 days pre-race. Don't run a heavy session of hills in the seven days prior to any race.
B. Doing only one (shorter) cross-training session.
C. Relax through your slightly shorter fartlek session.

There's no set rule saying you have to be running 18 miles twice a month at this early stage of marathon training. You can stay at 15s or up to 2 hours until you've finished your hill training, move up to 18 during Chapter Five, and reach a monthly or twice monthly 20 during Chapters Six and Seven.

Can't manage your long run in one go? Some would say that it would not be a long run, but consider these options.

1. Trusty walk breaks. One to 5 minutes of walking every 15 changes your form and allows you to hydrate easier. Don't use walking as an excuse to make your actual running faster than it should be.
2. Do part of your long run in the evening. Limit your morning run to say two and a half hours. 10 hours later your muscles will still be tired, but the remainder of the days mileage may be more enjoyable for you.

Your muscles will not get as much education at burning fatty acids by splitting your mileage, but you'll still practice running on tired legs. Because you've had two meals, your muscles will not get as much education about storing glycogen either, but as you progress through the next four chapters you'll run more of your 20 miles in the morning.

Triple European marathon champ, 1987 World Champ and 1988 Olympic Gold medalist Rosa Mota felt that she could race a half marathon almost every week because they are so easy to recover from. Being as bright as you readers are, she did not race every week, but most weeks she did run about 16 miles at 30 seconds slower than marathon pace. Most of you will need to run 60 to 75 seconds per mile slower than marathon pace to be at 60 to 70 percent of your max HR.

Mota also liked to start marathons conservatively because it helps to avoid the wall or lack of glycogen which will be covered on page 217 under carbohydrate loading.

Top marathoners such as 1992 Olympic Bronze Medalist Lorraine Moller from New Zealand share several things in common. Like Moller, they have a tendency to race every second or third weekend or run sessions such as 20 x 400 meters at 5K pace or 10 x 1,000 meters with a short rest. Just like your schedule, Moller then followed up her speed session the next day with a long run...up to 2 hours and 45 minutes for her, and generally on trails for strength and cushioning.

After an easy day, Moller repeats the formula of speed followed by distance, which is the same formula used in this book. The midweek long run is a modest 12 if you're on 45 miles per week, and adds vital additional endurance.

Half-marathon goal pace.

But we've got ahead of ourselves a little bit, so lets get back to the half marathon. Take the soft option for your first couple of half's. Double your 10K time and add eleven minutes. This is about 30 seconds per mile slower than your 10K race pace.

Run even pace, and the first 6 miles should feel easy. You'll be running a few seconds per mile faster than those 4 to 5 miles in the center of your midweek run; you'll be running much slower than in your fartlek training.

The remaining seven miles of the half-marathon will be a mental practice for marathon running. Just like in a marathon, these miles aren't fast, but you'll have sections when they feel harsh. Stay relaxed, maintain form, be positive and sustain your pace to the finish. You may run the whole marathon at this pace in a couple of years. Don't hurt too much in your first few half-marathons.

40 to 45 miles per week too tame for you? You can add a run at any stage...but be consistent. Liked 4 miles twice a week in addition to week one's training? By week 8 you may be doing two 5s. Other runners may wait until week 16 before adding a fifth run of only three miles. No matter. Do what works for you. 40 or 60 miles per week, you still get your finishers medal. You're almost one-third of the way to the marathon!

Preparation + Attitude = Achievement

is a corny phrase but appropriate for marathon running. You have to organize your life to get out running 4 or 5 times per week, to do long runs consistently and to incorporate several types of speedy running. Speed running will only give you benefits if you do it at the right effort level and with the best running form that you can muster.

Next up is 21 pages of hill training advice because most of you will be running hill repeats from week one of your marathon training. You should also be cross training twice a week with 30 minutes of weights each session and 30 to 60 minutes using a combination of pool running, elliptical training or biking, as shown in *Best Half Marathons* and *5K Fitness Run.*

CHAPTER FOUR

HILLS & STRENGTH TRAINING

Successful marathon racing requires three types of running in addition to simple mileage and long runs. You can complete the next three phases in any order. Namely:

1. Hill training;
2. Anaerobic threshold training;
3. VO2 maximum training:

According to Jeff Galloway, "Hill repeats, Anaerobic threshold sessions, and VO2 max intervals at 5K to 2 mile race pace, provide the edge to any runner who is trying to push beyond thresholds of current performance." The best marathon results, runners with the fastest times, train using all three types of running.

You can also train using the complex system…using all types of training at once. Using 1983 World Championships Marathon Gold Medalist Rob De Castellas' basic schedule:

Saturday: Race or tempo run
Sunday: Long (22 miles)
Monday: Recover 10
Tuesday: Hills
Wednesday: Medium Long (18)
Thursday: Track such as 8 x 400 meters at 2 mile race pace.

De Castella did one session of each type of training most weeks, with anaerobic threshold on Saturday, and hills and

VO2 max training mid-week. He also ran an additional 5 miles most days. It takes consistent training to reach your best level, with frequent running against resistance such as hills and sand. As with this book, his aim was not to overtrain in one session because you have to be able to run well the next day and "injury is the enemy." The long runs give skeletal strength, helps to avoid injury, and sets you up to further develop cardiovascular fitness from the quality running.

Alternating one 14 to 16 mile run with one 17 to 18 mile run per week should suffice until you're through the second phase of marathon training. Then sneak in 20s every other week, or every three weeks during phases three to five.

Many coaches, and this writer, believe that predominantly hill or strength training should follow the initial mileage and speedplay build-up. Page 75-76 showed you how to meld the hill training into the fartlek and base building phase to give you strength and endurance in one go.

The programs in Chapters 11 and 14 allow you to split the hill phase from base building, giving five training phases.

This chapter is your hill training guide for technique and effort level. During all phases you will actually be doing a little bit of all types of training. During the Interval training of Phase Four, you'll include some hills and hilly fartlek running.

You are now an experienced runner.

You should have raced numerous 5Ks and 10Ks by now, plus at least one half marathon. Whatever intensity you train at, you have some inkling as to what it feels like to reach nearly the halfway point in a marathon: the 20 mile point is closer to halfway physiologically speaking. Focusing for 6 to 10 weeks on each of the above three types of training will improve your potential to withstand the body assault which the second half of the marathon, those last 6.2 miles can provide.

Strength lays a solid foundation for you to build endurance and then speed. Hopefully, you've come from this author's half marathon training with its two sessions of weight training per week because according to the Centers for Disease Control and Prevention (CDC) researchers, weight training decreases your injury risk by about 44 percent.

Now then, lets ease this other muscle strengthener into your marathon running. After all, long distance runners gain muscle strength, stronger hearts and better knee lift with hill repeats.

If you went from recreational to dedicated runner following Chapter Three's program, you've already done hill training. You will know that hill repeats can be challenging, especially if you run them too intensely. Understand why you need hill training and you'll approach them with controlled gusto.

According to Jeff Galloway, "Hill repeats build leg strength better than any form of strength training, while giving a speed conditioning benefit at the same time."

As Mark Nenow, the former U.S. 10,000 meters record holder (27:20:56) said when asked by *Runner's World* for key training tips: "Hills, hills, hills."

Hill Running Develops the Neurological Pathways Needed for Fast Running.

Marathon runners tend to have a low knee lift and relatively weak muscles when it comes to strength tests. Running hills fairly fast with a high knee lift will:

* Add strength to your running muscles;
* Improve your coordination at high speed;
* Increase your confidence concerning hilly race courses.

As you read in the sarcomere section of page 30, strong muscle fibers allow you to run farther for every molecule of oxygen used and for each calorie which you burn. Improve your leg strength with hill training and you'll be able run your marathon using a lower percentage of your muscle power.

Run with good coordination and you'll be more efficient, using less oxygen per mile, leaving you with greater reserves.

Hill Training improves your racing speed by building strength in the quadriceps, hamstrings, buttocks, calves and back. Increased base speed makes it easier for you to maintain goal marathon pace.

Hill sessions develop strength in the lower leg muscles especially, which allows you to support your body weight farther forward on your lovely feet. Rapidly rolling the foot forward loads your ankle like a spring. As the ankle releases its mechanical energy, you get a huge push-off from the foot. Keep it flexible with stretching and make it strong with hill running, and the ankle is very efficient, achieving monumental amounts of work with minimal energy use. You'll be able run farther at any running speed such as doing a 10K at your old 8K racing pace or an entire marathon at last years 20 mile race pace.

Hill running also:

* Corrects your form: you can't run hills with bad form.
* Increases your aerobic and anaerobic efficiency.
* Strengthens your quads, resulting in fewer knee injuries. Hill reps cause fewer injuries because there is much less shock per stride.
* Opens your stride: Despite running fartlek and other fast running, excessive amounts of distance training can decrease your stride length. An economical short stride is effective for marathon running, but during hill repeats, remember to exaggerate the knee lift and the arm swing, while pushing off with your toes and calf muscles. Although this exaggerated running action would be inefficient in a race, it's perfect for strength training.

Enjoy these hill repeats. Work with the slopes and allow them to improve your muscle strength.

Confidence affects performance. Practice and perfect hill running, and you'll be confident on hilly courses: you'll also be faster on any type of marathon course.

Many runners hate hill repeats because they get a burning sensation in their chests and heavy legs and have achy arms afterwards from using them as pistons to drive their legs up the hill. Well gentle people, if you have those three problems, you're running the hills too fast. Run at 5K intensity, which is 95 percent of your maximum heartrate instead of mile intensity or 99 percent of max HR at the top; increase the number of repeats gradually and you'll avoid all three overtraining problems.

Only been running hills within training runs? It's time to replace some of the hilly courses with hill repetitions. You'll need to use 100 to 1,200 meter hills for these sessions.

Find a fairly steep hill, but a hill which you feel reasonably comfortable running up...3 to 4 degrees, or a 3 percent grade works well for most runners. Beginners could start with a one to two percent grade, and ease up at 10K intensity, or 90 to 92 percent of your max HR the first few weeks. While steeper hills do give you faster rewards, they place greater strain on the Achilles tendons and calf muscles.

Long time marathon runners may need to emphasize short, steep hill reps to improve knee lift and legspeed. Recent 10K or shorter race specialists may need longer reps up gentler inclines for speed endurance. All runners will benefit from running both types of hill repeat.

If this is going to be your first experience with hill reps, use a 100 meter section to begin.

Run one third of your planned mileage for this day as a warm-up, and then stretch. Then commence the first of about ten repetitions, by...running up the hill with a fairly high knee lift and a modified sprinters type arm action.

For the first few sessions raise those knees and work your arms just a bit more than usual. Don't make this a sudden change to your training or you risk injury.

The legs should not be going too fast; 100 stride cycles per minute is fast enough. The emphasis is on lifting the knees higher than in normal runs, but landing softly. Land closer to your toes than you usually do, midfoot is ideal.

Pick a focal point 50 meters ahead or close to the top of the hill to prevent yourself from leaning forward. Run perpendicular to the surface during hill repeats. Walk back down the hill for recovery, then stride up it again.

For your next effort, try shorter, quick strides, which allow you to stay close to the surface, avoid wasted effort, plus it's more akin to the way you'll run hills in a long race.

Run a variety of styles to practice knee lift, legspeed, full calf extension and arm movement. It will take several reps before you begin to feel relaxed running fast up the hill; it takes most runners months to learn the best style and running intensity to achieve the massive performance gains which hill training provides.

This hill training practice will improve your muscle strength, and from that added strength, your potential marathon speed. Aim for 5K race intensity during hill training sessions. Your heartrate should only reach 95 percent of your maximum at the end of the 30 to 90 second hill rep.

If you cannot fully recover in your rest period, stop. You can add more reps in future sessions. Warmdown thoroughly to relax your muscles and get rid of most of the lactic acid.

Hold back during your first hill sessions. Eighty to 90 percent effort is all you need to develop leg strength and sound cardiovascular endurance: it also avoids stressing your muscles too much. The leg tissues including the Achilles and calf muscles, plus the quadriceps and other hip flexors, the hamstrings, and your back may still get sore during your first hill sessions. Gentle stretching should clear them.

The second time you run hill reps, try about eight repetitions of 200 meters. The third time, try five at up to 400 meters. Early on, keep the hill sessions 7-10 days apart; later, if you're running the 50 miles or more per week required for a decent marathon, slip down to every 4-5 days by doing a hilly fartlek session once every two weeks.

The schedule on pages 75-76 gives you gradually increasing numbers of hill repeats at 200, 400 and about 600 meters. The short ones should usually be run at 5K to 2 mile race effort or 95 to 98 percent of your max HR at the end of each repeat. The 400s would be at 5K effort and the long repeats should remain at 10K to 15K intensity or about 90 percent of max HR.

It's not about Suffering

Respect hill training. Increase the number of reps and the grade in steps while running at appropriate intensity. Take care of your Achilles' with stretching. Don't strain your Achilles'. Use the calf stretches from pages 33 to 36.

Your entire hill session should feel no harder than a ten mile run. You should not take 2 to 3 days to recover from these sessions. You should be able to complete a long run in comfort the day after a hill session. If you can't, you did too many hills, or you did them too fast.

Be patient. You are stimulating:

* An increase in the size of your muscle fibers;
* The ability of those muscle fibers to contract rapidly;
* With short recoveries between each contraction;
* Hill reps will increase your muscle elasticity and the range of motion at the foot and ankle, which is vital for fast running and for running at marathon pace.

You are creating strength in your thigh, buttocks, and lower leg muscles: This strength and flexibility determines your stride length, which determines your speed.

If possible, finish some of the repeats just over the top of the hill, and then practice accelerating as the grade decreases. You can also practice this acceleration on steady runs when you're feeling fresh: pick up the pace by ten seconds per mile for 20 strides, before settling back to your steady pace.

When you're comfortable with hill repetitions, you can increase the quantity of reps and then your speed.

Your uphill speed when running at 95 percent of VO2 max, which is also 95 percent of your max HR, will increase as your muscles become stronger and as you learn running efficiency or economy. Of course, running speed can also be increased by training more intensely.

Running at 2 mile effort or 100 percent of VO2 max (and about 97 to 98 percent of max HR) is harsher on your muscles. Except for two sessions at the culmination of your hill phase, or for very short repeats, 2 mile intensity is probably overkill for marathon training. You will be much better off if you aim to increase the number of repeats that you do at 5K intensity.

Avoid exaggerated arm motions during other speed training. Exaggerated arm movements powering you forward, and up the hill or sand-dune is fine for hill reps. But when you move on to Anaerobic and VO2 max speed running, keep your arms under control. Allow your arms to balance you as you let your legs propel you forward. Arm power is only good for short distances; think running style for the rest of your speed training.

Hill Training Target?

20 to 25 reps of the short hill section is about right.

10 or 12 of the long section may be its equivalent.

10 to 15 minutes of actual hill reps works best for most runners, or up to 5 percent of your weekly miles.

As shown in Chapter Three's program, simply add a rep or two each session until you're on the hill for 30 to 40 minutes, including the recovery sections.

When you get stronger you can run easy for the recovery. This reduces your rest period. Land softly when running back down the hill.

You can also split the hill into sections. Stride up the first section of say 200 meters, and then run easy or walk up for thirty to sixty seconds, then stride up the second section. You will have a longer recovery going back down for your next set. You might run six sets of two efforts in a session, or your hill could be long enough for three or four repeats.

When you can handle a variety of hills in training, they will seldom be a problem in races. In a race or tempo run, always run them with economy, using a low knee lift and short but quite rapid stride rate. Tuck in behind someone, get 'pulled' up the hill, and then find the extra gear you've been practicing as you accelerate over the top.

Long Hill Repetitions.

Your short hill reps of 200 to 600 meters should be at 5K race intensity! Why? Because you'll be running with similar form to a sprinter. Long reps at 15K pace also give excellent results. During these reps though, you'll look like what you are...a distance runner. Anaerobic threshold pace is discussed at length in Chapter Five. You can get a jump on that Chapter, and gain huge endurance rewards, by running one hill session out of every three or four up a long gentle grade.

Half a mile to a mile hill repeats, or 800 meters to 1,500 meters is a reasonable range. Work on, or think about the elements of form as you run up the 2 to 3 percent grade.

Mud or other difficult surfaces give still greater strength gains. You can run reps with heavy, mud-crusted shoes. Adjusting your running style or stride length as you negotiate sections with uneven footing is easier at 15K pace than at 5K intensity. These longer reps mean you'll need to run at about 80 to 85 percent of your maximum heartrate in early sessions; gradually aim toward 90 percent of max HR.

You must increase resistance as you get fitter. The second or third time through this resistance training, find steeper hills, deeper mud or sand, or run longer reps such as 1,200 meters at the speed of your old 800s.

Seek a variety of hills to run reps on, or you'll become brilliant at one hill, but rarely see your hill in a race.

Practice accelerating over the top of the hill for your race situation. On race day, relax over the top of the hill, and pick up the legspeed by 2 to 4 strides per minute to find your steady rhythm again.

Remember: These hill reps increase your muscles' elasticity and the range of motion at the foot and ankle, which are vital for faster running.

Hills on the Treadmill.

Don't cheat the machine by pushing yourself up instead of forward when treadmill running. There is no point in setting the treadmill well beyond your natural speed limit because your running biomechanics will suffer.

Treadmill hill training advantages:

Treadmills allow you to set the grade accurately and to choose the hill length.

When you move city or State, you can run on the same hill for continuity.

No downhill running during the recovery, thus reducing your cumulative ground impact. Hill training on the treadmill reduces your potentially high impact sport to a low impact sport. For those of you who pound the running surface in preference to gently floating across the ground, kicking out those two to three miles of downhill running will reduce the wear and tear on your connective tissues.

Because you don't have to run back down, you can take shorter recoveries!

You can also recover by running at your usual training pace on the flat.

Treadmill Hill Training Drawbacks are the same as for all treadmill running! It's indoors and it can be hot, so use a fan to avoid overheating and set up your fluid bottle to make hydration convenient.

Sample Treadmill Session.

Start with at least a mile or greater than ten minutes warm-up. The running warm-up can be on the short side if you've done some cross training prior to commencing the treadmill training. Run enough to unwind from the cycling or weight training; run enough to get the blood supply where it belongs...concentrated in your running muscles.

Take your machine to marathon pace at zero percent grade for a quarter of a mile. Then, begin your hill training with a quarter mile up a 4 percent grade. Your running speed should remain at projected marathon race pace. A quarter mile at marathon pace is easy on the flat, but harsh when you have to raise the knees to account for the grade.

During the recovery quarter, maintain marathon pace at zero grade. Treadmill running at zero grade is 10 to 15 seconds per mile easier than asphalt running because there is no air resistance.

When speed training, runners tend to jog in the recovery. The treadmill keeps you honest because you have to keep running at the treadmills set pace. After a quarter mile of restive running at zero grade, repeat the 4 percent rep.

Then, run two reps each at 5 and 6 percent. To complete a two mile session of hills, finish with a half mile...but at only 5 percent elevation. You now have 3.5 miles at marathon pace, two miles of it being up-hill. Finish this time efficient training with a pleasant warmdown at one minute per mile slower than marathon pace.

Treadmill time limit at your fitness club? No problem. You can warmdown with pool running or cycling for 10 to 15 minutes at fairly high cadence and low resistance.

Beginners can start with hill reps up a 2 percent grade. As you get stronger, as your heartrate stays low enough at the low grades, ease up one percent each month toward 6 percent. Except for the last couple of reps, don't train more intensely than 5K effort for marathon racing.

On many treadmills, the belt goes faster when you run uphill. It may be that in addition to the motor's steady work, pushing off better with our toes propels the belt along. Whatever the reason, hill repeats at 6:50 mile pace, with the recovery at 7:10 pace should not concern you. It's better than the machine forcing you to run the hill reps slower. That would defeat the purpose of hill training.

Note: Provided the treadmill is set up properly, you can run precise workouts anywhere in the world. However, this author tested three treadmills at his health club recently using a heartrate monitor set at threshold pace. The treadmills ranged from 6:22 to 6:00 per mile at a HR of 162. In April 2,002, a major manufacturer recalled nearly 6,000 young treadmills, which had a tendency to speed up. That said, it's nice to work indoors on running form once a week.

If your machine gives you the same pace while recovering on the flat, running marathon pace will rid your muscles of their waste products from the hill reps. Depending on your weight, the grade and race pace, you'll be at 15K to 5K intensity during these treadmill hill reps. Yet you'll only be running at marathon speed. See the box on page 92.

It probably doesn't matter what grade of hill you use for hill training; the important thing is to run hill repeats. The effort is personal also: train at 15K and 5K intensity, plus a minimal amount at two mile race pace effort if you've been here many times before. Runners in their first three years of training should probably avoid two mile or 3K intensity.

Norwegian multiple world record breaker Ingred Kristiansen used the treadmill to good affect throughout her career, using it for much of her winter training.

Treadmill aims include:

* Feeling relaxed and comfortable on a moving belt;
* Teach yourself to relax at speed, perhaps with a large mirror in front of you to check your form: Which,
* Helps you to find a good rhythm to improve running form and expend less energy per mile.
* Quality training such as hill repeats and tempo pace or long Intervals at 10K to half marathon pace. Or program the machine for faster speed running.

Page 92 shows your equivalent intensity up a 1 to 6 % hill.

Grade or incline percentage					
1	2	3	4	5	6
6.03	5.52	5.42	5.32	5.24	5.16
7.01	6.46	6.32	6.20	6.09	5.58
7.59	7.40	7.23	7.08	6.54	6.42

6 min pace — 6.03, 5.52, 5.42, 5.32, 5.24, 5.16
7 min pace — 7.01, 6.46, 6.32, 6.20, 6.09, 5.58
8 min pace — 7.59, 7.40, 7.23, 7.08, 6.54, 6.42

Note: Running up a one percent grade on the treadmill roughly makes up for the lack of wind resistance.

* At three percent, you've reached half marathon intensity or the lower end of anaerobic threshold.
* 4 % takes most of you to the top range of threshold.
* 5 % is 10K effort or faster.
* 6 % grades, or 5K intensity stimulates your VO2 max or running economy…provided it's not ruining your form.

You can gradually increase the total amount of hill running, or do longer repeats. Two times a quarter mile at 4 percent is a nice way to ease your way into a session, but then build too:

A. One mile hill repeats at 3 percent incline, and 85 percent of max HR to run at anaerobic threshold;
B. Half mile hill reps at 6 percent incline, at 95 to 98 percent of your max HR to run at close to your VO2 maximum.

Both sessions will keep you in your desired heartrate training range for a greater percentage of the session compared to short repeats, but don't go over 3 miles.

Going above a 6 percent grade will probably ruin your running form, and strain your Achilles or calf muscles.

Maintain High Mileage.

You need to run mileage too during your strength phase. For those of you who follow Chapters 11 or 14, your long run and total mileage are unchanged during hill training. You'll get stronger, which means fitter for running a marathon, because the 2 to 4 of your miles which are hill repeats are harder, more productive miles. Chapter Three followers will still be building up their mileage while adding to the number of hill repeats.

Run at least eight sessions of hills in your build-up phase, then retain hills once every 10 to 14 days while training through Chapters Five to Seven. Try one hill session every 14 to 21 days leading into your marathon. Your last hill reps should be 14 to 17 days prior to your marathon.

Bounding and Plyometrics.

While the coach of many Olympic medalists Arthur Lydiard said the most beneficial resistance training for runners is hill training, 40 years have past, so we must admit that there's more to strength than hills. After at least eight sessions of hills you can add bounding: bring it in a few striders at a time.

When you're running on a soft surface or up a hill, bound forward with an exaggerated high knee-lift, and a fast running action. Bounce off the toes forcefully as you power your body up and forward. Go much higher and farther than during routine hill repeats, and land softly, toward the middle of your foot with a bent or flexed knee. Bound for 20 to 30 meters at a time with a walk down or jog back recovery.

If you have wide stairs or steps available, do double leg jumps up them. Hopping is an effective variation on bounding, and allows you to isolate each leg. Hop or jump up a grassy slope, in sand, or through mud. Land softly.

Stadium steps offer another bounding opportunity. Cruise up them at gentle pace the first few times. Don't overwork your calf muscles in your early sessions. Add additional repeats as the weeks go by, and when your calves and Achilles have adapted.

Find walking or running back down the steps a chore? The stair climber and elliptical trainer are options; you could also use the elevator in your favorite building.

Sand is an excellent surface for all jumping and bounding exercises because while your legs struggle to propel you forward, your arms have to work to maintain your balance, so you get a whole body workout. You also get a soft landing. Stay tall and relaxed.

Bounding develops hip flexors, calves and quadriceps, plus your tendons and ligaments. Stronger muscles will increase your stride, speed and running economy, while decreasing your injury risk. Bounding also gives you a maximum eccentric stretch to make you more elastic.

Include a few minutes of skipping rope for the calves. Deena Kastor credits the addition of skipping, plus other plyometrics for her 5 minute marathon PR and American marathon record. You need to build the power to enhance your endurance. You can only run a fast marathon if your muscles are strong, with the ability to contract hour after hour at sub-maximal effort. Avoid building the bulk of a sprinter.

Elasticity saves your energy.

Eccentric stretching is when a muscle elongates while it is working. On every stride, your calves, quadriceps and other muscles and tendons stretch at impact with the ground and store some of your incoming energy like pulling an elastic bands does. The Achilles and quadriceps in particular are stressed during this energy retrieval, though all your joints, tendons and muscles experience some stress.

At push-off on each stride your stored, elastic band energy is released. You maintain momentum with relatively little effort because 30 percent of your energy is in constant store and release, store and release…provided your muscle fibers and tendons are loose and strong.

Stretch regularly, include strength training with hills and plyometrics to maximize your ability to store and release power. Practice springing off the end of toes on soft grass with striders. Use your full range of motion.

Fast running improves flexibility and elasticity. When you are not doing hill repeats or bounding, that is, during normal running, power yourself forward instead of upward with the calves to extend your stride. Decrease your vertical bounce: the price of running half an inch too high on every stride can be 10 percent of your energy.

Other Resistance Options.

Grass, dirt trails and beaches without slope are perfect places to run. They're soft and uneven, forcing muscles and tendons to work harder than on a flat surface for the same speed. You become stronger by stressing your muscles. You also experience less shock on each stride, and work your stabilizing muscles, including abductors and trunk muscles.

Looking for 70 percent of max heartrate training? You can work your heart and lungs while running slower. Trail running at 8 minute pace may equate to 7.30 road miles provided you're at the right heartrate. It's easier to land softly at the slower pace, plus you're landing on a softer surface.

Achieving your training heartrate at slower speeds is one of the benefits you get from altitude training. The slower speed decreases injury risk, while giving you the potential for increased mileage. You'll also take 80 minutes to cover 10 miles instead of 75 minutes on the road, giving an additional 5 minutes of training for your cardiovascular system even if you don't increase mileage.

Gradually increasing the resistance is part of the overload principle: exercise to a modest degree of fatigue and rest to recover while your body adapts. You'll be able to train harder next month, or the next time through your marathon schedule.

Cross-country racing, and running long fartlek or
threshold pace intervals over cross-country style courses are a perfect adjunct to hill training for muscle strength.

World record breaker at the 1984 Chicago marathon, Steve Jones ran cross-country every winter as part of the British running tradition. Jones thus laid the groundwork for a 29:38 last 10K at Chicago, which was a mere two minutes slower than his 10K personal record.

Jones' training sessions included:
* 12 x 90 seconds at 5K pace (Chapter 6 training).
* 10 x 2 minutes at about 10K pace (see Chapter 7).

* 5 x 5 minutes at marathon pace…within a 90 minute run, which for Jones would mean 15 miles. This book suggests that you do 2 times one mile in some of your long runs, plus Chapter 5s threshold pace sessions.

Use low impact training to strengthen your legs by driving them through mud and soft grass. When you encounter mud on trails, you should look for a shine. Wet mud will let you drop into it, forcing you to work hard. However, if there has only been a very light rain, the wet stuff may only be a millimeter or so deep, and you'll slip on the dry under-surface. Mud with a dull surface is better during cross-country racing and trail speed running (if you wear spikes) because it's firmer and your shoes stay cleaner. Whether running on road or trails, watch for surface changes and uneven sections. While the frequent change in foot-plant on trails is good for running longevity, nasty cambers, curbs and other annoyances can lead to twisted ankles and falls.

Running tons of slowish mileage in resistive situations such as altitude, dirt and sand? You will need several sessions at slightly faster than marathon pace, and at marathon pace to practice your road running skills before racing. No problem. You've got weeks of gentle speed running coming up.

As page 95 says, on every stride, the calf and quads do an eccentric contraction as the foot lands and those sturdy muscle groups stretch and store some of the incoming energy. How much of your energy returns like a spring to propel you forward depends on your muscles and tendons elasticity.

Up to 30 percent of your propulsive power comes from the stored energy of your shock absorbers and springs. You convert the landing energy instead of wasting it. Keep your muscles and tendons flexible and strong with stretching and weight training and feed your collagen fibers well.

However, after only a few miles of running, our eccentric abilities decrease due to fatigue. We spend more time on our feet during each stride cycle. The braking effect and storing of elastic energy recoil takes longer, and the push-off on each stride takes longer. This combination gives a reduced stride rate, thus we slow down.

We do try to compensate by bending our knees a bit more, and by taking longer strides…but both changes makes us less efficient runners. If you try to keep going with fatigued muscles that are unable to stretch during the eccentric phase, you risk severely achy muscles afterwards from micro muscle strains or even a full strain or Achilles Tendonitis.

Our bodies do try to recruit the last of our muscle fibers to keep us going at 10K pace. You can help this recruitment with training, by:

* Doing sufficient mileage to develop your hearts capacity and the capillaries for fuel delivery.
* Sufficient up-hill reps for leg strength.
* Sufficient anaerobic training as shown in Chapter Five.
* The Intervals at 5K to 3K paces of Chapter Six.
* Longer Intervals at 5K to 10K paces (Chapter Seven).
* And of course, setting out at the right pace for your current days race or training run.

Mostly, you're learning to run with a short stride to delay fatigue. Learn to run upright with a minimal forward lean from hips to shoulders so that gravity is pulling you forward like the (nearly) perpetual motion machines which can move at 7.5 minute mile pace using low voltage.

You can also improve your eccentric skills substantially with downhill speed running.

Downhill Running for Strength.

Yes…for strength. This was covered in Best Half Marathons, however: Running striders and repeats on a soft surface down a two percent grade makes your running more economic: Downhills will improve your biomechanics.

According to renowned coach Jack Daniels Ph.D. the best stride frequency is 90 to 95 per minute. Increasing from 90 to 92 per minute can shave 4 minutes from your marathon time. Increase your cadence by practicing:

* Short, rapid downhill strides for 30 to 60 seconds.
* Fast leg action with short up-hills.
* Running form drills.

Downhills strengthen the hamstrings, gluteus maximus and minimus muscles to pull the leg rapidly through during the recovery phase, and to extend the hip behind the runner.

The main hip flexor muscles are the Ilio-soas group (Iliacus and Psoas major muscle), and the rectus femoris muscle (1/4th of the quadriceps femoris muscle). They lift or flex the upper leg, giving us our knee-lift.

Downhills also get your quadriceps used to their eccentric contraction or elastic stretch at landing on each stride.

If you're warmed up and stretched, proceed to:

Downhill Running to Improve Economy.

The slope should be gentle: one to two percent is sufficient.

The surface should be soft: Short grass, fairly even sand or dirt trails, or an old railroad bed, or:

Use a treadmill...if it has the ability.

The First Downhill Sessions.

Just like you would any other form of training, start with gentle strides. The first few sessions must be easy ones to get your muscles used to the faster legspeed. Your emphasis should be on increasing legspeed or stride turnover. An extended stride can place extra stress on tendons and bones, while giving your about to strain muscle too much to do. Eventually, you may naturally increase stride length by an inch or two, but think cadence first.

When you're loose, push off with the calf muscles to go faster and make full use of the hip extensor muscles to extend the work of the calf muscles.

Be conscious of your leg pull-through; whip the leg forward with the hip flexor muscles.

Think leg speed as you tear gently down the slope.

Work your hamstring muscles to speed the leg through; bring the lower leg closer to your butt than you normally do.

Do not run so fast that your butt muscles hurt.

Land softly, midfoot, and roll, then push rapidly off the toes after the support phase. Spring off your calf at nearly maximum leg speed. These sessions give the soleus muscle a bonus workout.

Run perpendicular to the Slope. Leaning forward can strain the gluteal and hamstring muscles. Leaning back puts pressure on the back and hip flexors. You'll be setting up a breaking action. You want a flowing, rhythmic biomechanically sound running style.

Think about your footstrike. Land on the outer part of your foot, half way up your shoe. As you grasp and pull back with your feet, the heel should drop down to support you and the feet roll over to a neutral position and then you roll rapidly off from the end of the foot between the two biggest toes. As always, push forward instead of upwards with the calf muscles for minimal vertical bounce.

Intermediate Downhill Running.
200 to 400 meter efforts or short intervals.

Run a modest amount of repeats to begin with - about two thirds of your normal interval session - because you'll be running them faster. You will be close to 2 mile or 3K race pace while putting in 5K pace effort.

Think about your running mechanics. Sprinting downhill with arms flying all over the place will not make you a more economical runner.

Push the arms back on each stride and allow them to move straight forward to their natural height; don't grasp for handfuls of air. Hands don't need to go across the chest, unless it's the perfect running form for your body. Straight back and forward to a just above waist height is best. The arms need to balance the legs.

Downhills teach you relaxation, good form and fast leg turnover. Swing those feet through close to your buttocks.

Advanced Downhill Training.

After three or four sessions of short efforts, move to:

Long Repetitions at VO2 max. 800 to 1,200 meter intervals at 2 mile pace. Again, you'll run 2 mile pace at 5K effort.

Running at 2 mile pace will be easier than on the flat. Enjoy flight during your training. Your heart and lungs will be at 5K pace, but the hip flexors and extensors get the benefit from two mile pace. Run one out of every four long repeat sessions downhill, and your track reps at 5K pace will seem easier because you will have the legspeed in hand.

Downhill Running Uses:

* Cruising a few strides is pleasant when you feel tired; you still get to run fast. However, don't substitute downhills for the rest which you may need.
* Race preparation at all distances, because you can run faster than race pace.
* Preparation for downhill race courses.
* Improved flexibility, increased elasticity of quads, calf and Achilles from practicing eccentric contractions, but stay with short strides to keep damage to the minimum.
* And finally, you can work on running economy without being under as much physiological or lung busting pressure as when you're running on the flat.

Don't want to devote an entire session to downhill running? Former masters champ at the Los Angeles and Big Sur Marathons, Greg Horner routinely includes downhill training. When running 2,000 meter repeats, the last 25 percent of it is down a gentle grass slope. Most of the first 1,500 meters is up a 2 to 4 percent grade.

CHAPTER FIVE

or, Phase Three to your Marathon

ANAEROBIC THRESHOLD TRAINING

Tempo running, or anaerobic threshold pace training is the third element for marathon preparation. If you follow Chapter 11 or 14s program, you may prefer to do this section before hill training. The order is not important; stimulating each type of physiological system is what's important. You'll be running some hills during this phase too, so although the emphasis is on improving your anaerobic threshold, you can run each type of training in your preferred order.

Anaerobic Threshold pace training means running at 15K to 10 mile race pace, or about 10 to 20 seconds per mile slower than current 10K racing speed. Threshold pace happens to be 20 to 40 seconds per mile faster than your marathon speed: It will teach you to stride rhythmically at good pace and improve your ability to run a great marathon race.

   Threshold is also the pace which you can sustain for about 50 to 60 minutes. For some of you it will be 10K or 5 mile race pace. For the elite, it's close to half marathon pace. For this Chapter we will assume it is 15K or 10 mile race pace.

You still need to practice running at marathon pace: Include two miles at marathon pace within your long runs. You also need slowish running at 65 to 70 percent of maximum heartrate to continue improving your aerobic ability, or your VO2 max. Running at one minute per mile slower than marathon pace still dominates your mileage.

However, running 20 to 40 seconds per mile faster than marathon pace will improve your ability to run at marathon pace...by improving your anaerobic threshold or turnpoint.

According to Jack Daniels Ph.D., researcher, coach of the State University of New York at Cortland cross-country team, "Anaerobic Threshold is the pace or intensity beyond which blood lactate concentration increases dramatically, due to your body's inability to supply all its oxygen needs."

Process More Oxygen

"Physiologically, threshold training teaches muscle cells to use more oxygen - you produce less lactate. Your body also becomes better at clearing lactate."

Threshold pace running conditions your muscle fibers to a faster pace. You build leg strength and improve running biomechanics by testing the limits of your aerobic system.

Because you're running at a fast pace for considerable distance, you develop speed endurance by bringing in more of your fast twitch muscle fibers and teach motor responses to more of the fibers used in racing.

Anaerobic Threshold Training Builds Stamina.

* Expand your capillary network.
* Increase your muscles' enzyme activity.
* Educate your muscle cells to tolerate higher levels of lactic acid.
* Yet you educate your cells to excrete lactic acid faster.
* You further increase your VO2 max.

Threshold Running Improves Form.

Concentration on form improves, giving increased running efficiency with less wasted effort, devouring more ground with each stride as your hip flexibility improves.

Further strengthening of your running muscles as you bring in more of your muscle fibers to maintain this fast pace.

Improved coordination at higher speeds...if you pay attention to your running form: you cannot just float effortlessly along. Threshold pace running also prepares you for the stresses of racing.

At threshold pace, the mitochondria in your muscle cells can no longer meet all of your energy needs. Your body partially switches to the anaerobic system and you produce energy in the fluid surrounding the mitochondria. Lactic acid is produced as a by-product to anaerobic running. Practice running at anaerobic threshold pace often enough and you'll adapt to running with a higher level of lactate or lactic acid in your muscle cells and circulatory system. You will also excrete more lactic acid.

The point at which you produce excess lactic acid is your red line or lactate turnpoint. If you run faster than red line pace, your body soon forces you to slow down. In the early stages of threshold training your red line will probably be 80 percent of max HR. According to Daniels, "As you get fitter, your red line rises from 80 percent of maximum heartrate to 90-95 percent. Race day red line speed rises."

How to start Anaerobic Threshold or Lactate Buffering Intervals and Tempo Runs?

You already have...provided you've raced 10K, 10 miles and the half-marathon. Those early races were not just to get you used to racing. They raised your anaerobic threshold limit. For many of you, the 10Ks were well over your red line. The races at 10 miles and half-marathon were at the low end of your threshold. All these races teach you pace judgment, while also stimulating your anaerobic threshold to rise.

Novice marathon runners.

Most of you will be visiting threshold pace for the third or fourth time; you already experienced a 6 to 10 week series of threshold pace sessions while training for 10Ks, and again for the half-marathon and twenty mile racing.

Those of you ignoring the shorter race distances are here for the first time: Do not worry. Threshold training is gentle speed running, and starts with innocuous sessions such as 4 times half a mile at your half-marathon race pace. That is slower than in your fartlek or hill running, and only 20 to 40 seconds per mile faster than marathon pace.

After each half mile effort, run easy for a minute or two before easing up to half-marathon speed again.

These intervals are often called cruise intervals because you cruise along at modest effort. While 10K race pace can be gruesome, long reps at half-marathon pace are a delight. You'll still feel fresh after a few repeats at this modest pace.

According to *Lore of Running*, half of your improvement in lactate threshold or turnpoint comes in the first 10.5 days, but it takes 12 weeks at X miles per week to reap your full gains. You can increase your threshold from 63 to 71 percent of your VO2 max, allowing you to run faster at your threshold and thus faster at 10K to the marathon. It will take another 12 weeks at X mileage to reach your VO2 maximum.

The next time you increase mileage by 5 to 10 miles per week it will again take 12 weeks for maximum threshold improvement and 24 weeks for max VO2 increase, but only 10.5 days to get half of your anaerobic threshold increase.

In the next 24 weeks you'll probably choose to run 2 to 4 of your extra 10 miles at good speed as fartlek, threshold intervals and some at 5K pace to further increase your economic running skills and endurance.

Gentle Transition to quality miles.

The trusty overload principle requires runners to increase training by adding mileage, or by running faster. While your long run may have increased by two miles in this phase, the real goal of the anaerobic phase is to get you running at sustained pace for several miles. Adapting to a faster running pace for 3 to 5 miles each week makes your legs, your entire running system stronger.

Run half-marathon pace before 15K pace, and add half a mile of threshold running each week until you reach 10 percent of your weekly mileage in one session. You should have been running fartlek and hills for 8 to 20 weeks by now. You're already used to running at fast pace. There's no excuse for running at the same pace day after day.

As stated in Chapter One, this training book takes exception to the training suggested for first time marathon runners. Most novice marathon schedules include no speed running. Low mileage or novice marathon runners will benefit even more from speed running than moderately high mileage runners. Fast running teaches you to run with good form. It's vital for low mileage runners to be economical with their energy. The low mileage runners schedule in Chapter Eleven contains the same percentage of speedwork as high mileage runners in Chapter Fourteen! There's no reason to deny yourself anaerobic threshold or the VO2 max sessions in future chapters simply because you run low mileage.

Though you've run at threshold pace in your fartlek sessions, these are your first serious sessions at threshold pace.

After a few sessions of half miles as described above, you can graduate to mile repeats. Mile repeats at 80 percent max HR, provided you run them in control, are a very relaxing way to get used to threshold pace running. Mile reps are a great benchmark for threshold training, and will prepare you for your Tempo runs, which are continuous runs of 3 to 4 miles at half-marathon pace.

You'll move up from that modest 4 times half a mile to 5 times one mile over a 12 week period. Meanwhile, your hills and fartlek sessions will complement threshold pace training.

Half-marathon pace is also Lactate Threshold Velocity, the fastest pace you can run without the build-up of lactic acid. You need to experience some lactate build-up, so after a few sessions you'll increase speed to 15K pace.

You'll produce less lactic acid if you run a few striders before the threshold repeats. Striders before speed running are even more important in Chapter Six. It will take a few weeks for your muscles to adapt to anaerobic threshold training. Give your muscles time to adjust by running half-marathon pace first, then apply the easiest training needed to raise your anaerobic threshold: 15K pace is best.

How Hard is Threshold Pace?

Threshold pace training should not feel very uncomfortable. This is far from all-out running. But threshold running is moderately hard. You will not improve your marathon fitness if you avoid these sessions due to fear of hurting. So don't let them hurt...moderate your pace. When you're a quarter mile into your warmdown, you should feel as if you could have run an additional mile or two at threshold pace.

Running too fast also makes you prone to injury due to excessive fatigue, especially if you bring the fast training in too much at a time.

The first time through this phase can give you a 10 second per mile marathon pace increase. That's over 4 minutes from your marathon time. Those of you who have been racing for years should expect less improvement, unless you've never done regular training at 15K pace.

Increasing your pace too often will increase injury risk; don't increase running pace more than once every three weeks. Instead, practice relaxing while running at the same speed, but with less physical effort, using fewer calories or less energy. Maintain the same intensity level in hot, cold or windy conditions, and on hilly courses. Don't worry about your running pace changing. Heartrate and how you feel at this effort level are the best indicators.

Fifty degrees today with 50 percent cloud cover and a 5 mile per hour breeze? Your pace at 80 percent of maximum heartrate may be just where you dream of it being: 6 or 7 or 8 minute miles. Really humid, or hot, or running into a nasty head wind, or using several layers of clothing to stay warm enough to run safely? You may be at threshold pace effort at 6.15 or 7.20 or 8.25 pace. You must run slower to get the right training effect. Run at the speed that gets your heartrate to 80 percent of your maximum.

After 2 to 4 sessions of Cruise Intervals, try, Continuous runs at threshold pace.

Run about 4 miles at half-marathon race pace - probably 80 percent of your max heartrate. Six to eight miles is the ultimate goal, or 10 percent of your weekly mileage; do whichever is the least amount. Increase your session by a half mile at pace every other week.

Early threshold sessions should be barely over 80 percent max heartrate because you need to get used to the effort involved during a continuous fast run. You'll also need to think about form on these runs.

Graduate to 15K Pace.

If it feels right, run one and a half mile or two mile repeats at 90 percent max HR: but you must not be too uncomfortable. You can also run longer reps of up to three miles to practice and perfect your running form and concentration.

After 3 or 4 tempo runs at half-marathon pace, you can try 4 miles at 15K or 10 mile pace: true threshold speed will take you to 85 to 90 percent of max HR. You should not accumulate much lactic acid because your body is learning how to break it down, and to rapidly excrete it.

Many physiologists recommend 90 percent max HR as the top range for these sessions. Most of these runs will be at 15K or 10 mile pace to hit that HR target. When your muscles are tired two days after your long run, or when weather is bad, it may only be half-marathon pace: It will rarely be slower. If your heartrate is over 90 percent of your max at half-marathon pace, you should add rest to the next few days. Difficulty maintaining half-marathon pace and aching quads could indicate overtraining, so back off on running pace.

Don't be concerned if you're able to run 10K pace at 90 percent of max HR. These good days are a joy. You're getting stronger, running more efficiently, or you sneaked in an extra rest day which left you feeling fresher. It could also mean that you're ready to PR at the 10K.

Faster than 10K pace puts most of us over the red line because it is too harsh. As Jack Daniels says, "86 percent of maximum heartrate is probably the best pace." Run 10-20 seconds per mile slower than 10K pace if you've never raced at 15K or 10 miles.

Here's another way to calculate goal HR for threshold:

205 minus half your age	*at age 50 gives 180*
minus resting HR	*40 gives 140*
times 85 percent	*119*
Add back your resting HR	*119 + 40 = 159*

The newer, 50 year old runner with a resting HR of say 60 gets: 180 – 60 for 120 x 85 percent, so 102 plus his resting HR of 60 to give a goal of 162. These three beats per minute can be the difference from running at 10K and 15K pace.

Calculate your goal HR at 90 percent of max to get your range for anaerobic threshold sessions.

Heart rate reserve (HRR) is similar to the above. HRR is max HR – resting HR

Target HR is the percentage of HRR you wish to work at, and adding back your resting HR. You will need to run a maximum heartrate test to use HRR.

High Mileage Runners:

Six to eight miles of long reps at anaerobic threshold or faster is a popular session for high mileage runners. Many Kenyans run eight times one mile at 10K pace or faster on dirt trails, with a 400 meter or a one minute rest at marathon pace, the ideal "restive" pace for muscles to deal with lactic acid.

World Record Holder at the Marathon in the 1990s, Da Costa often ran sessions such as 15 times 1,000 meters at slightly slower than his half-marathon pace, with only a 20-30 second recovery. He had 10 plus years of competitive training at the 10K and up before he set the world record.

1984 Olympic Bronze medalist Charlie Spedding did five miles at tempo pace followed by 3 x 2,000 meters a bit faster. This session was less than 10 percent of his weekly mileage!

Not had 10 to 20 years of competitive running?

Restrict yourself to 10 percent of your mileage in one speed session. If you run fifty miles a week, you're entitled to five miles of threshold pace reps. Try this four week rotation while racing once a month.

* 4 miles at half-marathon pace, then 2 x 800 at 10K pace.
* 4 x 2,000 meters at 15K pace, your true threshold pace. Take a quarter mile slow run recovery.
* 5 x one mile at 10K pace. The top end of threshold for most runners, but it helps your buffering system. Avoid this pace if you've recently hit 50 miles per week for the first time. Great session to run 2 weeks before a 10K race.
* 8 x 1,000 at 15K pace. Slower, yet shorter reps than last week, but keep the recovery to 60 seconds.

You need to train up to the point at which anaerobic energy production predominates. Try to avoid going over the red line. Avoid running too fast. While fast running is fun, you don't make greater gains on your changing anaerobic threshold speed by running at the faster pace. Generally, 15K pace is better than 10K pace; those of you on low mileage may feel the need to run some reps at 10K pace for psychological reasons. However, 15K pace makes you less tired, keeping your muscles fresh for a more worthwhile hill or VO2 max session later in the week.

Half-marathon pace is even easier on your body than 15K pace, causing less muscle fatigue. Half-marathon pace also gives you a closer feel to marathon pace, while still bumping up your anaerobic threshold.

Match each threshold pace session with some kind of speed at short distances. Run fartlek or hills each week.

Don't repeat training sessions more than once every three weeks. If you elect to run all sessions at 15K pace, the 1,000s and miles will need a 200 meter rest to make sure you give the muscles a chance to educate themselves: muscles need only a short chance to buffer and excrete the lactate. Long rests defeat your purpose.

Lets see how much of your training is likely to be at ideal anaerobic HR while running 1,200s with short rests. Our athlete runs 6 x 1,200 on a nearly straight section of grass and no undulations. Using a two minute rest, (200 meters of mostly jogging...HR down to 120) he averages 4.37 per repeat (slowest first at 4.40; fastest 4.35 in the middle and a 4.39 finish). His maximum HR is 180; because he is a seasoned runner of several decades, his goal HR for 15K pace is therefore 162 (90 % of max).

Repeat #	1	2	3	4	5	6
Point at which						
HR reached 162 at	900	550	350	250	200	150 meters
HR at 400	149	157	162	163	164	163
HR at 800	159	163	164	163	162	162
HR at 1,200	163	164	164	164	163	163

percentage of time the heart was at
| 15K intensity | 25 | 54 | 62 | 80 | 83 | 87 |

* The highest HR this day was 165, (950 meters into the 3rd rep) which would be 10K intensity, and not the goal of his session. He was at 165 for only a few seconds because the athlete reduced pace.
* The relatively slow first repeat contributed to only 25 percent of it being at 15K HR goals. However, the entire three quarters of a mile were at his 15K speed for the year, and the sensible start set up a pleasurable session.
* The 90 % level took 550 meters for the second repeat, with 54 % of his repetition at goal HR, and over three-quarters was above 85 % of max HR.
* As the session progressed, a pleasant fatigue set in and 90 % of max HR was achieved very early in each repeat, giving him 83 % of his time, or eleven and a quarter minutes at his 15K goal HR during the last three repeats.
* While he had the legs to do at least one more repeat, he saved himself for his long run the next day.
* He eased the pace just a little for the last two repeats to stop himself hitting 10K HR intensity.

How can we improve his anaerobic threshold?

1. Have him run another 4.5 mile threshold session every 4 to 5 days for 6 to 8 weeks.
2. Match each threshold session with short effort fartlek or 5K pace running alternating with hills.
3. Include tempo runs and longer repeats. When he does this session again, consider:
4. Running the first rep a bit faster and taking a one minute rest before the second repeat, which should get him to a 162 HR by perhaps 600 and 400 meters during those repeats, which would result in an additional 450 meters at a HR of 162. Then use 2 minutes rests so that:
5. He can add an additional repeat once a month. Or,
6. Increase length of repeats to one mile, which would give him an additional 92 seconds at his threshold HR on all six

repeats. This would take his current 47 % at goal HR during the first three repeats to 62 %. In total, he would get an additional 1.5 miles or over 9 minutes at goal HR.

7. Ask him to do a maximum HR test (fast uphill 200 to 300 meters) to make sure his max HR has not dropped to 178. If his max HR is 178, the training time at 164 HR would be in his 10K range. While that would be a very nice Chapter Seven session, unless he can race 15K at this intensity, it is too harsh for anaerobic threshold training. (Note: If he is training in his 10K range he will obviously not be able to race a 15K at that pace!)

Pages 263-265 shows what happens to a runner's HR while doing track Intervals aiming for VO2 max improvement.

A great proponent of heartrate monitor use is Dave Welsh, who coached wife Priscilla to a World Masters record (2.26.51) at London and to outright victory in New York.

Most of their training is guided by heartrate. Long runs at 60 to 70 percent of max HR develop aerobic and fat burning ability; the second longest run is at 70 to 80 % of max, but with 4 miles at 90 % of max HR (i.e., threshold pace). They also practice 5 mile runs at 80 % of max HR and monitor as the running pace gets faster over the months due to the increase in aerobic capacity, or ones maximum aerobic pace. You are also improving running economy, so you can run faster using the same amount of energy.

Like many top runners, one of their favorite sessions was 1,000s, doing ten or more of them. They also practice running form with striders and by experimenting at constant speed on a treadmill. The decrease in HR on the monitor shows the work effort decreasing.

Another way to do your second longest run each week is at **Best Aerobic Effort** or BAE. This is high end aerobic pace, just before anaerobic threshold so it's 30 to 45 seconds per mile slower than 10K pace; in fact, it's just a bit slower than marathon pace for most people. Because you build up to doing it for 10 to 12 miles, you'll learn to relax at good pace. The overall effort is fairly high, with your HR at close to 80 of max, so concentrate a little and enjoy the sensation of this hard, yet steady pace.

Your medium long run is the usual spot for BAE runs. This author sees little point in running 12 miles at marathon pace because it is too strenuous and does not develop a specific energy system. It has little purpose. The long run and all other mileage at 70 % max HR develop your aerobic ability. BAE pace runs, moving from 4 to 12 miles, teach you economic running and are less fatiguing than long runs at marathon pace. You can save your muscles for threshold sessions at half marathon to 15K pace.

Provided you include 2 miles per week at actual marathon pace, either in your BAE or your long runs, you should not need major sessions at marathon pace.

Long Runs: Maintain Mileage.

Your long distance runs increase only slightly during this third phase of marathon training. Run a fifteen on odd number weeks at 65 to 70 percent max HR. Run 18s to 20 on even number weeks. Some people like to do 20s during their entire marathon build-up, from the first weeks of fartlek training in Phase One, until three weeks before their race. Most of you should aim to reach regular 20s by the end of Phase Three, so that you'll get at least half a dozen 20s prior to your marathon. You'll also have a dozen 18s of course, but running 20s during Phase Four should be your goal.

You should probably run a quality speed session the day before each long run, because after all, you don't need fresh legs to run easy. After appropriate rest, you're ready for the second speed session of the week.

You should bounce back from speed sessions rapidly: if you cannot, then the speed session was too hard for your current fitness level.

How can you expect to run the 26.2 miles of a marathon when you _only_ do 20 or so in training? Because it's only training. You could actually run 26.2 miles almost any week during Phase Three of marathon training, but you're in training so you won't run that far.

Your legs should ache a bit during and after a 20 mile run because you did a 4 to 5 mile session of speed running the day before the 20. You'll hardly run in the 7 days before a marathon, and rest the day before it, so your legs will be fresh. You'll also have more glycogen in your muscles and liver and more fatty acids in your muscles on marathon day.

There is no need and no point in resting up for long training runs. You typically take a rest day on Friday to be fresh for speed running or a low-key Saturday race. Take your muscles through the long run the next day at one minute per mile slower than marathon pace and you'll soon be trained to race a marathon. Tapering before long training runs defeats the feeling you'd get from running with fatigued muscles.

Don't decrease your mileage while running the gentle speedwork at anaerobic threshold. Your mileage reduction comes in the peaking phase. If you had previously done most of your running at one pace, many coaches say that your legs would be "dead and lifeless" from too much pounding. However, you have been developing good running form while you float across the road or dirt and grass trails. You have been running with modest impact per stride. You have also developed a sense of pace with fartlek and hill running.

Your leg strength from high mileage and weight training will enable you to develop speed from a natural, flowing stride length and from high cadence. Don't reduce your mileage at this stage or you will lose that strength.

If you want more legspeed when running at threshold effort, run some of your reps with the wind or down gentle slopes. With downhill and wind running be careful about overstriding. In overstriding, your foot is still traveling forward as it strikes the ground. Your heel acts as a break, causing stress and connective tissue damage on every footplant. The damage could show itself as sore knees, aching soles of the feet, a tender back, or anything in-between. Overstriding also costs you speed because you lose momentum on every stride, so you'll fatigue earlier.

See the detailed schedules to see how threshold pace fits in to your training week. If you've run significant amounts of threshold training before, this phase need only last about 4 weeks; the runner entering threshold pace training for the first time would be wise to take a conservative approach to the marathon, and stay here 12 weeks while maximizing threshold gains.

Lets review the 4 rules of threshold running:

* Run 4 to 6 miles or up to 10 percent of your weekly mileage;
* Alternate one mile reps; two miles reps, with a continuous 4 miler;
* Ease down from half-marathon to 15K pace over 6 to 12 weeks.
* Make consecutive repeats a second or two faster (but note the heartrate for the athlete doing 1,200s on page 111). Gain a sense of relaxation at speed while being in control of your pace. Push back your anaerobic threshold.

You may find threshold pace to be the most enjoyable form of marathon training. You're running only a bit faster than marathon pace, yet you're fairly close to 10K pace so you get the exhilaration from near full-speed cruising. You're only running 4 to 6 miles at this gentle pace, so it's not exhausting. Your muscles should have a tingling freshness after you've showered. Limit yourself to one session every 5 to 7 days.

See page 373   for an "anaerobic point" analyzer.

Sample month during Threshold Training:

Retain your long runs of course. The long run is the cement which holds your training blocks together. This is the high intensity, three quality runs each week schedule.

	Day One	Two	Four	Six	
Probably	*Sat*	*Sun*	*Tues*	*Thursday*	
	hill repeats	Long	Fartlek	Anaerobic	Total
	(in meters)	run		Threshold	miles
Wk 1	12 x 400	15	8 / 5.0	T5	45
2	8 x 600	20	32 / 4.0	CI5	45
3	20 x 200	18	8 / 5.0	T4	44
4	12 x 300	14	24 / 3.0	CI3	35

5   Race at 10K, cruise 13 to 15 miles the day after and a gentle fartlek session midweek, then repeat the first four weeks.

T5 means a 25 minute to 5 mile tempo run at half-marathon pace with a 3 mile warm-up and 3 mile cool down.

CI5 means 5 miles of cruise intervals at about 15K race pace, but with only a short recovery between reps.

Because two of the fartlek sessions (e.g. 8 / 5.0 is 8 efforts to give 5 miles at speed) are still long efforts, you'll have 6 threshold pace sessions per month. As always, those 300s the week pre-race are on the flat, though you could practice gentle downhills if the next race is downhill.

Most runners will prefer to train moderately hard only twice a week, and switch a few sessions around. You'll still get four threshold pace sessions per month, and two hill sessions.

	Day One	Two	Four	Six	Total
1	H 12 x 400	15	T5	12	45
2	F 32 / 4.0	20	CI5	12	45
3	H 20 x 200	18	T4	10	44
4	12 x 300	14	CI3	8	35

Reminder: H and F stand for hills and fartlek respectively.

Lest you've forgotten or skipped pages, you will all cross-train two days per week.

Day Six on page 116 could be at 45 seconds per mile slower than marathon pace, but include 20 to 60 minutes at BAE. (Best aerobic effort is typically 15 seconds per mile slower than goal pace for your marathon.) Add about 5 minutes every 2 to 3 weeks at BAE.

Pre-marathon build-up races.

Anaerobic threshold training, if practiced for a long enough period, should allow you to race the half-marathon at 25 seconds per mile slower than your current 10K race pace. If you feel good at 10 miles, increase pace by a few seconds per mile for a strong finish.

Try to arrange your 10 week phase at anaerobic threshold to culminate in a half-marathon race. Your last week pre race will be really easy, such as week four above. Cutting down to 11 on Sunday and 5 on Thursday would be wise.

After your 10 weeks at threshold, run a session every ten days or so to maintain your gains and for the joy of running long repeats at 15K pace. If you've been used to 5 to 6 miles at threshold, two times 2 miles is a great session the weekend before almost any race. Also, run a few races at 10K to the half-marathon while working on the final aspect of your marathon training in Chapters 6, 7, 10 & 12.

Note: The usual advice on windy days is to run into the wind on the way out, so that if you feel bad, you'll be pushed back home on the return. On hot days, the better option is to run with the wind on the way out and enjoy the cooling affect of running into the wind on the way back. For chilly days it's probably best to have the easy running in the second half of the run.

You can also run at easy pace with the wind on the way out, and then do hard efforts at threshold intensity into the wind on the way back. You'll be running slower while doing your quality threshold running, so ground impact will be less on each stride.

Think lactic acid is bad for your running? Then why do nearly all of our body systems produce it?

According to George A. Brooks Ph.D. Director, Exercise Physiology Lab, at Berkley, "Lactic acid is not just a useless by-product of exercise. Lactic acid is an energy source involved in using glucose and glycogen. Oxidation of lactic acid is one of our most important energy sources. Don't let this important metabolite scare you. But do still:

"Use a combination of long sub-maximal training and quality training to minimize the lactic acid production and enhance its removal."

Studies by Brooks suggest that Lactate is an important energy source which allows you to preserve glucose and glycogen.

How to use the Speed Table on page 120.

Your best recent 10K is the starting point. Your base threshold training pace is 15K speed, or 10-20 seconds per mile slower than 10K speed for most runners.

The slightly less accurate starting point is to find your current 5K time in the left column, then read across for your ideal training pace for long cruise intervals and tempo runs of 20 to 25 minutes.

The 5K personal record (PR) line also shows you if you've done sufficient strength and mileage training. For example, if the 17.11 5K runner cannot run 35.27 for 10K, he or she should add more steady runs, long runs, hills, fartlek and threshold, before moving to Chapter Six. You have to develop enough endurance to stay relatively close to 5K pace at the 10K, which will give you the endurance to stay relatively close to 10K pace at even longer distances.

The 15K time is the projected PRs based on the 10K time...provided you're running sufficient mileage. As stated in this Chapter, you should also do threshold training with longer repeats such as 2 miles and with tempo runs of up to half an hour or 5 miles, whichever comes first.

Use 85 to 90 percent of your maximum heartrate as an additional guide to the upper limit of your training pace.

Note: one way to move up the table, with improved PRs is to train for that upper line. Currently doing 6.51 mile repeats with a 90 second rest because your 10K PR is 41.15, and because 15K pace is fast enough to improve your anaerobic threshold while leaving your muscles fresh for other running? At some stage you'll increase speed toward 6.39 miles and feel relaxed doing it, and with your heartrate well below 90 percent of maximum. 6.40 is 15K pace for the next level.

When you can run 4 or 5 repeats at 6.39 without a rest week leading into the session, you may be ready for some PRs. Moving up a line can take months. Try 5 seconds per mile steps rather than jumping up a line. Don't cheat yourself into thinking you're in PR shape by taking an easy week prior to mile repeats. Do rest up once a month for a 10K or 15K race to check your progress though.

As ever, when increasing mileage, run your repeats at the slower end of your range. Run half-marathon pace if you're in the top two-thirds of the table; run 15K pace if in the lower third. Increase pace by 5 to 10 seconds per mile or closer to 10K pace as you get used to your new mileage.

Lactate Threshold Velocity incorporates elements of threshold and VO2 max and running economy. It's the highest rate of using oxygen without the build-up of lactic acid. It also equals half-marathon pace. Use this pace as preparation for 15K pace sessions, or while resting up. Half-marathon pace also saves your legs for the long run, which is the most vital run each week. Two and three mile reps work well at half-marathon pace. Use a mixture of sessions to meet your needs and the freshness of your legs on a particular day.

Anaerobic Threshold training pace table

PR at 5K	PR at 10K	10K pace	Best 15K	15K pace	Half-marathon pace	finish time
14:57	30.54	4.59	48:19	5.11	5.24	70:45
15:31	32.02	5.10	50:02	5.22	5.37	73:34
16:05	33.10	5.20	51:34	5.32	5.47	75:46
16:39	34.20	5.32	53:27	5.44	5.59	78:23
17:11	35.27	5.43	55:09	5.55	6.10	80:47
17:45	36.37	5.54	56:51	6.06	6.24	83:50
18:20	37.50	6.06	58:44	6.18	6.36	86:28
18:54	39.00	6.17	60:26	6.29	6.47	88:52
19:27	40.09	6.28	62:09	6.40	7.00	91:42
20:00	41.15	6.39	63:51	6.51	7.11	94:06
20:34	42.23	6.49	65:24	7.01	7.21	96:17
21:07	43.29	7.01	67:34	7.15	7.35	99:21
21:41	44.40	7.12	69:17	7.26	7.48	102:11
22:18	45.56	7.24	71:09	7.38	8.00	104:48
23:06	47.35	7.40	73:38	7.54	8.19	108:57
23:56	49.18	7.56	76:07	8.10	8.35	112:27
24:46	50.41	8.10	78:56	8.26	8.51	115:43
25:36	52.44	8.30	81:43	8.46	9.16	121:24
26:33	54.41	8.48	84:30	9.04	9.34	125:20
27:24	56.26	9.05	86:50	9.19	9.54	129:41
29:10	60.06	9.41	93:12	10.00	10.40	139:44
30:25	62.42	10.08	97:33	10.28	11.08	145:51
33:36	69.16	11.09	107:12	11.30	12.15	160:29

Anaerobic Threshold Pace for Mile Repeats or training speed for longer efforts, at 10K pace (roughly threshold if your 10K PR is slower than 45 minutes), 15K pace, and Half-marathon pace (threshold for top runners).

CHAPTER SIX

Phase Four to your Marathon

INTERVAL TRAINING

at close to your

VO2 MAXIMUM PACE

Increase your basic speed by 10 seconds per mile and you can lop four and a half minutes off of your marathon time. You'll spend less time under the sun or in the cold, and get under or closer to that magical time barrier you've been grafting toward. Training faster than marathon pace will make you a more efficient user of oxygen and glycogen, while making you a more economic runner and less likely to injure yourself. Running at 5K race pace and up to 3 seconds per 400 meters faster than 5K pace will help you to master fast marathons.

Running economy and oxygen uptake or VO2 maximum is nicely developed with long runs at easy pace because you keep your feet close to the ground for mile after mile. You also improve economy by running faster miles at the right pace. But don't sprint to find speed. Sprinting will leave you with injuries. 1972 Olympic Marathon Gold Medalist Frank Shorter was world class at 2 miles and up, in part because of his marathon training, and partly due to his 2 to 3 sessions of quality speed training most weeks. He typically did three miles of Interval training on Mondays and Wednesdays.

Runners with a high VO2 maximum absorb more oxygen into their blood stream and efficiently deliver the oxygen to the muscles: they can run faster marathons.

Economic runners need less oxygen for a given pace: they're frugal with oxygen use. They run faster marathons.

Here's a surprise: The fastest marathons are run by athletes with a combination of high VO2 max and good running economy: Training regularly at 2 mile, 5K and 10K race pace improves your VO2 max and your running economy.

The aims of Interval Training then, are to:

* Improve Maximum Oxygen Uptake Capacity or VO2 Max, which is the amount of oxygen you can absorb.
* Get more efficient at utilizing that oxygen...by improving leg turnover and running efficiency.

Strong enough for Interval Training?

The easy running and long runs in Phase One to Three did not develop your neurological pathways needed for fast running, or use all the muscle fibers needed for fast running: which is why you ran fartlek, hills and anaerobic threshold during the first three phases of your marathon training. Your fast twitch muscle fibers are now strong; they possess speed endurance and are ready for the rigors and if you run too fast, the rigor mortis, of Interval training at VO2 maximum.

You need a good base before commencing serious speed running. Never lose sight of the strength phase. Keep your long runs and the modest paced fartlek sessions in which you stride up some hills and down others.

Your mileage and strength base increased the number and size of your mitochondria, the organelles inside the muscle cells that make ATP (adenosine triphosphate), which fuels your muscles. The strength you gained from Chapters 4 & 5 will allow you to run this sub 10K pace training. Your patient strength build-up facilitates your shift to speed running.

Phase 4 takes your running speed to a much higher level, while improving your running economy. You can run hills and threshold pace after this phase if you wish. The order in which you do the types of training is less important than the act of using all three types. Now lets sneak in some science.

What does VO2 MAX mean?

VO2 max, or Maximum Oxygen Uptake Capacity, to use its formal name, is the amount of oxygen we can absorb into our cells in one minute while working at full capacity. It's a measure of fitness expressed in milliliters per kilogram per minute.

You can predict your VO2 max with 95 percent accuracy by running around a track on a windless day for 15 minutes. The distance run to the nearest 25 meters is noted, and Bruno Balke's formula is used to predict VO2 max. After a base of 6.5, this follows a linear pattern of 5 mls/min/kg. for every extra 400 meters covered. For example, if you run 10 laps (4,000 meters), it predicts 56.5 mls/min/kg. 4,400 meters gives a 61.5 VO2 max.

If 4,450 meters is run, VO2 max would be:

VO2 Max = 6.5 + 0.0125 x (distance run in 15 minutes)
          = 6.5 + 0.0125 x 4,450
VO2 Max = 62.125
World class runners reach 80 (male) and 70 (female).

Frank Horwill, The British Athletic Federation coach and advisor to many top British runners, says, "The best way to improve VO2 max is to run between 80 and 100 percent of

VO2 max. One hundred percent equals the athlete's 3K or 2-mile race pace; 95 % equals 5K speed; 90 % is 10K speed.

"Work physiologists believe training at 95 % VO2 max brings the best results - though one Russian physiologist of note - Karibosk, thinks 100 % (3K or two mile pace) is better because it tunes up the anaerobic pathway.

"Physiologists are agreed the percentages at the higher level (100 - 95 %) should be done for 3 to 5 minutes' duration, repeated many times in one session, with a short recovery. The lower percentages (90 to 80 %) should be for 10-20 minutes, also with short recoveries."

Already worked through Chapter Five? You've trained at 80 to 90 percent VO2 max while running threshold pace sessions. Chapter Seven deals with 90 percent of VO2 max training with running at 10K pace, and is a vital element before your first marathon. Chapter Twelve deals with long repeats at 3K to 5K paces, which is for very experienced runners...save Chapter Twelve until after your first marathon.

This chapter deals with fairly short intervals at 95 to 100 percent VO2 maximum. Stay here for months and perfect the art of short reps at 3K to 5K paces.

The last 9 months have increased your VO2 max substantially. Now it's time to make additional VO2 max gains by training at close to your maximum oxygen uptake pace. Applying this modest stress to your lungs, muscles and circulatory systems will stimulate your VO2 max to rise: you'll be able to race faster.

The Track.

Interval training is a precise and progressive form of training. You change one of 5 variables once a month to:

* Further stimulate your VO2 system;
* Force yourself to run more economically;
* Use all your muscle fibers - making you stronger; and,
* Develop pace judgment.

These goals are best achieved on a flat surface of known distance. The advantages to track sessions are:

1/ Same distances all over the country. A quarter mile track is a couple of yards or meters longer than a 400 meter track!

2/ A smooth surface. Even the ruttiest high school dirt tracks have a good surface much of the time.

3/ You get away from traffic, dogs and pedestrians.

4/ Tracks help you keep interval training precise in any city; you can measure your progress more easily.

Here's a few track running guidelines.

Look before you change lanes; avoid lane one if possible; don't assume someone will move to the inside of the track after his fast interval. Assume everyone else's brain is malfunctioning, and you should stay safe.

Rest During Interval Training.

Technically, the rest period is the Interval! Generally, you should take less than 90 seconds rest during interval sessions. The greatest stimulation of heart development occurs in the first 10 seconds of the rest period. If you're running short repeats such as 300s at the appropriate pace for you, it should only take 30 seconds for your heartrate to get below 130. The extra minute of rest is for your mind, not your body. Let your HR reach 110 to 120 while you maintain a decent recovery speed. Run at a steady pace during your recoveries to bring in nutrients and to help the muscles rid themselves of the lactic acid from fast running.

VDOT refers to velocity or running speed at your VO2 maximum and is the same as 3K to 5K pace for most people. Entire books are devoted to training at a percentage of your VDOT. The results are the same as this book: Steady running at low intensities mixed with training at threshold and percentages of VO2 max or percentages of max heartrate. The good books also include hill training.

<u>Running Speed at Maximum Oxygen Use</u> (RSMO) measures how efficiently you use oxygen. It's the same speed as 100 percent of your VO2 max, or about 3K pace.

Maximum work rate is one predictor for performance at middle distances, but your best speed for a 3K race is a better predictor for the marathon (lactate turnpoint is an even better predictor of performance as demonstrated by the way we use 10K to half-marathon bests to predict marathon performance).

The fastest 1,500 meter runner has the potential to become the fastest marathon runner due to his or her speed advantage. In practice, few fast 1,500 or mile runners have enough slow twitch or Type I muscle fibers, let alone the <u>will</u> to train for the marathon. This years 5 best runners at the 10K and perhaps the 5K are more likely than this years 5 best milers to win the major marathons in 4 to 6 years time.

Interval Training Basics.

* Run a warm-up and stretch because flexibility determines your range of movement, your potential stride length.
* Muscles are 10 percent longer when warmed up. Muscles work better when they are long - exerting the same amount of force with less effort.
* Don't jump straight into long sessions of intervals.
* Feel as comfortable in the last 500 meter rep as you did in the first 500 and start with 5K pace intervals.
* Run the last few reps as fast as the early ones.
* Sometimes, run the last few reps a couple seconds faster.
* Don't feel wasted afterwards. Feel as if you could have run another interval or two when you've finished.

For marathon runners who have never trained for a 10K, and did not follow this authors half-marathon training advice, here's how you can progress if doing formal VO2 max training for the first time. See page 142 for the table of suggested training speeds at 95 and 100 percent of VO2 max (5K and 2-mile race pace).

* <u>Week One:</u> Bends & straights. Stride quite fast along the straight then jog the bends at a steady pace. Run 8 to 12 laps, which gives 16 to 24 striders. You should not feel exhausted. Short striders of 20 to 30 seconds need little concentration, yet you'll improve running form, and your muscles will get used to the new running surface.

* <u>Week Two:</u> 16 x 200 meters with a 100 interval recovery. The nice surface may tempt you to run fast; hold back at 5K pace to decrease injury risk. How do your hold your speed back? Keep the rest periods to 30 seconds.

Or, instead of the 100 jog, ease to a stop at the end of the 200 meters, jog back to your finish point and do a small circle to begin the next rep from there. You'll be using the 200 and 400 meter start points, whereas faster runners will have 4 different start points for their 200s.

* <u>Week Three:</u> 10 x 300 meters. Keep the 100 recovery. Run two straights and one bend for the repetition; jog one bend for the recovery. Use lane 4 or 5. This reduces the strain on your knees and hips from leaning into the curves.

* <u>Week Four:</u> 8 x 200 and 4 x 400 meters with a one minute rest after your 400s. Run 400s at 5K pace.

Gradually take the 200s down to 3K speed, which is 100 percent of your VO2 max. Aim for 12 seconds per <u>mile</u> faster than the speed of your best recent 5,000 meters. This modest pace stimulates your leg muscles and your heart. However, your first time through this schedule, 5K pace is better than 2 mile pace. Don't hurt during these early sessions.

Use the sprinters start point when running in the middle lanes. Your start point for a 400 meter effort in lane 5 is about one third of the way through the curve. If you run a whole lap in lane five, starting and finishing at the same spot, you'd add 26.8 meters per lap with the lanes at 42 inches wide. That's about 5.4 seconds for the 80 seconds per 400 meter runner.

* <u>Week Five</u>: 12 x 300. Pace judgment should improve with practice; aim to run your reps at even pace. Many

runners blitz the first 100 then stagger through the last 100 of each rep. Comfortable interval sessions require even pace for the individual reps, and even pace for all reps.

   * <u>Week Six</u>: 4 x 200 and 6 x 400 meters. Run too fast and this session is hard. Maintain good form for the entire lap. Monitor your running form. Quarters have the advantage that you start and finish each effort at almost the same place.

   * <u>Week Seven:</u> 4 x 300, and 3 to 4 x 600 meters. You'll have to concentrate a bit to keep your running form in the last third of the 600s, which is why you're here.

   * <u>Week Eight:</u> 4 x 200, and 8 x 400 meters.

Then alternate sessions using mostly short reps at 3K or 2 mile pace, with sessions of longer reps at 5K race pace.

   Interval sessions should be as long as you can handle them in comfort. No hurting because you need to be able to run 14 miles or more the next day, i.e., to recover easily. When you've done a few Interval sessions, your exercise capacity will increase, so you will be able to run more repetitions.

Match each interval session with a hill training session or fartlek run to give yourself two sessions of short efforts a week. Do retain a tempo run or a session of long reps at anaerobic threshold each week.

   Intervals fine-tune your body, helping you get the best out of your muscles. Measure the real progress in tune up races. Don't just become good at running interval sessions.

   Interval running is the second most likely form of running to be social. Most people like to do their longest run with company. A three hour or more run is usually more pleasurable with a few companions who have similar goals...provided they run at your pace! Interval training, especially when you run at 2 mile pace, is more fun and easier to achieve in a group. Most running clubs and marathon preparation groups have a track night. Or you can bring 2 or 3 like minded runners together for your own sessions.

Practice good running form, and intervals at 95 to 100 percent of your VO2 max will:

Improve your flexibility and running efficiency or economy...enabling you to run faster marathons.

Recruit even more of your fast twitch Type II fibers, more of your total muscle fibers to move your legs fast, which:

* Improves your leg strength and potentially your stride length, which allows you to run faster.
* Raises your leg turnover or cadence.
* Improving overall speed and economy.
* Your smoother running requires less ATP, so that means your energy lasts longer. You can run farther at a set pace.
* You improve your neuromuscular coordination even if you forget to work on form.
* You breathe deeper and your intercostals and diaphragm muscles develop tone.
* The body's ability to process oxygen improves.
* Your aerobic capacity and VO2 maximum rises.
* You're able to run longer before you reach oxygen debt. You'll be able to handle that oxygen debt better.
* You'll improve pace judgment and run faster marathons.

VO2 Max Intervals are Progressive.

Apply an appropriate load and your body adapts by getting stronger and more rhythmic at running: You're better able to handle that load a few weeks later...provided you include sufficient rest. You can also measure your progress.

You can run the speed of race distances you've no desire to race, which will improve your marathon times. Few runners race at two miles, but interval sessions at 2 mile pace will help your half-marathon and marathon times.

You make gigantic early gains with relatively few interval sessions at 2 mile pace, provided you have enough background endurance.

This economical, yet fast and controlled running is great preparation for races at all distances. It gives you a huge amount of speed in hand compared to marathon pace.

Training at 5K to 3K paces makes anaerobic threshold sessions seem like jogging. When jogging those threshold reps you'll be running 30 seconds or more per mile slower than in your interval sessions, yet you'll still be 20 to 30 seconds per mile faster than marathon pace!

High mileage runners can run 10K of reps at 5K pace (95 percent of VO2 max). Because of the rests, each repeat will be no harder than a small section of a 5K race. Your legs will get the training benefits of much more than a 5K race.

Provided your rest periods are short enough, and the length of your repeats are long enough, your heart will also get the benefit of more than a 5K race (see page 120 for mile reps at 10K speed). With good base, you can do an intense workout, yet you won't feel as if you've punished yourself.

Have a Naturally High VO2 Max?

Runners with a natural ability to run a fast mile should probably work on their endurance to maintain the fast pace longer. They'll do more anaerobic threshold and steady runs to improve base endurance, but also run plenty of these VO2 max intervals to maintain running form. Your emphasis should be on long 5K pace intervals.

You runners who feel very relaxed at 15K pace, yet lack speed, should do strength and short hill reps to develop your 3K race potential to the limit. Increase your VO2 max by running a higher percentage of your intervals at 3K pace.

However, all runners should train at weak areas in moderation while continuing to practice their strengths. Follow the rule of alternating 15K pace running or hills, with 2 mile to 5K pace sessions, and you won't go wrong.

To Make Progress with VO2 Max Training.

Vary your Interval workouts according to:

* Rest period: gradually shorten your rest.
* What you do during the rest period (walk or jog).
* Running intensity or speed. 5K or 3K pace, which are 95 and 100 percent of your VO2 max respectively.
* Workout volume: increase the number of efforts which you run at 300, 400, 500 or 600 meters.
* How hard you train in the days before an Interval session. How fatigued you are from yesterdays training affects your ability to run economically at 3K to 5K paces.
* Length of repetitions: Longer reps are more stimulating.

Long Intervals produce much higher lactate levels than short repeats. Long Intervals improve the ability of your muscle fibers to contract in the presence of muscle acidity. The lactate you produce is used again and again in energy metabolism, even if there is a good supply of oxygen. Long Intervals also force you to run economically.

Stimulate your mind and muscles by changing one or more of these factors for each session. As Frank Horwill suggests, the best results are obtained between 5K and 2 mile race pace.

To improve your VO2 maximum capacity, your running economy and your potential at the marathon, make these changes over months or years, not every week. You can:

* Run faster in your speed effort: run 3K race pace instead 5K pace, or 100 percent VO2 max instead of 95 percent.
* Take a shorter recovery: As your body adapts to fast running, your heartrate will recover to under 120 beats per minute faster than it used too. You may only need a 200 meter run instead of a 400 jog to recover from 600s.
* Put more effort into the recovery (running at marathon pace for a minute instead of jogging).
* Increase the number of efforts steadily toward 10K at speed, or up to 10 percent of your weekly mileage.
* Run longer reps as shown in Chapters Seven and Twelve.
* Do 12 miles the day before Interval training instead of 10.

Prudent runners change one of the factors at a time. Intending to run a few 5K races? Increase speed to 3K pace, then steadily decrease the recovery period month by month.

For marathon racing though, once you've achieved relaxed running at 5K speed, decrease the recovery period a bit, but focus on increasing the number of repetitions at that pace.

Your body, that is:

*   The level of fatigue in your muscle cells;
*   Your mental approach and determination to do long sessions of intervals because you believe in them;
*   Your previous history and experience with intervals;
*   Pace judgment for the first repeats on any particular day;

Set the limit on the number of repeats which you will run.

Running at 5K pace? Aim toward 10K of speedwork.

Training at two mile speed? Few runners will attempt 10K of intervals at 100 percent of VO2 max. Four miles, or 6,000 meters is the limit for most runners at 2 mile pace. Like four miles? Run 16 x a quarter mile, or 8 half miles. Prefer 6,000 meters (it's about 400 meters under 4 miles!) Run 20 x 300 meters, or 15 x 400, or 10 x 600, or 6 x 1,000.

Or stick with three miles at speed like Bill Rogers did with his 12 x 400 meters at 2 mile race pace. He called it a great weapon for marathon training.

Interval Training Limits:

The 1952 triple Olympic Gold medalist, including the marathon, the late Emil Zatopek showed the running world that there is no limit to how many intervals you can do. 50 x 400 meters at 5K to 10K pace is daunting, and is not recommended to any readers of this book, yet Zatopek had phases when he did this session twice a day for a couple of weeks. He also set three world records during his back to back sub 30 minute 10Ks for a 59.51 20K at a HR of 168.

Arturo Barrios, one of Zatopeks' successors at holding the 10K and 20K world record was content with 20 x 400 in 63 seconds, or about 3K race pace. Of course 2.08 marathoner

Barrios trained in a more enlightened time, (1980s and 90s) and balanced his Intervals with long runs and sessions such as 10 x 1,000 meters at his 10K race pace with 60 seconds rest, and 5 x 2K repetitions. Barrios was also keen on bounding like a long jumper over a puddle of water, lifting the forward knee quite high while extending the back leg.

Note on 400s. When aiming for say 90 seconds, some of your efforts may be closer to 88. If you make a conscious effort to run every fourth rep faster, that is, to intentionally run an 88, the transition to 88s for your training pace will be easier. The occasional faster rep also helps to break up the session.

Avoid running 400s or 300s week in, week out. Doing the same session repeatedly will only make you good at running that session. The 600s do something for you which the 300s won't. Don't miss out on their benefits.

Relax at Speed when Fatigued.

Race pace running with weary muscles, if practiced with good running form, teach you how to run fast in the middle to the end of a race. It will improve your race day concentration.

When you begin to lose form, run several striders on grass while fatigued. Any marathon runner can run a fast quarter mile. It takes practice and patience to run efficiently in the 80th to 104th quarter mile of a marathon. Practice running relaxed at 5K pace when you think you're drained.

Running 4 to 6 times 200 meters at 3K pace is a great way to conclude a session of 400s at 5K pace. When you've trained through the next chapter, try 2 to 3 times 300 meters at 5K pace after your sessions of long reps at 10K pace.

Striders at the end of sessions are great preparation for increasing the volume of your interval session. Don't sprint or rush through these short reps, and don't make them hurt. Run relaxed with tired muscles to stimulate your cardiovascular system; don't risk straining your muscle fibers by sprinting.

How Many Weeks for Intervals?

Marathon runners new to interval training will make big improvements in running economy over the first few sessions. Most runners striding out their 200, 300 and 400s for the first time find it very easy to speed up their 400 meter pace by 2 to 3 seconds per lap after two or three sessions. This would give 10 seconds per mile off your marathon pace. Four minutes off of your marathon is a large carrot!

Incidentally, carrots protect your muscle cells from damage and getting sore. Beta carotene can help you to run faster or with the running seeming to take less effort. Eat a few yellow or orange fruits like peaches, apricots and of course, carrots. But lets get back to Interval training.

This pace increase will not translate to 10 seconds per mile off of your marathon time unless you retain your strength and endurance by continuing long runs and threshold pace sessions while also improving your running form.

Some marathon training programs recommend only six weeks of interval training, because coaches fear burn out.

But why stop interval training after only six weeks?
*   You've just got used to the sessions;
*   Your running economy has improved;
*   You're now beginning to reap the secondary benefits from these repeats, the enzyme and muscular changes inside your body, which added to the improvements in your physical running form will allow you to sustain a fast pace for more time, or to run faster.

Marathon runners should enjoy and benefit from interval sessions year round. The main reason runners become jaded with Intervals is because they run them too fast. Run them at 5K to 3K pace and they will be pleasant training sessions.

Ignore the six weeks, then take a break idea. Improve your endurance by adding more repeats. Get away from the track for a few weeks twice a year, but continue fast running elsewhere to keep your improved running form.

Keep these speed sessions fun by running in tranquil environments when possible. Enjoy the ambiance which nature offers and avoid the distractions from people. Got a nice park close to home? Run 12 times 90 seconds, instead of quarters at the track. The next week, run 500s and 300s at the track. Seven days later, head to a golf course for tee to green running on the edge of the fairways.

Experienced with interval training? Try this nine session progression:

* 12 times 300 meters at two mile pace with 200 rests.
* 10 x 400 meters at 5K pace with 200 rests.
* 8 x 600 meters at 5K pace with 400 rests.
* 15 x 300 at two mile pace.
* 10 x 400 ONE second per rep faster than 5K pace.
* 10 x 600 at 5K pace.
* Either 18 x 300 at two mile pace; or, 15 x 300 at 5K pace with a much shorter recovery.
* 10 x 400 at two mile pace.
* 12 x 600 at 5K pace.

Note how each distance progresses in a different way. Gershler, the great German coach who described five variables to adjust interval sessions, would be proud of us.

* The speed of the 400s increase;
* The number of 300 reps rises,
* Before the recovery is shortened; and,
* The quantity of 600s increases.

Once you're satisfied with the number of repeats, decrease the recoveries toward 60 seconds or less.

You Don't Need Pain.

While a little discomfort is good for you because it indicates a modest degree of intensity, only the last quarter of your reps should feel hard: it's these harsh feeling reps which will make you stronger.

Get through your interval sessions by thinking about running form on each rep. Run each rep, and the entire session at appropriate pace - a pace which allows you to run well the next day for 10 to 20 miles. Count the number of repeats you've done, instead of counting the number of repeats you have left to run. Counting up inspires achievement; counting down is negative.

Think about the purpose of this session while you're experiencing modest discomfort or aching, which is from exercising at 5K to 2-mile race pace, not from sprinting.

You can add variety by running ladders or pyramid sessions, running several distances at roughly the same pace. It could be 200, 400, 600, 800 and then back down. If you do 2 x 800 at the top, you'll have a 2.5 mile set and probably run two sets with a 200 jog after all repeats, and an extra 5 minutes between sets. The 800s would be at 5K pace, the 400s at 3K pace. The 200s are mere striders at 3K pace. If you do one 800 in each pyramid it's a 2 mile set. When you've done Chapter Twelve, you can add mile repeats. You can also start with the long repeats and run the short stuff in the middle.

A study has shown that athletes recover 79 to 92 percent of their muscle strength within a mere hour of a difficult training session. Unless you injured yourself with the speed running or low-key race on Saturday, you should be 95 percent recovered, but yes, just a little achy for your long Sunday run. Recharge your muscles with carbos in moderation and rehydrate, then run long and at a sensible pace for a complete training weekend on nearly 24 hours recovery.

Don't decrease mileage yet. Most studies which show interval training to be the most effective way to improve running speed while improving running economy have also included a huge reduction in training volume.

Reducing mileage gives an enormous performance boost to race times at distances such as the 5K. The improved race times are a combination of the rest and the interval training.

Most of those studies take a group of runners who have done steady running for only about 10 weeks to develop base. They don't take a group of runners who have run fartlek, hills and anaerobic threshold pace training for several years...because their gains would be more modest. You already have good running economy from other types of speed running, and a fairly high VO2 max.

However, you are now easing an extra bit of VO2 max and running efficiency into your body. This takes time.

You will rest and peak for your marathon in due course. Keep your current mileage and long runs during this phase or you'll lose your base aerobic capacity and strength. For now, practice good running economy on moderately tired legs.

You will take an easy week every three to four years. Just kidding. Easy weeks are every <u>3 to 5 weeks</u>. Resting a bit to run a 5K to 10K race every few weeks is great for speed training and also lets your muscles adapt.

By this stage in your marathon preparation you're in excellent shape. Even if you rest up to race a 10K at close to a personal best you should be able to cruise 400s at 5K pace four days later. True, your muscles will not have fully recovered from the 10K, but 5K pace with short intervals is not hard training. Simply relax at this important training pace to enhance your ability to run fast on marathon day with fatigued muscles.

Of course, this post 10K race session would not be the week to increase your interval session; you'll be better off doing a mile less than usual. Also:

* Run short efforts instead of long ones;
* At 5K pace;
* Don't try a new session;
* Don't attempt 3K race pace intervals.

Races, either with expectations of coming close to a personal record or simply as hard training runs, adds excitement to your training. Speed sessions at the right pace, especially with friends, also add excitement and satisfaction to what would otherwise be a long buildup to one race.

Longer repeats do stimulate your physiological systems for a greater percentage of your running time, but short reps make it easier to relax at speed. Restrict yourself to 300 to 400s for your post race sessions.

You set the limit on the number of reps.

You can ignore the 10 percent mileage rule once a month. Rest up to peak with a six mile training session. Or, ease through more reps at 10 to 12 seconds per mile slower (10K pace). Half the reps should still be close to 5K pace. Run the second half of your intervals faster, or alternate a 5K pace with a 10K pace rep. When you've done a particular session three or four times, ease more reps toward 5K pace.

Note: your reps should be 3 seconds per lap faster than 10K pace to represent 5,000 pace; 5 to 6 secs a lap faster than 10K pace to equal your two mile potential.

Rob De Castello, the 1983 Gold Medalist at the World Championships did fairly short Interval sessions. 8 x 400 meters at 3K race pace is not demanding...unless it's two days after a session of hill repeats, and one day after running 18 miles at 6.15 per mile. De Castello's recovery was a 200 meter "float" in 45 seconds (six minute mile pace) so you'll realize his short Interval session was very stimulating.

Chapter Seven shows a 24 session rotation for long repeats. Do one session most weeks, plus a few races at 5K to 15K and you'll get 7 to 9 months of variety and progress.

Match each session of the long reps with a session of short repeats using hills, fartlek and the true interval training as outlined in this chapter. Incorporate the 18 sessions on page 139, plus sessions of 600 meter reps to give yourself 9 months of fun with short reps.

* Session One…10 x 400 at 3K or two mile pace.
* Two…Hill repeats from Chapter Four. Use mostly 200 to 400 meter hills or 45 to 90 seconds, and run mostly at 5K intensity, though your last four repeats could now move up to two mile race effort. Relax at high effort.
* Three…Fartlek: Focus on short efforts because the long efforts will come from Chapter 7. You need 10 percent of your mileage at speed in this session, but no faster than 5K pace. Take short rests if you're tempted to run faster. Fartlek is a bit more relaxed than the first two sessions and is more likely to be on trails or grass, and is therefore the ideal session the day before your 20 mile run.
* Four…12 x 400 at two mile pace.
* Five…Add one more hill repeat.
* Six…Got some sand close by to run some of your fartlek in? Use it to build strength with bounding and jumps.
* Seven…14 x 400 at two mile pace with 200 rest.
* Eight…Add another hill repeat.
* Nine…Stressed out? Replace hills or 400s with fartlek any time you feel the need, such as when you're on vacation. It's fun to do a fartlek session in unfamiliar parks.
* Ten…16 x 400 at two mile pace with 200 rest.
* Session 11…Do 6 of your hill reps at 2 mile intensity.
* Session 12…Fartlek.
* Session 13…Alternate 400s with 500s at two mile pace. The extra 100 meters in a 500 will all be at 98 % of your max HR, a high reward change to your session. Do 7 reps of each distance to keep yourself to 4 miles if you wish.
* Session 14…Run half of your hill reps at 5K and half at 3K effort.
* Session 15…Fartlek.
* Session 16…8 x 500 and 6 x 400 (3K pace).
* Session 17…Perfect your relaxed hill repeats. It does still feel hard toward the end of each repeat and toward the end of the session. Run no harder than 98 percent of max HR.

* Session 18…Your resting up session once a month for a race could be 3 miles of fartlek instead of 5 miles, or 10 x 500 meters at 2-mile pace (only 5K of training).

Here are progression hints for 600 meter reps. You've made it to 12 x 600 at 5K pace with 400 meter jogs so:

Begin to reduce the recovery by increasing the speed of your jogging or decrease the distance jogged to 300 meters. Next time, speed up the last 4 x 600 by 1.5 seconds, which is only one second per lap or 4 seconds per mile.

Then, alternate a 400 jog with a 200 jog for the recovery. Graduate to running the last 6 reps 2 seconds faster than the first 6 and move toward alternating one rep at 5K pace with one rep closer to 3K pace.

Play with your form and change the session according to your progress and tolerance. Please, no killer sessions. Run no faster than 2-mile race pace.

Long Runs for Economic Running.

It's not only Interval training which improves your running form or economy. It's unfortunate that long runs are the best way to improve running economy. However, it's not until you do 12s, 14s and 16s on a regular basis that you learn to:

* Curtail your stride length to reduce jarring and fatigue from overstriding;
* Maintain high cadence on long runs while using those short strides at 90 per minute for each foot;
* Land close to the rear of your foot with the knee flexed at about 15 degrees and keep a slight knee bend during the support phase;
* Keep your feet close to the ground with minimal knee lift to conserve still more energy;
* Move the arms just enough to avoid shoulder roll;
* Yet push off from your calves with a forward motion to propel yourself forward while saving the quadriceps;
* With a very slight forward lean;

*   Thus making you a smoother runner.

Intervals at 5K to 3K paces also teach you the above skills, but long runs teach your muscles to use fatty acids, thus conserving your limited glycogen supply. Balance your training with hill repeats to build calf and quadriceps strength and also emphasize these muscle groups in weight training.

The VO2 Max Pace Chart on page 142 is based on

2 mile or 3K pace, which is about 12 seconds per mile or 3 seconds per 400 meters faster than 5K speed, and gives you training at 100 percent of your current VO2 max. This is also training at your VDOT. 3K pace is the maximum speed to run at for significant training benefits. 5K pace is fast enough for most of your long repeats.

If the 400s feel easy, but you find 600s difficult, you may lack background endurance or need more practice to relax at 2-mile pace. Do 300s before trying the 600s again. Relaxed running at 3K pace takes practice. Don't let 400s dominate; run 500s to get a much higher percentage of your session at 98 percent of your maximum heartrate, to get three straights per rep, and a nice transition to 600s, which are your goal.

<u>300s</u> allow you to run two straights and one bend on the track, and encourage you to take a 100 meter rest between reps. Eventually, take shorter rests at all distances to make your sessions harder and more stimulating.

Your 5K time not on the chart? Divide your 5K time in seconds by 12.5 to find your 5K pace for 400 meters. Take off 3 seconds to find your 3K pace.

Multiply your 400 meter pace by 0.75 to get your time for 300 meter reps and by 1.25 for your 500s.

Don't try to power yourself down the track or you will tense up and waste energy. Think relaxation and good running form to keep your biomechanics smooth.

Interval training paces at 100 percent of VO2 maximum and 98 % of max HR.

Run 3 seconds per 400 meters faster than your 5K speed.

Current 5K time	Reach 98 % of max HR with...				
	200s in	300s in	400s in	500s in	600s
15:00	34.5	51.8	69	1:25.7	1:43.5
15:37	36	54	72	1:30	1:48
16:15	37.5	56.2	75	1:33.8	1:52.5
16:53	39	58.5	78	1:37.5	1:57
17:30	40.5	60.8	81	1:41.2	2:01.5
18:07	42	63	84	1:45	2:06
18:45	43.5	65.2	87	1:48.7	2:10.5
19:22	45	67.5	1:30	1:52.5	2:15
20:00	46.5	70.8	1:33	1:57.3	2:19.5
20:37	48	72	1:36	2:00	2:24
21:15	49.5	74.2	1:39	2:03.7	2:28.5
21:53	51	76.5	1:42	2:07.5	2:33
22:30	52.5	78.7	1:45	2:11.2	2:37.5
23:07	54	81	1:48	2:15	2:42
23:45	55.5	83.2	1:51	2:18.7	2:46.5
24:22	57	85.5	1:54	2:22.5	2:51
25:00	58.5	87.7	1:57	2:26.2	2:55.5
25:37	60	1:30	2:00	2:30	3:00
26:15	61.5	1:32.2	2:03	2:33.7	3:04.5
26:53	63	1:34.5	2:06	2:37.5	3:09
27:30	64.5	1:36.7	2:09	2:41.2	3:13.5
28:07	66	1:39	2:12	2:45	3:18
28:45	67.5	1:41.2	2:15	2:48.7	3:22.5
29:22	69	1:43.5	2:18	2:52.5	3:27
30:00	70.5	1:45.7	2:21	2:56.2	3:31.5
30:37	72	1:48	2:24	3:00	3:36

Note: If you prefer your intervals at 5K pace, find your PR for 5K on the left and drop down one line for your repeats. Example: A 22:30 5K runner will run 54 seconds for 200s.

CHAPTER SEVEN

LONG INTERVALS at 10K RACE PACE or 90 % of VO2 MAXIMUM

You may recall from Chapter Six that 10K pace or 90 percent of VO2 max is one of the best training intensities to improve your VO2 max, and of course to improve your running economy. For sub 40 minute 10K runners, it should be about 92 percent of your maximum heartrate. Closer to 60 minutes for 10K? You'll be at 90 percent of max HR.

* Improve your max oxygen uptake capacity and you'll use a lower percentage of that max at marathon race pace.
* Make additional running economy or efficiency gains and you'll decrease injury risk, plus conserve energy. Your glycogen supply will last longer. Maybe you'll conk out at 26.2 miles instead of at 22.6 miles.

Runners who have spent years training for and racing fast 10 kilometer races and half marathons usually run the fastest marathons. Grete Waitz and Ingred Kristiansen of Norway did so in the 1980s; Tegla Loroupe and Catherine Ndereba of Kenya, and Paula Radcliffe continued the habit with marathon world records in the 1990s and in 2001-2003.

While these runners were born with relatively high VO2 maximum capacity, they then developed still higher VO2 maximums to absorb even more oxygen into their blood stream. They spent years developing their efficient running form while forcing their cardiovascular system to efficiently deliver huge amounts of oxygen to their running muscles.

When training intensely, Ingred Kristiansen, the World record holder at the marathon and 10,000 meters in the 1980s, usually did three sessions at 10K pace or faster, and tended to focus on the 10K for major championships.

During the year leading up to her World Record at the marathon, Catherine Ndereba trained extensively to improve her 10K time. You can do like-wise even if you never race a 10K: Run long repetitions at 10K pace consistently and for many years and you'll run faster marathons.

The universal rules of Marathon Training

To decrease injury risk, run at the slowest speed which gives a significant training effect.

Running a mere 60 percent of maximum heartrate improved your aerobic capacity in your early training, and it still improves your aerobic capacity on your long runs.

Half-marathon to 15K pace developed your anaerobic threshold.

Interval training at 10K pace is easier on your body than 5K pace, and offers huge improvements to VO2 Maximum, or the amount of oxygen that you can utilize.

One blessing about training for the marathon is that you can run most of your interval training at closer to 10K pace. Most of you will still be running a whopping 40 seconds per mile faster than marathon pace.

Several months of short interval training and preparation races have increased your VO2 max and running economy. Now you can stimulate greater gains while changing three of interval training's five variables:

During this chapter you will:
* Run slower than in the last chapter...10K pace, but
* Increase the length of your interval runs; and then
* Increase your workout volume.

Decreasing speed to 10K race pace but with longer repeats:
* Further stimulates your oxygen uptake ability or your VO2 max system;
* Forces you to run even more economically;
* Keeps your heartrate in the training zone for long periods and for a greater percentage of your training sessions.

Strength and Speed are required to run long repeats at

10K pace. In one sense, these long repeats will be easier than a 10K race because you get a recovery break every 5 to 15 minutes. However, you will not generally be resting up for five days prior to these interval sessions, and you will not have that pre-race adrenaline surge either, so they may feel as hard as a 10K race. Which of course is one of the main purposes of interval training!

When you break a session into manageable bits, you can complete a goodly volume at current 10K pace on slightly tired legs. One easy day prior to these sessions should enable you to handle mile repeats and longer at 10K pace.

10K running is easier if you've already done the 5K interval running of Chapter Six, or many 5K races, or a dozen fartlek sessions. You also need long runs for your base.

Interval speedwork at 90 percent of VO2

max helps you get the greatest possible amount of energy from your highly trained marathon muscles. Use the form hints from Chapter Three: Short, fairly fast strides are usually better for the marathon. Think about the elements of good form to help you maintain efficient form for longer periods.

Ideally, you will not run long reps at 10K pace until you have worked through Chapter Six and can (and have) run 4 miles of reps at 5K race pace on several occasions. However, provided you can run 3 miles of 600 meter reps at 5 mile pace, longer reps at 10K pace should be tolerable for you.

The Three Best Sessions.

The simplest way to improve VO2 max is to run long reps at about 90 percent of max VO2. Alternating sessions of Miles, 2,000s and 2 mile repeats at 10K pace gives excellent variety and apart from 10K races, maximum stimulation.

Very experienced marathon runners may want to run the miles and 2Ks at 5 mile race pace. Although 5 mile pace is only one second per lap faster than 10K pace, at about 92 percent of VO2 max, it's more stimulating than 10K pace.

Less experienced runners can cheat. Run laps 3 and 5 of your 2,000 at 5 mile pace.

Still not raced 10K? Have someone slap your wrists, go back to the beginning of this book, then enter a 10K to check your training pace. Or add 2.5 seconds per 400 meter lap to your 5K pace. Former milers will benefit immensely from these long reps at 10K pace. All runners should continue to run some short reps at 5K pace.

Ready for long reps at 90 percent VO2 max.

These long intervals at 90 % VO2 max will:

* Improve your pace judgment. Run that first lap of 5 too fast and you will not want to experience it again.
* Make you work on running form. You'll hug the ground with your feet to avoid wasted energy.
* Enhance your anaerobic buffering system; your lactate tolerance goes up. Your muscle fibers will contract despite the presence of high levels of lactic acid.
* Allow you to miss 10K races if you don't have many in your area.

You can run 10K of reps at 10K pace. Your legs won't get the full benefit of a 10K race, but you'll get most of the training benefits of a 10K race.

Mile Repeats.

Mile intervals are the simplest way to start your long repeats. You've run these reps at anaerobic threshold many times, so you're only looking for a 10 to 15 second per mile pace increase to reach 90 percent of your VO2 max or 10K pace. You've also run at least 5 mile race pace and hopefully 5K race pace with short Intervals so you have some legspeed in hand compared to 10K pace. Your two problems are to run at the right pace and to keep going for the entire distance.

Long reps at 90 percent of VO2 max keep you in oxygen debt for a greater percentage of your running time compared to short reps: This gives your cardiovascular system and muscles more stimulation than short intervals, thus making, indeed forcing your muscles to adapt.

Because you're running slower than 5K pace, you'll also be able to run more miles at 90 percent of your VO2 max than you could at 95 percent of max.

Running fast for 5 to 15 minutes at a time instead of only 60 to 200 seconds will make you think about your running form. You have to keep your arms relaxed because you can't get away with wasted motion. Relax your way through the most difficult minutes or 400 meters of each rep while maintaining the same steady 10K race pace.

Interval training with long repeats places greater mental strain on you than short repeats: You have to concentrate on running form at high speed for greater than 5 minutes at a time. It may also place you under more physical strain than you've been used to.

Keep moving during recovery periods: movement brings in oxygen, stops your blood from pooling (which can cause you to faint) and replenishes your energy supply. Don't suddenly stop on long runs either. Ease to a jog or keep walking.

Current fitness 12 x 400 at 5K pace?

Run some 5K races and then get used to 800s at 5K pace in training while alternating these 3 sessions of long repeats at 10K pace every other week. Take up to 5 minutes rest between repeats.

Week one: run 3 x one mile
Session 2 - Repeat week one. Run even pace and relaxed.
Session 3 - 2,000 meters; then an 800 rep; then a 2,000
Session 4 - 2 x 1.5 miles or 2,400 meters.

Then transition to 5 mile pace or one second per lap faster as shown below.

Able to handle 20 x 400 at 5K pace? Take 2 to 3 minutes rest while doing these.

* Week one...5 x one mile at 10K pace.
* Session 2...As week one but run the last lap of each repeat at 5 mile pace, i.e. 1 second faster than prior laps.
* Session 3...4 x 2,000 meters at 10K pace.
* Session 4...5 x one mile with 2 laps at 5 mile pace.
* Session 5...2 miles at 10K pace; then one mile; then 2.
* Session 6...4 x 2,000 with the last lap at 5 mile pace.
* Session 7...5 x one mile with three laps at 5 mile pace.
* Session 8...2 miles at 10K pace; then one mile; then 2.
* Session 9...4 x 2,000 with two laps at 5 mile pace.
* Session 10...5 x one mile at 5 mile race pace.

Ready to increase your training volume?

Add a quarter mile at 5K to 5 mile pace to the end of your session every other session. After 8 sessions over about a 12 week period, you'll be ready to run an extra mile repeat at 10K to 5 mile race pace instead of the 4 x 400 meters. The formerly 3 miles of long reps person will be ready to rotate:

* 4 x one mile, with
* 3 x 2,000 meters, with
* 2 x two miles.

The formerly 5 miles of reps person can rotate:
* 6 x one mile at 5 mile pace, with
* 5 x 2,000 alternating between 10K and 5 mile effort, with
* 3 x 2 miles at 10K pace.

Think these sessions are tough? They are. But so are marathons if you're going to run them remotely fast (for your level). Think about one or two aspects of your running form on a part of each lap or quarter mile, and these sessions will feel tamer. Increase the volume and pace of these long reps gradually as your muscles' capacity for work rises and you will have tamed these sessions. Develop confidence from having run these sessions many times, and you will have conquered long reps at 10K pace.

Too many laps of the Track?

You don't have to run all of your interval sessions at the track. Once you've learnt how to do them, one session a week of intervals can be done anywhere. You can use a watch with a beeper for those short reps in Chapter Six, doing one or two minute efforts with a minute rest...on grass, or paths and road.

These long reps at 10K pace are still better off the track. Find a field or park and work out a pleasant course or two that takes you 5 to 15 minutes to run. The exact distance is not important. Alternate reps in this tranquil environment with the somewhat less interesting, but often more physically stimulating and rhythmic track environment. Then return to the ambiance which nature offers the following week to avoid the boredom of track sessions.

When training in the park, woods, on the edge of a golf course or on your favorite slightly undulating but smooth trails, you must train at the same intensity as during your track sessions. If you don't, you'll be at threshold training pace from Chapter Five. 15K pace is a vital training intensity for marathon running, but try not to do it accidentally while avoiding your 10K pace session.

You can run all these 90 percent VO2 max training sessions at the track and never get bored. Run a variety of interval sessions as out-lined above, at a variety of related paces, with a variety of company.

Training companions are a huge asset at 10K pace. You don't even need to be at the same level.

The more accomplished runner can do his or her 2 mile repeats at 10K pace with a three minute rest; the soon to be accomplished runner can run 3 times one mile at her 5 mile or 5K pace with up to a 10 minute rest.

The slower person would be wise to run 2 to 4 striders at relaxed tempo half-way through that 10 minute rest to maintain deep muscle warmth. Your other job is to encourage your companion through the second half of his or her two miles. You could run the second mile with your partner, or the middle four laps, or do a variety so that he or she is self reliant for a different part of the repetition each time. This works even better if there are 6 to 8 runners in your group.

Make sure you have the endurance to run a 10K within 3 seconds per lap or within 12 seconds per mile of your 5K speed. Your half-marathon pace should be within 25 seconds per mile of your 10K pace. If you have problems, consider:

Long runs for aerobic base.

Hills and anaerobic intervals for strength.

Long reps and lots of short reps for VO2 max endurance and lactate buffering capacity.

One of the finest ways to improve your endurance is to run 10 percent of your weekly miles in one interval session. Your warm-up and cooldown will be another 5 to 10 percent of your weekly mileage. Twenty percent in one session is short compared to the 30 to 35 percent of miles which constitute your longest run, let alone the 50 to 60 percent which your marathon will be.

Run a Mixture of Training Sessions.

You might decide to run 2,000s at 10K pace every four weeks. Your second Interval session could be 400s and 600s at 5K pace. Your third, another of the sessions discussed above at 10K to 5 mile pace, and your fourth, a mixture of 800s at 5K pace with 300s at 2 mile pace.

The 12 sessions of each would give you a full year of progression. Reduce the recovery to 100 when running 300s, and to 200 for your 600 to 800s. Mixing in a quality fartlek session every 5 weeks will add to your variety.

One of the best ways to train for a race is to run the entire race distance as intervals. Not a sound choice for marathon runners, but certainly attainable for the half-marathon. Threshold pace intervals at 5 seconds per mile faster than half-marathon pace for 10 to 13 miles of repeats is a great substitute for a 10 mile or half-marathon race if done about 8 and 4 weeks prior to your marathon. You would need to rest up for these sessions, but they will stimulate race type fatigue.

When you're a master of 10K of reps at 10K to 5 mile pace training, insert an occasional session of 800s or 1,200s at 5K pace with a 3 minute rest.

Don't race to take great chunks off your fastest time for any session. Running relaxed at up to 5K pace is the goal, not increasing speed to 2 mile pace. In the warmdown, your legs should feel re-energized, not wasted.

Don't turn off the pain during these long sessions. Pain warns you to slow down. Don't mask the pain with pills, or you will lose the body's warning sign to stop exercising. Ignore pain at your peril, or you will get what you deserve, which is a long break from running.

Which Pace?

Runners on high mileage might eventually run these interval sessions at 5K pace, or 95 percent VO2 max. Most of you will find 8K pace plenty hard enough for the longer repeats. Catherine Ndereba ran her 1,200 meter repeats between 5K and 10K race pace, but on a cinder track. Ten times 1,200 meters is not for many readers of this book, but 10 percent of your weekly mileage as 1,200s at 5K pace, or mile reps and longer at 10K pace are great sessions.

Try not to run these tough Interval sessions three days after a half marathon, or you'll increase your injury risk. Try not to race a fast 10K the week after your marathon either. Use Yakovlev's rule (*Best Half-Marathons*). Give muscles a chance to heal and get stronger before running fast again.

You can cheat your Heart and Lungs though.

If you have a longish section of smooth grass at one to two percent grade, run downhill at 5 to 10 seconds faster than 5K pace, which will be two mile race pace. Your heart and the rest of your cardiorespiratory system will only be working at around 5K effort level. It's the opposite for up-hill reps. Legs are at 5K speed, and your heart will be at 2 mile intensity.

The pace to run your VO2 max intervals is current 5K race pace, not your dream pace. This will be 10 to 15 seconds per mile faster than recent 10K pace, and about 40 seconds per mile faster than marathon pace.

Think about your running form during these intervals. Though it's difficult to run this fast without decent form, this is your chance to correct little faults.

Yasso 800s help to make dreams come true.

Runner's World Race & Event Promotion Director, Bart Yasso, came up with his "Yasso 800s" many years ago, and as far as I'm aware, until now no one has come up with an explanation as to why they work. But first of all, what are "Yasso 800s".

Simple. Start week one with 4 x 800 meters at the same time in minutes and seconds as you intend to race the marathon in hours and minutes: Examples.

Marathon goal	mile pace	800s time	speed per mile	speed diff secs per mile
2:37:19	6:00	2:37	5:14	46
3:03:22	7:00	3:03	6:06	54
3:36:18	8:15	3:36	7:12	62

Add one interval each week until you reach 10, then taper for your marathon. *The reason this session works is because whatever your marathon goal time is, your intervals are between 5K and two mile race pace.* You'll be training between 95 and 98 percent of maximum heartrate and at 95 to 100 percent of your VO2 maximum, which stimulates economical running.

Provided you also have sufficient mileage, long runs and anaerobic threshold pace running ability, you should achieve your marathon goal. For example, a 3:36 marathoner will race at about 8:15 per mile, so he or she should have done:

* 4 to 6 runs of 20 miles at 9:15 pace, and over a dozen 18s at the same pace and with 2 miles included at 8:15 pace. These were of course preceded by numerous 15 mile runs.
* 18 to 24 threshold sessions at between 7:30 and 7:45 per mile for 4 to 5 miles or long repeats at the same pace.
* A series of 10 to 12 hill sessions on a weekly basis, followed by hill reps every 14 days to maintain strength.
* Then peak at 10 x 800 meters in 3:36 about three weeks before the marathon.

You're probably better off varying your intervals as shown in this and other chapters though. Run mile repeats at the same speed (7:12 for the 3:36 marathon runner) and you'll stimulate your heart for a greater percentage of each interval, plus you'll have to concentrate on running form to stay at that pace for those last two quarters.

My problem with Yasso 800s is that the recommended recovery is the same time that it took you to run the interval, which means three and a half minutes for our 3:36 marathon runners. Take that recovery and it takes an entire lap to get your heartrate up to 95 percent of your maximum on each repeat. Sure, your legs are at 5K pace and you're improving your running economy, but your ticker isn't in high octane mode for very much of your session. Take 90 seconds or less recovery for this session and you'll be up to 95 % of max HR in the first 200 meters of all except the first repeat. You'll then get almost 75 % of your 5 miles at 95 % of max HR.

How can you achieve these short recoveries? Start 10 weeks earlier. Achieve the 10 repeats 10 weeks before your marathon, and then gradually reduce your recoveries by 15 to 30 seconds per session.

Bear in mind the rule about not repeating sessions too often, and you'll have to consider alternating:
* 800s at 5K pace, with
* 400s at 2-mile pace, with
* 2 mile reps at 10K pace.
You'll also need hills, threshold pace and long runs.

This author disagrees with training schedules that use the same session for weeks on end. Don't use 800s at 5K pace for 10 weeks in a row or miles at 10K pace, or even 2 miles at 15K pace. All three are great sessions. It takes about three weeks for your muscles to complete their physiologic changes from the stimulation of a particular session, so why not do each session every three weeks.
* Add an 800 or decrease the recovery every 3 weeks;
* Do 2Ks instead of mile reps at 10K pace;
* Or take shorter rests for the mile repeats as described earlier in this chapter;
* Mix in tempo runs…
And you can have a lifetime of training with these sessions. You'll also run fairly long once a week, really long once a week and do repeats at 2-mile to 5K intensity…on the track, trails or uphill, i.e., a Chapter Six interval session, or Fartlek session, or hill repeats.

One week in four or five you'll do a half session to rest up for a race. Ignoring those easy sessions, a combined series of quality mid-week runs could go along these lines.

* Week one…5 x one mile at 10K pace.
* Session 2…3 x 2 miles at half marathon pace.
* Session 3…8 x 800 at 5K pace with 4 minutes rest. If you are used to 2 minutes rest, use it and then gradually reduce by 15 seconds per session starting at session 12.
* Session 4…4 x 2,000 meters at 10K pace.
* Session 5…30 minute tempo run at half marathon pace.
* Session 6…9 x 800 at 5K pace.
* Session 7…5 x one mile starting at 10K pace but with half a mile at 5 mile pace.
* Session 8…3 x two miles at 5 to 10 seconds per mile faster than half marathon pace, but slower than 15K pace.
* Session 9…10 x 800 meters at 5K pace.
* Session 10…4 x 2,000 with the last lap at 5 mile pace.
* Session 11…30 minute tempo run at 5 seconds per mile faster than half marathon pace.
* Session 12…10 x 800 at 5K pace with shorter rests.
* Session 13…5 x one mile, with three laps at 5 mile pace.
* Session 14…3 x two miles at 10 to 15 seconds per mile faster than half marathon pace, or at 15K pace.
* Session 15…10 x 800 meters at 5K pace.
* Session 16…3 x 2,400 mostly at 10K pace but the last lap of each repeat at 5 mile pace. Finish with one 800 at 5K pace to reach 5 miles for the day.
* Session 17…30 minute tempo run at 10 seconds per mile faster than half marathon pace.
* Session 18…10 x 800 with two and a half minutes rest.
* Session 19…5 x one mile at 5 mile pace.
* Session 20…3 x two miles at 15K pace. Reduce your rest periods toward two minutes.
* Session 21…10 x 800 with two minutes rest.

* Session 22...3 x 2,800 (7 laps) mostly at 10K pace, but the last lap of each repeat at 5 mile pace.
* Session 23...30 minute tempo run at 15K pace.
* Session 24...10 x 800 with 90 seconds rest.

Note: A short repeat rotation was shown on page 139.
Add a monthly race and you've got about 32 weeks of training with long repeats here. Notice that:
- The 800s increase to 10 reps and then the recovery gradually drops. Next, you could incorporate a series of sessions to get used to running 1,000 meters at 5K pace by going the extra 200 meters for one rep, then for one additional rep every three weeks. The initial goal is 8 x 1,000 meters at your 5K pace. 8 x 1,000 gives you a greater percentage of your session at 5K heartrate level than 10 x 800.
- Anaerobic threshold pace gradually comes down from half marathon to 15K pace as described in Chapter Five. You've probably already had a 10 week phase working predominantly at threshold training.
- The mile repeats at 10K pace gradually convert to 5 mile pace, and in your next session you should begin to reduce the rest periods toward two minutes as you do with 800s.
- The 2,000 meter reps at 10K pace gradually lengthen toward two miles (your next session would be 2 mile reps or 3,200s), then you would reduce the rest periods.
- For all types of repeats, you will gradually spend more and more time with your heartrate at its ideal training point to reap the huge rewards of VO2 max and threshold pace running.
- For all types of repeat you'll have to practice controlled running with fatigued muscles. The shorter rests duplicate the physical and psychological stress of racing, and teaches your body to get oxygen and sugar to where it can be used...your brain and your muscle cells.

Recovery sessions pre-race would include 6 x 600 meters at 5K pace, which is a nice change from 800s. 5 x 1,000 at 10K pace is a nice break from 2Ks at 10K to 5 mile pace; 3 times one mile at 15K pace is much easier than 2K at 10K pace or tempo runs at 15K pace. It's probably best to run the 600s if your up-coming race is a 5K. However, miles at threshold pace will also leave your legs fresh for the 5K!

You'll also run short repeats or hills most Saturdays to set yourself up for the long run. Seven days before your monthly race, you'll do about two-thirds of your usual speed session. The long run is going to be 5 to 7 miles less than usual too, on a flatter course and 5 seconds per mile slower than usual.

You don't have to run short reps on Day One (usually Saturday) and the long repeats midweek. You don't have to run long repeats every week on Day One either. You can do a month with short stuff on Day One, then a month with the long stuff on Day One for variety. The decision could be based on which day you're able to train with a group, and what session they usually do; it could be based on which type of running is easier or more relaxing to do while watching part of your daughters soccer game.

Because you do a different session every week, you could run long reps on Tuesday of this week, then run long reps again on Saturday of the next week. Because you're training slightly different energy systems it should work for you.

Example: with the above 3 session rotation, you'll run at 5K pace to practice relaxed running at 95 % of VO2 max with your 800s, but your next session of long reps will be miles or longer at 5 mile to 10K pace. Just done 2Ks at 10K pace or 90 % of VO2 max on Tuesday? 2 mile repeats or a tempo run at threshold pace would be great on Saturday.

After a 15 mile run on Sunday, many high intensity runners run fartlek sessions or short hills on Mondays, and run 800s to 1,200s at 5K pace on Tuesdays, yet still have the legs or fast enough recovery to run 12 miles at 30 seconds slower than marathon pace on Wednesday. These runners are usually in their fourth year or so at 40 to 60 miles per week. However, in the days following their 20 mile Sunday run, they usually take an easy run or cross train, then do the three quality, yet nicely balanced runs on Tuesday to Thursday.

Here is a sample of how your sessions from this Chapter and Chapter Six can be melded to make a five week cycle which you can repeat 3 to 6 times to prepare you for your marathon. It allows two restive weeks (4 and 5) and a race.

	Sat	*Sun*	*Tues*	*Thur*
Week 1	5 x mile	18E	16 x 400	12
Week 2	3 x 2m @ An	20E	5F	12
Week 3	10 x 800 @ 5K	18E	Hills	10
Wk 4	3 x 2,000 @ 10K	15E	6 x 600	7
Wk 5	Race 10K to Half M		3F	12

The Sunday after your race, cross train or walk if the race was more than 10 miles. Run 5 easy miles if the race was 10 miles; run 10 to 15 miles easy if the race was 10K or below.
*   Week Ones mile reps can be 5 mile to 5K pace depending on your fatigue from the previous weekends race.
*   Both 18 mile runs will include 2 miles at marathon pace.
Repeat the schedule while making slight changes to the speed sessions as out-lined in the last two Chapters. 400s in Week One will transition to 500s or to 3K pace. Cross train of course; higher mileage people will do 5 to 8 mile runs most days - probably 8s in weeks 1 to 3, and 5s or less in week 4.

Great races in your town only three weeks apart? Reduce your Tuesday quality session by 25 percent and cut 4 miles off your Thursday run and you can race pretty well at 5K to 10K on any Saturday. The race is a nice break from training, but start 5 seconds per mile slower than usual, and don't expect personal records. Don't race too often or you'll never build the base required for your marathon.

You'll rest up more significantly for your marathon, and perhaps for a major half marathon 6 to 10 weeks before your marathon. The details are in Chapter 10, 11 & 14.

Fast Running without injury requires:

- Strong calves from calf raises three times a week; push yourself up on your toes while holding dumbbells.
- Sound hip flexors, from hill repeats, bounding and using the captain's chair at the gym.
- Balanced arm power from a few bicep curls, press-ups and the overhead dumbbell press.

Using a Heartrate Monitor

Set your lower and upper alarms at…

For easy runs including 20s	65 and 75 %
Anaerobic threshold sessions	86 to 92 %
Long reps at 10K pace	92 to 94 %
5K to 3K pace Intervals and Hill reps	95 to 98 %
or when racing a 5K	95 to 97 %
a 10K	92 to 94 %
half marathon	85 to 88 %
and of course the marathon	80 to 85 %

You should reach the lower end of the training zone in the first quarter of each repeat to make them effective; even in the last 200 meters, don't go beyond the high rate.

You should not go much beyond the low rate in races until past the first quarter of the race. You should not flirt with the upper limit until you reach the last quarter of any race.

Run the same training sessions regularly, at the same fitness level, and the times of your reps will vary according to how tired you are, (mental or physical), your food intake and hydration status, and the weather. Run at your planned intensity level and it's bound to be slower than 5K or 10K pace on some occasions. Don't worry about the pace changing, but try to find the reason for your fast days. These factors can be used to increase your fitness if you plan for the conditions or go with the flow when they arrive. Aim for ideal conditions on race days and see pages 160-161.

Conditions and situations which will slow your repeats and your Racing:

Higher humidity or temperature: wear less; run reps in a shaded area; do recovery stretches in the shade; take in 5 to 8 ounces of liquid between repeats; run miles instead of 2,000s; or see how perfectly you can pace yourself to one second per lap slower than usual, while your heart and other muscles work at their usual intensity due to the heat.

Windier: adopt a very slight forward lean into the wind while working the arms just a little more; maintain a solid effort when the wind is behind you, yet don't run much faster than usual. Practice landing lightly as if onto hot-coals with bare feet. Kiss the ground and roll rapidly through the ankle. Don't turn it into a fartlek session where you work like a dog into the wind and allow yourself to be pushed on the other half of the lap. Think relaxation but work your muscles just a bit with the wind; think relaxation and put in slightly more effort than usual when running into the wind.

Wearing more stuff on cold days: you have to stay warm, especially the legs. Keep your upper layers to the minimum even if it means taking shorter rest breaks during Intervals to maintain warmth.

It's Raining: Running in the rain is a joy, but until you've done so at race pace, you will not know how much your shoes slip on wet asphalt, how much to shorten your stride to actually stay on your feet, and how much extra clothing to wear at each training or race pace. Metal manhole covers are very slippery when wet and ice up rapidly!

Heavier training shoes make you work harder for the same pace compared to wearing racing shoes. This is a good thing. Do wear your lightweight training or performance shoes or your racing shoes once a week though.

Stress: relax through the first few reps a little slower than usual. Finish with a few reps at your desired pace if you feel calm enough. 75 percent of your training benefits come from the first one third of your repeats; 90 percent if you achieve two thirds of your goal session. In high stress weeks, 75 to 90 percent will keep you on track for a great marathon, while resting your muscles for better sessions next week.

<u>Trained too hard or fast</u> on your recovery day...if you did it on purpose, it's called the overload principle. Running back to back harsh days make you concentrate and work to run VO2 max pace with slightly achy legs. Do run your desired pace because you have a rest week planned...don't you! If you trained too fast by accident, run a few seconds per mile slower for the speed session, but do run slower on those recovery days next week.

<u>Ran more than usual</u> the last week. See above.

<u>Ran too far yesterday</u>: The whole idea of marathon training is to prepare your muscles to run fairly fast, relatively soon after a long run. This combination of training prepares you for marathon race pace. 15K pace should be manageable the day after a fifteen mile run; 10K pace two days after; and at least 5K pace three days after. For weeks with an eighteen mile or more run, add an additional day of recovery prior to speed running. A very gentle fartlek session also does wonders to aid recovery the day after a long run!

<u>Avoid the following diet errors</u>:

Ate too much food over the last few days.
Ate too much food over the last few hours.
Lower than usual carbohydrate intake.
Insufficient liquid intake...dehydration.
See Chapter Eight and Nine for more information.

<u>Relax When You're Tired.</u>

When you begin to lose form during your long reps it's time to stop, or to regain concentration with some easy running. Cruise a few 300s at 5K pace after your rest. You'll find these 300s pleasant because they are faster than your long intervals were: You will also find that those long reps did not completely exhaust you! Keep these 5K pace reps comfortable to avoid injury.

Post speedwork you're after a pleasant, satisfying tired feeling. If you feel completely stuffed after an easy mile and a shower you probably ran the session too fast, or it was too much volume for your current fitness. Achy muscles for days after any VO2 max session indicates overtraining.

Change the variables of interval training a bit at a time. Don't jump from 400s at 5 mile pace to running 600s at 5K pace. Transition over many weeks and numerous sessions to reduce injury risk. You will not be able to prepare for a marathon when injured. Mileage is the best predictor of injuries: Training mistakes are the second best.

When you've mastered 800s at 5K pace, slide in one 1,200 and then change one more 800 to a 1,200 each month to get the entire third lap at 95 percent of your maximum heartrate, while focusing on relaxation at 5K pace. Longer repeats will improve your running economy more than short repeats.

However, many coaches recommend you run no more than 5 minutes for long reps. Page 163 is your table of times for training at 5K to 10K paces. Note the three bold face times. A 4:58 rep lets our fast runners complete a mile at 5K intensity; slower runners are working just as hard with 800 meter reps in 4:55. Most of you can use 1,200s at 5K pace. After all, <u>long reps give you more time in Oxygen debt, more time at the ideal heartrate and require greater concentration and effort.</u>

Prefer a more simplistic approach to your speed training. Run short reps at about 45 seconds per mile faster than marathon pace. Run medium reps of 800 meters to one mile at 35 seconds per mile faster than marathon pace. Run really long reps at 20 to 25 seconds per mile faster than marathon pace. You should find yourself training at 5K, 10K and half-marathon race pace! You'll be incorporating VO2 max and anaerobic threshold pace training.

Long reps at 95 to 90 percent of VO2 max, or 5K and 10K paces.

5K pace is 95% of VO2 maximum.   *10K pace is 90 % of VO2 max.*

Splits per 400	800s @5K pace	PR at 5K	1,200s @5K pace	1,600s @5K pace	PR @ 10K	mile at 10K pace
71.8	2:23.6	*14:57*	3:35	4:47	30:54	4:59
74.5	2:29	*15:31*	3:44	**4:58**	32:02	5:10
77.2	2:34.4	*16:05*	3:52	5:09	33:10	5:20
79.9	2:39.8	*16:39*	4:00	5:20	34:20	5:32
82.5	2:45	*17:11*	4:08	5:30	35:27	5:43
85.2	2:50.4	*17:45*	4:16	5:41	36:37	5:54
88	2:56	*18:20*	4:24	5:52	37:50	6:06
90.7	3:01.4	*18:54*	4:32	6:03	39:00	6:17
93.4	3:06.8	*19:27*	4:40	6:14	40:09	6:28
96	3:12	*20:00*	4:48	6:24	41:15	6:39
98.7	3:17.4	*20:34*	**4:56**	6:35	42:23	6:49
1:41	3:22.8	*21:07*	5:04	6:46	43:29	7:01
1:44	3:28.2	*21:41*	5:12	6:56	44:40	7:12
1:47	3:34	*22:18*	5:20	7:08	45:56	7:24
1:52	3:41.8	*23:06*	5:33	7:24	47:35	7:40
1:55	3:49.8	*23:56*	5:45	7:40	49:18	7:56
1:59	3:57.8	*24:46*	5:57	7:56	50:41	8:10
2:03	4:05.8	*25:36*	6:09	8:12	52:44	8:30
2:07	4:15	*26:33*	6:22	8:30	54:41	8:48
2:11	4:23	*27:24*	6:34	8:46	56:26	9:05
2:19	4:39	*28:59*	7:00	9:18	60:06	9:41
2:27	**4:55**	*30:29*	7:22	9:50	63:13	10:13
2:36	5:12	*32:20*	7:48	10:24	66:50	10:47
2:45	5:30	*34:22*	8:15	11:00	70:48	11:25

Chapter Eight

Liquids for Hydration

and for Food.

Please excuse me if some themes from Chapter Two get repeated.

Lubricate and feed your muscles and they'll be kind to you. Dehydration makes you prone to cramps and increases your risk of injury...to your running muscles and to your cardiac muscle! Dehydration increases your risk of micro muscle fiber tears, often the beginning of stiffness and injury. Additional hydration information is in Chapter Two.

Research shows that long distance performance is improved by taking in 200 calories per hour during the event. 32 ounces, or 4 full cups of Gatorade just happens to be 200 calories. No prizes for guessing which institute sponsored the research. 13 ounces of apple juice also supplies 200 calories, and it's easier to carry a sufficient supply on long runs. Drink 5 ounces of water at the fountains on route, plus 3 ounces of juice each time, and you'll take in your 200 calories per hour. One 24 ounce bottle with juice (plus half a teaspoon of salt) will cover you for two hours if you find 8 sources of water: You don't have to lug round 64 ounces of sports drink. You can use the same water sources twice on out and back routes.

Juices contain many antioxidants and vitamins, but sports drinks and goos do not. Goos also raise your heartrate as your body struggles to absorb the energy, which is not a good thing when you're already working at close to 80 percent of your maximum heartrate at mile 15 of a 20.

Marathon performance is also improved if you complete five 20 mile runs instead of only one prior to your marathon during the last 12 weeks of your build up; you'll also improve your marathon performance if you:

* Run several sessions at anaerobic threshold, and
* Run hills or do some running at 5K pace.
* Drink 5 to 12 ounces of liquid every 15 minutes.
* Rest up for your marathon.
* Run the first 10 miles at *slower* than goal pace.

Sound preparation will give you the optimum performance. While taking in liquid, plus a few hundred calories (from 100 to 400 per hour depending on your needs) will help, they will not make up for poor preparation.

Mans' most crucial nutrient is water.

Your body is 60 to 70 percent water, so stay hydrated: During our everyday activity we get about 10 percent of our water needs from our own metabolism. We get about 30 percent of our water needs from food, especially if we consume citrus fruits, the melon family, tomatoes and many other fruits and vegetables. You'll have to drink the rest of your needs.

Dehydration decreases running performance and

leads to cramps which can cause muscle injury. Recommendations to consume 8 glasses of water per day are cute, until you realize that an hours running can burn those 64 ounces! So:

* Start your exercise sessions well hydrated.
* Make drinking before runs a habit.
* Make drinking during your long runs routine.

* Drink before you feel thirsty during the day and during your runs (but see hyponatremia pages 58-60).
* Continue re-hydration within minutes of finishing your runs.

After your run, find a cool spot and keep moving slowly while taking several refreshing drinks. Include carbohydrates and a little protein in the first half an hour post run. Do a few gentle stretches pre or post shower, then drink some more liquid while taking in calories to rejuvenate your muscles.

As dehydration increases muscle soreness and decreases athletic performance, drink persistently throughout the day. Keep water and other low calorie and low caffeine drinks close by. Then also drink:

More than sixteen ounces one hour before exercise and again half an hour before exercise. Drink smaller amounts 20 and 10 minutes prior to running. Include some electrolytes and calories via diluted juices, or by eating a piece of fruit. If you really must use sports drinks, go ahead. Drink based on your sweat loss rate every 10 to 15 minutes during the run.

You can include a caffeine drink in the last 30 minutes pre-runs. Once you start running, its diuretic or urine stimulating powers are 95 percent lost. Caffeine, if taken 2 hours pre-running can give a short-term dehydrating affect, but when you factor in a 24 hour period it is not dehydrating.

A cup of coffee 30 minutes pre running does not dehydrate you, and the caffeine in one cup of coffee will not usually improve your running performance! Unless of course you're comparing your performance on one cup of coffee verses no liquid in the hour prior to running.

The caffeine in twelve ounces of coffee or a 20 ounce soda increases heartrate and the hearts irregularities while increasing your body temperature. All three are bad for runners. Caffeine also decreases the absorption of Iron, one of many substances which you need to transport oxygen, and calcium uptake is decreased. Coffee, like tea does have some antioxidants. Sweeten your tea with honey and you'll take in still more antioxidants. The tannic acid in tea also reduces iron absorption. Black tea relaxes arteries, increasing cardiac blood flow for 2 hours.

In some studies, caffeine has been shown to improve performance. Take it in your favorite beverage 30 minutes before hard runs to get your system going. Caffeine:

* Stimulates the nervous system;
* Makes you more alert and motivated;
* Decreases your perceived effort;
* May increase fatty acid burning ability;
* May allow you to exercise for longer without fatigue (mostly due to a delayed perception of fatigue).

Don't use caffeine to overtrain though. The experimenters use 2 mgs of caffeine per athletes' pound. Check your caffeine source and your weight. A 150 pound brewed coffee drinker needs about 20 ounces of java, plus other liquids. Most sodas take 64 ounces (4 pints) to give the same amount of caffeine.

Louise Burke Ph.D. of the Australian Institute of Sport showed that coke, containing about one-third the caffeine of coffee, worked wonders when combined with the sugar in the coke and its abundance of liquid. So Frank Shorter's de-fizzed cokes of the 1970s finally get scientific support.

Dark sodas usually contain phosphorous, which because it competes for the same transportation site as calcium, results in less calcium being absorbed, so watch out for those shin pains in the summer!

Asthmatics are particularly sensitive to dehydration. Their oxygen uptake decreases significantly when dehydrated. If you are lactating, keep yourself well hydrated too.

All people lose about two pints of water from the lungs and perspiration per day. Your level of water loss from perspiration or sweating depends on how much heat you need to get rid of. Your urine output is dependent upon your hydration status. Well hydrated? Your urine will be pale yellow. Hyperhydrate in the hours pre training until your urine is almost clear. Your kidneys are quite talented; they will keep most of your electrolytes in your system. When you start training, consume some sodium and potassium in your liquid to help maintain your blood volume.

As shown in Chapter Two, lose more than two percent of your body water and your blood gets thicker and your heart has to work harder on each stroke. Your blood volume will be lower, so less blood will be pumped out of the heart with each beat. Fewer nutrients will get to your muscles, and your training <u>intensity</u> will need to go up to maintain your current speed. More likely though, you'll continue at the same working effort and be forced to slow down.

Dehydration decreases your core blood volume. Blood flow to the skin decreases and sweating also decreases as your body tries to maintain body fluids in its central core. You'll get even hotter because you can't lose much heat from your body surface. Running performance declines.

According to a study in Medicine and Science in Sports & Exercise, dehydration lowers your lactate threshold, which makes you feel exhausted earlier in a run. For hot days:
* Dress sparingly and use white cloth;
* Make small changes in exercise duration or intensity;
* Educate your system to cope with the heat;
* Replace the fluid lost based on the "sweat loss test" (page 53) using a variety of liquids.
But do all that is possible to avoid dehydration:

Only commence races which you are fit enough to complete. Start at appropriate pace and start well hydrated.

Heat exhaustion is brought on by excessive amounts of exercise in extreme heat or simply by lack of fluids (page 57).

Quote from a rocket scientist. "The hotter or more humid it is, the more liquid you should drink." Plot your running circuits to include reliable sources of water. Time how long a water fountain takes to fill up a 12 ounce bottle. Then drink for twice as long to allow for the water which does not go into your mouth. While 3 or 4 swallows of water is pleasant, and gets rid of that dry mouth feeling, it does little to prevent dehydration. After a deep and complete drink, stretch and walk in the shade, then you'll be ready to continue your run.

Have a ton of supermarkets on a favorite running route with soda machines? Take some quarters and get the generic drinks. Don't worry about the caffeine. During exercise it has minimal effects. Sugared or diet? It depends on the duration of your session. It's prudent to take in some calories if you'll be out more than 90 minutes, or if you're covering more than 15 miles. Match each sugary soda with a diet soda to get the sugar concentration right. Keep a couple of plastic wrapped salt sachets in your key pocket just in case you need it.

Making liquid or hydration stops every 2 to 3 miles or every 20 to 30 minutes will give you a chance to assess yourself while resting for a minute and stretching, and then to practice exercising with liquid in your stomach.

Death as we nurses say, is quite fatal. Overheating, or its usual precursor, dehydration, can be fatal or merely debilitating.

Training for more than one hour, or for half an hour longer than you are currently used to? Plan your fluid intake. Include carbohydrates and electrolytes in your liquid. The electrolytes or salts will decrease your risk of muscle cramps. Sport drinks are the easiest choice, but their empty calories can help to keep you overweight.

Some studies show that a 6 percent solution empties from the stomach faster than water or more sugary solutions, though on balance, there is no advantage. Use any flavoring to make the ingestion of liquid more enjoyable, and thus more likely to happen.

If you use gels or goops for your carbo, drink plenty of water too. You will probably drink more fluid if the liquid is cold. The colder liquid also helps to cool you because your body uses energy to bring it up to body temperature.

So-called "Fitness Water" and low sugar waters with a flavoring add very few calories to your waist, and often give you the electrolytes which water lacks. A little flavor also stimulates you to drink more of it, which decreases your dehydration risk. However, an orange plus water from the faucet will provide more antioxidants and healing vitamin C for less cost than "enhanced water, fitness water" or whatever the marketing people wish to call it this week.

Liquid Food:

Eating to run before the event? Due to their faster gastric emptying time, liquid meals can be taken closer to training or race time than solid food.

A cup of skimmed or non-fat milk, a cup of vegetable juice, plus an orange zip out of the stomach fast, especially if you add a pint of water. They provide about 38 grams of carbohydrate, plus over 10 grams of protein. Add these calories to the solid food of two hours prior, and your meals from yesterday and you've got plenty of fuel to burn. Liquid meals work well after training too; then munch on a bagel.

Drinking excessive amounts of simple sugars just before the event does not provide an energy boost. It does not raise your glycogen levels. However, for a few people it can result in excessive blood sugar fluctuations. Those little energy drinks with caffeine are your enemy here. Sure they'll wake you up a bit, but the marathon is not a sprint.

Many regular exercisers suffer from chronic dehydration, putting themselves at higher risk for urinary tract infections, and decreased performance during long events. Drink every 10 to 15 minutes during long training sessions or races. Drink cranberry and apple juice every day to further decrease your urinary tract infection risk.

Weigh yourself daily in the morning and check your urine color. Don't be surprised if your weight is up two pounds the morning following a rest day. Your non-training day has not made you gain two pounds of fat; it has allowed you to cover your liquid shortfall or chronic dehydration. The rest has also allowed your muscles' glycogen and fatty acid stores to be replenished!

Staying Hydrated.

You'll still need to drink early and often during your marathon. Your thirst center is not reliable enough, so don't wait for it. Thirst comes on too slowly to be a reliable indicator that it's time to drink. Drink before you get the call to drink or you will already be dehydrated when you take your first drink. You will also have missed the chance to drink during the first 60 minutes or so of your run or race. You will never make up this fluid deficit.

Drink at the first water and all other fluid stations. Those half-filled eight ounce cups don't give you much to throw over your face, which is what often happens as you try to find your mouth! Here's a few drinking hints.

* Cold liquid is generally best: many studies show it is absorbed faster than warm liquid. However, some studies show that warm liquids are absorbed just as fast. Most of us are more likely to drink cold liquids though, especially if they taste good.

* Cold liquids give an additional cooling affect because once it gets inside of you, your body uses its heat to warm the liquid to 98 to 100 degrees. But it needs to get inside of you, rather than being splashed over your body.

* Take more than four hours for the marathon? Walk through the aid station, pick up two cups of liquid and drink it down. The 15-second walk relaxes you to run the next two miles. If liquid stations are every mile, one full cup of liquid may be enough; it will give the 10 minute mile person 48 ounces intake per hour if the cups are 8 ounces each. Take two cups if they are smaller. Match intake to your sweat loss rate.

* Expecting a sub four hour marathon? Ease the pace by a few seconds per mile as you pick up a cup from the second or third table (the first table is often crowded).
* If people are handing out the cups, try to make eye contact and say, "yes please" as you approach.
* Learn the left hand pick-up. Most of us are right handed, so tables on the left can be easier to get at.
* Squeeze the top of the cup and cover the upper half to prevent spills. While the lungs are quite adept at absorbing water, snorting liquid is not the best way to get it into your circulatory system, so practice drinking from cups in training. Carry a large bore plastic straw if you have problems drinking at close to race pace.
* Discard the cup to the side of the road and pick up a fresh one from toward the end of the liquid station.
* If the water cups are completely full, after checking to make sure that it is water, pour half of it over your head so that you can squeeze the cup and actually get the remaining four ounces inside of you.
* However, the basic rule is liquid goes inside of you first. It has a greater cooling affect than pouring it over yourself.
* Sports drinks should also go inside of you for the sugar to reach your muscles!
* Feeling full after one cup, which was usually half a cup? Fold over the top of your cup and you can carry a couple ounces of liquid while you decide if your stomach contents are sloshing around too much to warrant this extra couple of ounces going inside you. Offer it to a companion if you elect not to take it.
* Taking an energy gel pack? Consume it a quarter mile before the liquid station, and then flush it with 8 to 12 ounces of water at the station.
* PS. Don't try any new sports drinks on race day. Instead, try most of the sports drinks on the market prior to your race. Find out which ones will be on your race course. Used in moderation, sports drinks only give bad effects to

a few sensitive people. Their fructose can make bowels hyperactive.

Don't overhydrate with water or sports drinks in the second half or at the end of the marathon or you'll risk hyponatremia (See page 58). Include minimal sugar (200 calories per hour) and electrolytes each hour during the race, and consume a variety of liquids and fruit after the race.

Practice in training too: You'll need to carry this liquid. Hand held water bottles change your running form. So:

Carry your liquid bottle or bottles in a waist belt. It allows you to keep running while drinking. Stashing liquid on your running route works too. A one-third strength apple juice mixture with a little salt in a 16 to 24 ounce plastic water bottle allows you to trash the bottle at the next bin. Tip: Place them in the freezer for an hour before you drive out to drop them off in shady spots close to known landmarks.

Marathon hyper-hydrating.

The well trained runner who rests up while carbo loading will store extra glycogen in the muscles for a dry day, AKA your endurance event. The side effect of glycogen storage is water storage and weight gain. The weight is water, not fat. This extra weight will encourage a sedate first 10 miles for your marathon as the glycogen is efficiently reduced to its constituent parts, releasing energy to run and supplying water to keep your blood volume up.

The sensible early pace also allows you to burn more fat, thus conserving your huge glycogen store.

You can add to your carbo loaded water supply by using glycerol, which helps you to retain water and reduce urine output. However, according to Tim Noakes, studies show that this hyperhydrating does not improve marathon performance.

You don't need much glycerol, and you still may not like to drink it. Olympic marathoner and writer Ed Eyestone was recommended to use .012 fluid ounces of glycerol per pound of his body weight by David Martin Ph.D. an exercise physiologist at Georgia State University.

Gastric Emptying Rate.

To decrease the sloshing in your stomach from taking liquid on the run, you need to train your stomach. Well, actually, you'll have to train your mind to feed your stomach the best stuff for you.

* Low fat liquid meals empty faster than fatty liquids.
* Nonfat, fruit flavored yogurt gives you liquid and sugar (about 42 grams of carbo).
* Smoothies empty faster than solid foods, especially if they are low fat smoothies.
* High water content fruits like bananas, grapes, oranges and the melon family are absorbed fast.
* The sugar in energy gels is taken up rapidly if you include water with them.
* Low sugar drinks at about 5 to 6 percent sugar have been shown in some studies to be absorbed faster. The 14 grams of carbohydrate in an 8 ounce serving of Gatorade gives a 5.8 percent solution, 110 mgs of sodium and 30 mgs of potassium.
* Potassium is important to decrease cramps, so consider a half strength orange juice (4 ounces of OJ and 4 ounces of water) once an hour to get: roughly the same carbo concentration as a sports drink at 5.6 percent, a very nice 225 mgs of potassium, 7 mgs of sodium, plus, a gram of protein, 65 percent of your vitamin C needs, and a bit of thiamine, niacin, B6, Folate, magnesium, all of which are needed for energy metabolism. Use sports drinks or other juices and water for your other 5 drinks each hour.
* Add a small salt sachet from fast food restaurants to give your fruit juices sufficient sodium.

Note: Carbo percentage in a liquid is: the number of calories in your drink, divided by the volume of your drink, times 100.

Calorie saving tips to Lose Weight Part One.

Most milk servings contain 30 percent of your daily calcium needs, plus a ton of Vitamin D to aid in the absorption of calcium, yet non fat or skim milk has only 86 calories per cup; Chocolate milk has 208. Regular milk packs 80 calories from fat into its 150 calories per cup. Drink non fat milk and use it in your coffee or tea also. One milk serving also gives you 8 to 9 grams or about 16 percent of your daily protein needs.

Soda. Unless you're within one hour of exercising, the only soda to drink is diet. Or drink more water. Twenty ounces of regular soda contains 250 empty calories. 250 calories is a good pre-run snack. Soda is probably the poorest way to get that snack. Slush a small bagel down with 12 ounces of tomato juice instead. You'll still get about 250 calories, but tons of nutrients, with electrolytes and 8 grams of protein.

Use ice and plenty of it. It takes one calorie to warm one liter 1 degree centigrade. Your typical 2 pints of ice water will take 37 calories to reach body temperature. Drink 3 liters or 6 pints of icy liquids per day and in theory, you'll burn 112 calories. In practice though, you'll simply sweat a little less to lose your body heat. The ice itself takes 80 times as many calories to melt, compared to bringing water up one degree centigrade, but even when munching on some while you wait to eat, you'll not be chewing down a huge quantity. You will use more of your calories with ice drinks than if you drink predominantly hot drinks though!

A pint of flavored sparkling mineral water has no calories, whereas one pint of juice or lemonade or a snapples, "weighs" an average of 200 calories. Substitute one sparkling water per day to take off 20 pounds a year.

Eat an orange to fill you up with 65 calories instead of 8 ounces of orange juice with 112 calories to save 49 calories.

A cup of grapes has 58 calories, yet a cup of grape juice has 96, which is another 38 calories saved.

An apple gives a more modest saving of 30 calories over its juice (111 versus 81).

A cup of cantaloupe has 57 calories; a cup of cranberry juice has a massive 147. Tomato or other vegetable juices have only about 50 calories per cup, a ton of vitamins, a little fiber, and save you 46 to 97 calories compared to the three juices above.

Substitute real fruit for juices four times a day and you'll save about 150 calories and lose 17 pounds per year!

Match each piece of fruit or fruit juice with one to two cups of water to maintain hydration. Don't waste your calories on fruit punches, cocktails or blends. They usually contain fructose from corn, plus water as the first two ingredients, and so little actual juice that they add vitamin C to con you into believing you've got a decent fruit serving.

Drink lite beer instead of regular beer, or drink fewer beers. Alcohol increases the affect of drugs like Ibuprofen. The gastric irritation increases your potential for ulcers.

Heavy (alcohol) drinking is bad for your health. Moderate drinking is only unhealthy if done in the company of smokers. Alcohol increases your risk of mouth and throat cancer if done in a smoky place, or while socializing or dating smokers. Plus you're more likely to smoke a cigar!

Four to 8 servings of alcohol, if spread out over the week, can actually bring health benefits. The flavonoids in grapes (and thus wine, especially red wine) protect arteries from cholesterol. But alcohol calories can make you fat: The 1,200 to 1,500 in 8 servings per week means 18 to 22 pounds of fat put on per year. Or you can save 78,000 calories per year from elsewhere in your diet to allow yourself alcohol without weight gain! That excludes the calories from mixers. Rum and diet coke costs no more calories than rum on ice. Note: the U.S. Dietary Guidelines is one drink for women or two for men.

Besides the potential for weight gain, there are also unhealthy side effects from alcohol if you intend to drive home. Don't drink any alcohol if you're driving. That first drink makes you six times more likely to have an accident. The second drink makes you 12 times more likely to be in an accident. The only safe level of alcohol consumption if driving in the next 12 hours is Zero.

Quick Fix Weight Loss.

Think you'll be able to lose five pounds in five days on the THREE shakes a day diet, or Hollywood style diets? No problem. You can lose a pound every day provided you burn 4,250 calories each day.

Most people who need to lose weight burn about 2,000 per day; this is part of the reason they are overweight. The second reason is over-consumption of food.

To lose one pound of fat you need to burn 3,500 calories. Add in the 750 calories from those three shakes, and you can see where the 4,250 calories came from. Yet advertisers keep a straight face when they make their weight loss claim. The actual weight lose is from the shunting of fluid which occurs when you deny yourself food. You'll use up some of your glycogen stores, which contains lots of water.

The day you re-commence normal eating, the glycogen stores and the water is restored. Make subtle changes to your drinking and eating habits.

However, smoothies can still be part of a steady weight control plan to prevent you from pigging out and as healthful snacks between meals or before runs.

Perhaps the ideal snack is a smoothie made from low fat yogurt plus blueberries and cranberries, followed by eating another piece of fruit to enjoy the sensations from chewing food one day; munch on a bagel for your chewing pleasure the next day.

Use any two to four fruits that you like for the smoothie, and you'll get a more balanced combination of carbohydrate, minerals, fiber, antioxidants and phytochemicals. Use any low-fat protein source to add creaminess. Add crushed ice for a cooler smoothie. Iced milk, sherbet or frozen non-fat yogurt are other ways to cool it.

For instance, on the second day your smoothie may actually be made with non-fat milk, strawberries and a banana. Your third day would probably be a low fat energy bar with a pint of water and a piece of fruit. Fortified soy milk works well instead of non-fat cows milk or yogurt. Consume soy in other products too in order to get its isoflavones and to reduce your animal protein intake, thus decreasing risk of cardiovascular disease, breast and prostate cancers.

Prefer fruit only smoothies? Use whole fruit instead of juices for the fiber and to reduce the calorie intake. If this is a meal substitute, you'll need a protein source. A chicken drumstick works well, a couple ounces of very low-fat ham or turkey slices, or a slice of beef are other options; or knock back two egg whites for 12 grams of protein. Otherwise, this could be the one occasion when a protein powder fits your nutritional needs. But only because it is convenient. Don't use it in addition to your non-fat milk or yogurt. There's no need to pay a fortune for protein powder. Nonfat dry milk powder or slim fast in its variety of flavors work well.

Smoothies are great meal substitutes and pre or post run snacks because of their energy and liquid content. In the 60 minutes post exercise, muscle cells suck up sugar and protein, provided you put the stuff in your stomach. Including protein in your first post exercise food increases the amount of glycogen in your muscles. A one to four ratio is all you need. The protein in your bread, plus a glass of non-fat milk or a yogurt will *meat* your needs. So will a balanced smoothie.

Meal in a can or in a plastic bottle make a great snack as they usually give 10 to 15 grams of protein, and are fortified with vitamins, but you'll need to chase them down with a piece of fruit or carrot sticks and a bottle of water.

Chapter Nine

Solid Food &

Nutrition Issues

Note: You should also consider water and other fluids to be food! See Chapter Eight. There's so much information here that we had to decrease the font to 12.

Your Ideal Running Weight is the weight at which you feel most comfortable. However, it's difficult to run a good marathon if you're overweight. Carry too much weight and you'll place extra strain on your joints, especially the hips, knees and ankles. Extra pounds slow you down in marathon running too. Two pounds per inch of height works best for competitive running. One kilogram or 2.2 pounds per inch should be your maximum running weight if you desire a decent marathon. Very few runners should weigh less than 1.8 pounds per inch.

Prefer it as fat percentage. Top runners get down to 5 percent body fat; most of us are comfortable at 10 %; you'll become ungainly at running, and approaching unhealthy for life at greater than 15 % body fat. Ladies can add 5 % to each of those three levels, giving you 10 to 20 % as your range.

Officially, 15 to 18 percent body fat for men and 18 to 22 percent body fat for women is the ideal range for healthy living for non-marathon runners. Remember that for a 150 pound runner, every additional one percent body fat is 1.5 pounds of actual fat which you have to lug around all of your running courses, including the marathon course, and will cost you about 2 seconds per mile for every 1.5 pounds or roughly one minute for the marathon.

According to the American College of Sports Medicine, for general living, the optimal level is 19 to 22 percent body fat. Most gyms and health clubs can measure your body fat percentage using painless calipers or an electrical impedance device. Digital scales also come with a fat percentage gismo and may be accurate to within 0.1 percent.

Once you have an accurate starting number for your body fat percentage, you can reduce your daily calorie intake slightly and weight train twice a week to decrease the percentage! The extra muscle increases your lean percentage, and burns 35 to 50 calories per pound every day to keep your body fat percentage even lower. A weighing machine does not tell you the changes in your fat percentage; it only shows you your weight.

Calorie burning tip: Add two pounds of muscle mass with twice weekly weight training and you'll burn an extra 70 to 100 calories every day. That calorie burn excludes the calories used during weight training. It is the calories burned by owning extra muscle mass, which has a high metabolic rate. That's 7 to 11 pounds of fat you can lose each year. Weight training also reduces your running injury risk. Keep the weight training simple and you'll actually do it. Use dumbbells to exercise the arms and shoulders, and use step-ups, lunges and half squats for the legs.

Internal fat or the fat which surrounds your organs can predict your health status. It's usually expressed as the waist to hip ratio (W/HR). Divide your waist measurement by your hip number. A waist of 30 and hips of 38 gives a W/HR of 0.79. Under 0.80 is ideal for health and you'll run better marathons. Greater than 0.85 is considered unhealthy.

Under 35 inches for the waist is also better for your health. Greater than 35 inches puts you at higher risk for fat related diseases such as heart disease and diabetes, and of course will slow your running. Every extra pound slows you by 1 to 2 seconds per mile. Being 10 pounds overweight on race day will slow you down by over 8 minutes. If getting rid of the extra 10 pounds gets you closer to ideal race weight, do it months before the marathon so that you train at your ideal weight, then run your marathon 8 minutes faster.

One argument for losing fat is that you will then have more blood, oxygen and other nutrients for your muscles. However, fat uses only about 2 percent of the energy which muscles use: it takes minimal resources to keep fat happy. Perhaps that's why some people don't notice their fat. However, the real cost to runners is the cost of carrying the extra weight. If you want to carry a backpack or hikers waist pack with ten pounds in it all day, go ahead, but it will fatigue you just like a bag of flour or sugar tied to your hips would.

Lose the fat slowly with a mere 250 calorie per day deficit compared to what you burn and you'll sift away 10 pounds in 20 weeks. Exercise too though to maintain your muscle.

The fifth number you can use as a weight guide is your:

Body Mass Index, or BMI, which measures your composition based on height and weight.

Divide your weight in pounds by

The square of your height in inches

Multiply the tiny result by 703

For example, this author is 145 pounds and 5 feet 9 inches or 69 inches.

69 squared is 4761

so…145 divided by 4761 = 0.03046

0.03046 x 703 = a BMI of 21.4

His BMI when at his racing peak of 140 pounds was 20.7, but his body fat percentage was only 5.

The healthy BMI range is debatable. A BMI below 20 implies low body fat, but if you're a non-exerciser, it does not mean that you're lean and healthy. You could have small muscles due to inactivity.

A BMI above 25 implies a degree of fatness, but you could be very fit or muscle bound from weight training and running 40 miles per week. If your BMI is above 25, take a look at your waist measurement and body fat percentage too.

Most runners should not look like Olympic marathon champions. Don't try to be skinny if it does not suit you. Weigh yourself regularly and get a feel for your ideal living and running weight. If your weight sneaks up because you've decreased your training, get back on the trails. If your weight moves up due to increased calorie consumption...get control of your intake again. Get used to portion sizes. You don't need 6 or 8 ounce steaks.

Don't allow one high calorie meal or one extra day off from running turn you into a softy. Get straight back to good habits. Plan for some wicked treats within your 2,500 to 4,000 calories per day; plan for days off from exercise.

Don't starve yourself before running. A 250
calorie snack an hour or two pre-run helps you to maintain energy levels. If you're running longer than 90 minutes, liquid food on the run helps too. Side stitches and nausea result if you eat too much before or during the run. Liquid is still your most important nutrient. Even skinny people have sufficient fuel stores to run several marathons without eating.

Eat to run, but don't pig out. You need carbohydrates to exercise, so eat some 2 to 3 hours before exercise, and again soon after finishing. Include a little protein with your carbos.

How much carb and how close to the race depends upon how active your stomach is. The range is wide: One to two grams of carbohydrate per pound of your body weight, taken one to four hours pre-race is your goal. You'll need that "experiment of one" to find your level. Avoid the empty feeling at race time. Remember that most of the food which fuels your race or training run was eaten the day before; the fuel is already in your muscles.

A bowl of cereal with non fat milk, or pancakes, or toast, or a bagel with half of a low fat sports bar plus a banana works well pre-training or racing. Drink too of course. Eat the other half of the sports bar with an orange after the run. These 200 to 400 calories each time should suffice. Your post-run snack should include more protein than the pre-run snack for muscle repair. Use your remaining calories for a balanced diet of about 60:20:20 (carbo, protein, fat). Those carbo snacks give you the potential for a 65:20:15 diet.

Staying well nourished with a balanced diet sustains your healing capacity to recover from each run. The snacks help to maintain your blood sugar levels, enabling you to maintain your training pace more easily.

Eat a balanced diet with modest amounts of protein from low-fat sources, and plenty of grains, vegetables and fruit. The only supplement you may benefit from is a multi-vitamin with iron. Their iron content is modest compared to iron pills, which you should only take to treat anemia. Complex athletes need complex carbohydrates: Keep simple sugar intake to a minimum and you'll have the energy to run.

As *Running Dialogue,* says, there's really no debate on diet: eat a sensible, balanced diet, and the person living in western society will get all the nutrients he or she requires.

Eschew all fads, especially if they are at the heart of a book. Avoid "Protein" or "Fat" diets that try to make carbohydrates the villain in weight gain.

The villains are on both sides of the calories absorbed versus calories used equation.

The only guaranteed ways to lose weight are to absorb fewer calories than you use, or, to burn more calories than you absorb: which of course means the same thing. If you absorb more calories than you expend...you will gain weight.

HOW CAN YOU LOSE WEIGHT?

First you have to make the decision to lose weight. You cannot be pushed into weight lose, though support from others such as a running group can help. Knowing that weight loss will decrease your risk from over 3 dozen diseases is nice, but it still takes an active decision to lose weight slowly to give yourself a chance for permanent success. Lose one to two pounds per month with exercise and minor changes to your eating habits instead of shocking your system with the cruelty of a diet.

Five years after this author (and Registered Nurse) recommended that people do not diet (Chapter 22 of *Running Dialogue*), a study came to the same conclusion, saying that dieting was depriving yourself and was hard to maintain. The study recommended an hour of exercise per day instead of dieting, and as the average person watches TV for 2 to 3 hours, finding 60 minutes for physical activity will be easy! You'll have to exercise at very low intensity early on, and build up over several weeks or you'll be done-in and retired after one session. The goal is to keep going for an hour almost every day. But how to get your weight loss started.

Place an ad in the paper or get together with like minded people with similar goals to begin a group, or join an established group for support early on. Training buddies will help you to lose those last few pounds. Walk or jog some 5Ks and meet people at similar levels. Join a walking or running club.

More exercise is an option for some people who are ready to lose weight, but you are or soon will be marathon training, so how much can you add. One mile of walking or running burns about 100 calories. Move up from 33 to 40 miles a week, and these one hundred calories per day will take off one pound of fat every 35 days.

Keep your food intake unchanged, while doing the extra mileage, and every 5 weeks you will lose one pound, which will make 11 pounds per year until you reach your goal.

When you've got your heart into fairly good shape you can start speed running. Running a bit faster than marathon pace for 2 to 4 miles during a session increases the body's production of human growth hormone, pumping up your metabolism and burning calories. Fast running for 20 to 25 percent of your mileage will make you leaner.

* Ten times a 30 second strider will increase your calorie use by about 100, but you should only do this twice a week, and lose 3 pounds per year.

* Twice a week after an easy run, do two sets of press-ups, crunches and step-ups or lunges to lose one pound a year.

* Then jump rope for five minutes to work the calves and lose another pound per year.

* Change your weight lifting routine slightly every 6 to 8 weeks by lifting a bit more or doing a couple more reps on each machine, and lift a bit slower so that you're working the muscles for a longer period.

* Take short rests between machines so that you're doing three times as much exercise as resting, not the other way around. After all, you'll be exercising a different muscle group at the next machine. Do aerobic cross training too.

* Add one mile to one of your mid-week runs and one mile to your Sunday run each week for five weeks, and then run these

extra 10 miles each week for a year to burn over 1,000 calories per week or drop 15 pounds. Mid-week run already at 12 and long runs already at 20? Do the extra miles as a second run for the day. Still not close to marathon weight after a year?

* Drink water during most training sessions instead of a sports drink (or the one-third strength fruit juice recommended by this author) and you'll save 200 calories per 32 ounce bottle. The only exception would be sessions lasting longer than 2 hours, during which you could take in more water than you used to, but still consume a little energy with the water.

Take off your weight sedately to join the <u>minority</u> of Americans (35 percent) who are not overweight! The reason some people stagger around at 300 to 400 pounds is because they put on five to ten pounds per year for two or three decades. If you consume 100 calories per day more than you burn, you'll gain 11 pounds every year. So consume 100 calories less each day to lose 11 pounds per year.

Address any life issues which are stressful, make you angry or depressed. All three can cause you to overeat. Food is not an anti-depressant. How is making yourself even heavier and unhealthy going to make you happier? Take a contemplative 5 minute walk or do something constructive instead of snacking and figure out a better solution.

Expect and plan for setbacks as you regain 2 to 5 pounds of lost weight occasionally. Weight loss, like running, is a process. Steady amounts of sensible eating or training lead to good results. Some weeks you will not train as wisely or eat as sensibly. Get back on track within a few days and you'll be back to your pre set-back weight in a mere days. Most days, make your basic 40 to 60 minute exercise session one of your highest priorities. You make the time for 8 to 10 hours of work 5 to 6 days a week, you can find 40 minutes to exercise most days.

Don't let vacations be 5 pound weight gaining weeks. You don't have to run every day. In fact, you probably shouldn't be running every day. Find other exercises which will excite you for two or three sessions while on vacation and you'll exercise most days, and keep the weight off. Frisbees and badminton rackets take up little space. Enjoy the new scenery on foot. Share a special entrée instead of eating it all yourself and eat small desserts.

Vacation eating is the same as at home eating: Start with a protein and calcium containing breakfast and you're less likely to snack later. Include fruit to fill you up and whole grain products too. Pack some fruit, pretzels and nuts to keep you away from snack bars, but have your small size hot chocolate made with non-fat milk if that's your passion.

Drink plenty of water. Make your own sandwiches using low fat goodies, or use the mayo-free, low-fat chain store version. Eat a small bag of baby carrots or half a pound of strawberries.

Still short on time? Exercise in short bursts during the day. Three times 10 minutes will give you most of the benefits of your 30 minute session. But also:

* Add longer walks from your car to your next activity.
* Stand while you stretch.
* Use the stairs instead of elevators.
* Do food shopping soon after a meal: you're less inclined to buy junk food if your stomach is full.
* Use a food basket instead of the cart while shopping: you're exercising and you're less likely to buy too much.
* Do your own gardening and cleaning.
* Put the clock back a hundred years or only 15 years by walking to your colleague instead of telephoning or e-mailing across the office.
* There are numerous other options for an active lifestyle, instead of the inactive lifestyle perfected by many people.

Set modest goals for your weight loss. Record your food intake for a few days to see your eating pattern and you'll be less likely to eat certain things. Keep a log to record your successes and your less successful days.

How can you decrease your calorie intake by 100 calories a day to lose 10 or 11 pounds per year. Finding 100 calories is easy for most of you. In addition to the liquid suggestions in Chapter Eight, check the calories per serving of your:

Premium ice creams compared to iced milk, sorbet, or low-fat yogurt. The latter three save you calories, fat and cholesterol. Note: A serving size is one scoop, or half a cup of ice cream, but most people consume 2 to 3 scoops. A typical serving of chocolate sorbet saves 100 to 200 calories compared to chocolate fudge ice cream.

One low-fat chocolate-covered frozen yogurt bar has 80 calories whereas a premium chocolate-covered ice cream bar packs in about 260 calories. Cost to you is 180 calories. A Starbuck's Frappuccino coffee bar combines two pleasures for a mere 120 to 130 calories.

The next time you buy a gallon of ice cream, multiply the calories per serving by the number of servings in that container. Divide the calories in that gallon by 3,500 to find the amount of fat (in pounds) which will be added to your waist, thighs or elsewhere.

Cream of soups and chowders. Check the labels or the contents if you make them.

Potato or corn chips typically cost you 150 calories per serving, with 90 of them from fat. Pretzels are far cheaper at 110 calories and zero fat. Most people cannot restrain themselves to one serving of chips; dips are usually riddled with calories too of course.

Dried fruit usually has a cheaper calorie count than chips. Keep some at your workplace to avoid the vending machine; drink water with your fruit. Ask your vending machine company to put bags of dried fruit next to the chips column! However, due to the added sugar and oil in dried fruit, fresh fruit is better for you.

Eat a jacket or baked potato (*sans* butter) instead of fries.

Corn on the cob with a spray of butter-flavored oil is 165 calories. A cob with 2 tablespoons of butter to clog up your arteries is 335 calories, saving of 170 calories, while maintaining the current lumen of your coronary arteries.

The chicken sandwich in restaurants usually has fewer calories; but: Take the Mayo (100 calories per tablespoon) and cheese from hamburgers and it's close. Take the mayo off of the chicken sandwich too. There are plenty of non-fat dressings to add flavor to your sandwich. You might like to actually taste the animal once in a while. Request extra veggies on those sandwiches to make them more filling.

Exchange a veggie burger with 110 calories for your average hamburger (a 3 ounce, 73 percent lean beef has about 360 calories) to save 250 calories. Say no to the mayo or you've wasted your time and another 90 calories!

Avoid chicken nuggets with their 17 grams of fat per three ounce serving. Never supersize a fast food meal. Order the kids meal for yourself to save 200 to 300 calories, and drink diet soda. Or pay a couple dollars extra for McDonald's "Go Active Meal" which is essentially the same.

Choose lean meat and vegetables for your deli sandwiches instead of animals soaked in dressing or fat.

Trying to fatten yourself up? Start with baked beans at 225 calories per cup, corn at 150 and green peas at 105 calories.

Want to lose a few pounds? Carrots have 45 calories for 3 ounces; green beans, spinach and broccoli each have 30 calories per cup, and celery has even less.

And eat low-fat hot dogs (50 cal) instead of regular hot dogs (140 cal) to save 90 calories.

While one cup of potato salad with low-fat mayo still has 210 calories, a cup with regular mayo has 370. Save 160.

Take your lunch to work, but pack it with healthful stuff. Include one quality protein source such as non-fat milk or 3 ounces of lean meat such as tuna! 3 ounces of tuna in oil has 75 more calories than 3 ounces of tuna in water! No mayo.

Take fresh fruit to work and also take some into restaurants instead of eating two sandwiches. Can fast food chains please stock apples, bananas and oranges for 50 cents each as a gesture to their patrons' good health?

Eat whole fruit instead of drinking juice. You'll save calories and take in more fiber while satisfying your appetite.

A cup of granola is 340 calories before you put the non-fat milk on it. A cup of Wheat Chex is only 180 calories. One serving of each is nice after a 10 mile run.

Eat an egg white, plus one whole egg, instead of two whole eggs to decrease the fat & cholesterol and to save 50 calories.

Get used to serving sizes. Most of us drink from 12 to 20 ounce cups and much bigger soda containers. Play with a set of serving cups and see what a quarter cup of cottage cheese, a half cup of baked beans, and a cup of cooked rice actually look like. If in doubt...measure it...especially the high calorie stuff. Use a spoon to measure your occasional topping.

*   Half a cup of fruit or veggies is the size of a small fist and counts as one serving.

* Half a bagel is usually one serving, so most people eat two servings at a time.
* An egg-sized muffin is one bread serving, so your typical muffin is 4 to 5 servings.
* A one serving size pancake is 4 inches, or the size of a CD, not the size of your plate.
* A medium apple or orange is the size of a baseball, not a softball, for one serving.
* One small potato or a three ounce cooked meat portion is a normal size computer mouse or pack of playing cards.
* If you want to ruin the taste of bread with peanut butter, two tablespoons is the size of a golf ball and about 225 calories, mostly from fat, and most commercial brands contain artery-blocking hydrogenated trans fat.

Ready for a snack. Eat a large carrot and drink a glass of water and wait ten minutes. Still need to eat? Walk around the block while eating a small apple...you'll burn 25 calories and take in some good fiber. Then it may be time for your 200 to 400 calorie healthful snack, 25 percent of which could be from a snack size candy bar. The energy boost from a short run lasts longer than a candy bar. A yogurt or banana most days will do you more good than a candy bar.

Snacking at work? Walk slowly up the stairs. You'll burn 11 calories for 6 flights, and you can take the elevator down to save your knees. Do this twice a day and you've got another 1.5 pounds of fatty tissue off of your body per year, while building lovely butt muscles.

Snacking at night! Popcorn without butter, plus a glass of non-fat milk keeps you under 150 calories. A 12 ounce can of V8 has 70 calories, plus sodium and potassium to help your muscles contractions. Or don't eat at night. Pick an arbitrary time such as 8 pm and take in zero calories until morning. On days that your training finishes at eight or later, you'll need to delay your eating rule clock until you've finished dinner.

Place jelly on your toasted bagels instead of cream cheese and you'll save a hundred calories. Or use Philadelphia fat free to get some animal protein.

Do you have to fry food? Use no calorie or low calorie cooking sprays instead of oil or butter. Soak up excess fat from hamburgers with napkins before placing them on a bun.

Consume the so-called unhealthful foods in small amounts.

Dump the chicken skin because it has half of your calories; eat baked instead of fried chicken to save 75 calories per serving.

Eat low fat, non-fat or light versions of milk, yogurt and cheese. Note: All cottage cheese is not low fat, but you can buy low-fat versions!

Minimize high fat veggies such as olives and avocados.

Use low fat and non-fat spreads on your potatoes, breads, pasta, rice and cereal group. The croissant family of breads gets their taste from their fat content.

Love chocolate? Accept it and eat the stuff on a regular basis. It's the same as skipping meals if you don't, because you're more likely to pig out. Partial to chips or pretzels? Buy small bags and allow yourself one bag per day. Or place a handful on a plate and put the bag back in the cupboard. Then look forward to tomorrow's portion as you enjoy an apple to finish your snack. Then, despite the fact that apples and its juice have tannins, which have anti-adhesion properties and help prevent periodontal or gum disease, clean your teeth to decrease the tendency to keep munching. Drink some more water.

Got kids in the house? Move house. No, no. Have them buy their own cookies and store them in their spot. The kitchen is for healthful food choices. Oatmeal cookies are less detrimental than chocolate chip cookies. Balance each pair of cookies you eat with an orange or apple and a pint of water and you'll be unlikely to eat more than four cookies.

No ice-cream parties. The kids can eat ice cream when they are out. If there's no ice cream in the freezer, you cannot snack on it.

Start your day with a calcium source and a high fiber source and you'll consume fewer total calories. High fiber cereal with fresh fruit and non-fat milk is better for you than a bagel. Save that coffee for a couple of hours later so that it does not decrease the absorption of iron.

Eat alone instead of with others, while listening to relaxing music instead of fast or loud music, and in front of a mirror so that you can watch yourself eat: any of these three factors decrease the amount that you eat.

There are two key rules to eating:

* Include fiber with each meal or snack to make you feel full early in the meal. The oil free side salad, or an apple prior to your meal, or two to three veggies with each meal, or fruit on your cereal all qualify. Check for truth in advertising. One brand of fiber tablets claims to contain more soluble fiber than 6 apples. Very nice, but apples contain mostly insoluble fiber, which is the stuff that does you more good and there are only 80 calories for the 5 grams of fiber from a medium sized apple.
* Include quality, low-fat protein food with each feeding to keep you satisfied longer & defeat the glycemic index.

Plus, see the smoothie section in Chapter Eight.

Plan For Perfection.

Cook healthful low-fat entrees to freeze for your "hunger pain" days. Keep several meals available to microwave instead of ordering pizza. An empty fridge is an invitation to pig. Keep several healthful choice meals available, including low-fat yogurt, pasta, bread and rice.

Crack open a bag of frozen veggies to go with your frozen entrée, add some carbs and your dinner is set. Fruit and vegetables fill you up with fiber and micro-nutrients. Don't put oils on them and they will not fatten you up. A large baked potato (the near perfect endurance food with carbs, potassium, vitamin C, iron and water) is better for you than a large bag of chips.

Store bought foods have to obey certain laws, but:

* Lean meals or foods can still contain up to 9.9 grams of fat. (Which is 89.1 calories from fat!)
* Extra lean can still have 4.9 grams of fat per serving, and often have 2 to 4 servings per box, giving you 175 fat calories.
* Reduced or less or fewer only means 25 percent fewer calories or 25 percent less fat than the original.
* Light versions must be 33 percent fewer calories or half the fat of the original.
* Low, few or little contain a modest amount of the nutrient in question, and it usually takes 15 to 20 servings to reach your daily limit. Low sodium items can contain up to 140 mgs per

serving, so if it's your only food for the day, it would take 17 servings to hit your limit.

On the plus side, however.

* <u>Fat free</u> only contain a trivial amount of fat per serving such as with Philly fat free cheese (30 calories and 5 grams of protein per serving)
* <u>No calories</u> means almost no calories - the one calorie cokes.
* <u>Good source of</u> means the food contains at least 10 to 19 percent of the RDA for said nutrient.
* <u>High in</u>…means it contains 20 percent or more of the RDA or daily value for the nutrient.

Light ice cream often breaks the philosophical law by calling itself light ice cream. Yes, they have cut the fat in half to qualify for Light status, but they add extra sugar for consistency, giving almost as many calories as the original version.

Peanut butter starts off with so much fat and so many calories per serving that even its reduced fat version contains 12 grams of fat and 60 percent of its calories from fat. Of course, most people don't need a full serving on a bagel or in a sandwich! High fat comfort foods do decrease the release of stress hormones, but the extra weight on your hips increases your stress, so take a walk instead of eating a candy bar.

Plan social outings around activities instead of sitting in a restaurant. However, restaurants can cook healthful choices too, even if they need coaxing at times by you. Take half of your oversized entrée home to save 400 or more calories.

Unless you've just done your 22-mile run, avoid all you can eat buffets! Even then, start with fruit or a beany salad.

Don't attempt to lose weight with diet alone. Don't diet at all! Make minor adjustments to your food intake. You've decided that exercise is good for you so use exercise to help you lose weight. Don't start with a marathon.

If you lose weight by diet alone, 25 percent of the loss will be from your muscles. The human body is 50 percent muscle, so retain most of it by exercising while losing weight - then you'll lose only 5 percent from your muscles - mostly the fat which was stored in them anyway. Better yet, incorporate weight training during your weight losing phase to increase muscle size and speed your body weight loss.

Adopt a combination of changes that will work for you. Find hobbies which keep you physically active. Find out which foods you have a weakness for and learn to manage the craving for that food. Train for 5K to 10Ks until your weight and therefore the ground impact while running is at a reasonable level.

Take responsibility for your weight. Unless you're suffering from advancing dementia or dependent upon others for some other reason, you're the person putting food into your mouth. You have to take charge of your energy intake.

Vitamins.

Organic compounds called vitamins are coenzymes which facilitate the action of enzymes to achieve most body functions. Each vitamin has some of its running related tasks listed below.

Vitamins are classified as:

* Fat-soluble (A, D, E & K), which are stored in our fat, and usually are consumed in fat. The liver can store 6 months supply of A and D and we can overdose on either, especially when taking supplements.

* Water-soluble (Bs & C) are easily excreted in urine and sweat and need replacing almost daily. Very difficult to overdose on B or C.

* We can make vitamin A from its precursor carotene, vitamin D from ultraviolet light on the skin, and vitamin K courtesy of the bacteria in our intestines.

Taking a vitamin to ward off cancer will not work unless you also eat the fiber and healthful food which pushes the carcinogens out of your intestines. The main disease fighting benefit from consuming a vitamin or mineral is from the food you eat, not the vitamin. A healthy lifestyle is superior to pills.

When meat is listed as a good source, it implies beef, pork, chicken, fish or any other creature with muscles which helps it to swim, crawl, fly or run.

Vitamin A is needed to make new tissue and build bigger running muscles, decent bone growth for your running skeleton, prevent night blindness so that you can run at any hour of the day, and improves resistance to infection so that you can run 52 weeks each year. Liver, meats, milk and milk products have plenty of

Vitamin A. Green, yellow and orange veggies are your best source of Vitamin A...courtesy of beta-carotene, which is converted to Vitamin A, negating the overdose potential. Try to avoid retinyl or retinal-derived vitamin A because overdosing is easier.

The numerous B vitamins assist in energy release from glucose and fatty acids, cell growth (including RBCs), protein and fat synthesis & hemoglobin synthesis. Insufficient B-vitamins will lead to anemia. Whole-grain products contain most of the B-vitamins. Other sources:

B1 or Thiamine: Brewers yeast, milk, enriched bread or cereal, pork, kidneys, peas, pecans and other nuts.

B2 or Riboflavin: Liver, heart, milk, cheese, yogurt, collard greens, broccoli, asparagus, enriched bread, meats.

B3: Liver, meat, poultry, peanuts.

B6 or Pyridoxine: Meats, whole-grain cereal, egg yolk (sorry, that's the fatty part), bananas, nuts.

B12 or Cyanocobalamin: Liver, kidneys, meats, eggs, dairy products and is synthesized by the gastrointestinal flora. Unless you've had a stomach transplant, consider a supplement after you reach age 50 because old stomachs absorb less B12.

Biotin: Egg yolks, peanuts, peanut butter, liver, kidney, cauliflower, yeast, oranges, carrots, salmon.

Folic acid or Folate: Needed to keep the number of circulating RBCs up. Folate also decreases depression. Eat fortified grains or whole-grains, green leafy plants, apples, citrus fruits and the white veggies cauliflower, sweet potatoes and parsnips, plus liver. Many fortified breakfast cereals pack 100 percent of your daily needs, and as marathon runners may eat 3 to 4 servings, overdosing is possible, especially if you also take vitamins each day. Decrease the problem by eating three different types of cereal one day (at least one of which should not have folate added), while rotating real oatmeal and other breakfasts. Many whole wheat breads do not add folate, so toast, plus one serving of cereal would work.

Niacin facilitates glycolysis, including the first stage of tissue respiration in which glucose is broken down and releases ATP or energy. This cellular energy production allows your muscles to contract. Niacin is also needed for fat synthesis. Consume whole-grain or enriched grain products, legumes, milk, eggs, meat.

<u>Vitamin C</u> or ascorbic acid is needed to make collagen, the adhesive which binds our connective tissues and gives it strength; vitamin C also facilitates iron absorption. The trusty citrus and melon family are your friends for Vitamin C, plus peppers, beets, tomatoes, broccoli, mustard greens and kiwi.

Vitamin C from natural sources (5 to 9 servings of fruits and veg per day) is an excellent antioxidant; it deactivates free-radical molecules which harm all cells, including muscle cell membranes. Vitamin C helps to heal tissue and prevent muscle damage. Vitamin C from food will also give you folic acid and biotin: Vitamin C pills generally do not. Decent Vitamin C intake reduces bladder infections; 500 mgs daily can extend your life by one to 5 years. Deficiency causes joint tenderness, decreased resistance to infection.

<u>Vitamin D</u> is needed for calcium and phosphorous absorption, bone growth and neuromuscular activity. A shortage will increase muscular pain. Vitamin D is satisfied by milk products, egg yolk, fish liver oil, fatty fish or from about 15 minutes of noon-time equivalent sunlight if not wearing sunscreen. Unless you do all your running indoors or always wear SPF 30 sunscreen or you're dark skinned, making enough Vitamin D shouldn't be a problem.

<u>Vitamin E</u> is needed for red blood cell function which helps you to run fast, and is an antioxidant, which decreases the damage to your muscles from running fast; find Vitamin E in high calorie vegetable oils and nuts, sunflower seeds, or wheat germ, whole-grain cereal, liver or leafy green veggies. Consume 200 to 400 IUs per day for speedy muscle recovery, and consider popping a 1,000 IU capsule after a particularly grueling race or training session.

<u>Vitamin K</u> is needed for the synthesis of clotting factors, but is only stored for a few days. So, consume dark-green leafy veggies, broccoli, cabbage, tomatoes, liver or eggs regularly.

Minerals.

<u>Iron:</u> A good source of vitamin C should be consumed with products high in iron. Vitamin C increases the percentage of the iron absorbed, thus decreasing your potential for anemia: you'll

also increase your training, healing and racing potential. Avoid milk (or calcium supplements) or caffeine at the same sitting as your main iron source: both decrease your iron absorption.

Plasma Ferritin levels (an indicator of your iron store) below 25 ng/ml may be a warning sign of impending anemia: it's also a warning sign for overtraining with injuries increasing by a factor of three with low ferritin levels. Get your plasma ferritin level, your Transferrin level (an indicator for your transporting iron), and your hemoglobin level checked once a year to see where you are.

Good vegetable sources of iron include beans, peas, dark green leafy vegetables (spinach is champ), grain products, apricots, and iron-fortified cereals. A large potato contains 20 percent of your daily iron needs and comes pre-packaged with plenty of vitamin C.

A greater percentage of the iron (called hemi iron) from animal sources gets absorbed. Liver and red meats, which include pork and chicken's dark meat, supply goodly amounts of iron. Oysters contain huge amounts, but it will take 3 to 4 weeks before it shows up as improved endurance in your other athletic event!

<u>Zinc</u> enhances enzyme activity, collagen production, wound and muscle healing. Seafood, meats, whole-grain products, eggs and cashew nuts are good sources. Calcium at the same sitting interferes with zincs absorption.

<u>Copper</u> also enhances enzyme formation, energy release, plus hemoglobin production, protein and cholesterol synthesis, and cell respiration. Sources include Liver, oysters, nuts, cocoa, cherries, mushrooms and whole-grain cereals. A copper shortage can show itself as anemia, weakness and the poor utilization of iron. Copper is stored in the liver.

<u>Chromium</u> is vital for getting glucose into the cells and for lipid metabolism, is also found in your trusty whole-grain foods, plus meat products, cheese and veggies.

<u>Calcium</u> is the most abundant mineral in our bodies, and is needed for rapid release before every muscle contraction:
* It regulates many of the body's chemical reactions;
* For strong bones;

Exercise and sweating does not increase the bodies calcium needs. Low fat dairy items (which increase your metabolism…burning more calories) plus dark green veggies like broccoli, kale, collard greens and mustered greens, plus, seaweed, wheat or barley grass, nuts and watercress are great sources.

Consume calcium from low fat sources. People who take in adequate calcium are more likely to lose weight and to keep it off. They lose more abdominal or visceral fat. Aim for 1,200 mgs per day. Not much of it should come from supplements, and none should come from coral. Check your multivitamin and fortified cereals and juices to make sure that they don't push you toward kidney stones.

Runners develop 40 percent more bone mineral than non-runners, but you need to take in the calcium and vitamin D.

Phosphorous is also needed for bone and tooth development, plus energy release (from ATP), fat transport via phospholipids and the synthesis of enzymes. Soda drinkers tend to O/D on phosphorous. Better sources include animal protein, cereal products and peanuts.

Magnesium regulates muscle contractions, is involved in the conversion of carbohydrates to energy, and protein synthesis and nerve transmission...and is found in nuts, whole grains, and dark green veggies. Low magnesium levels in the muscle cells can cause chronic fatigue and muscle cramps. Dr Kenneth Cooper showed it is the only mineral whose bloodstream concentration is lowered by heavy exercise. Low blood magnesium usually means low muscle magnesium. Magnesium deficient people use 15 percent more oxygen during exercise.

Sodium is good for you. You need this basic e.g. table salt for water distribution, but by eating a variety of fruit and veg, you should not need to add it to food (unless you're outside during a heat wave, or you only drink water during a long event). The body has an in-built warning system to ask you for salt. Too much salt can give you hypertension.

Pretzels and vegetable juices are great ways to top up your sodium level, which helps to maintain your hydration status and blood pressure. See hyponatremia pages 58-60. Too much sodium intake can lead to weak bones due to calcium loss; high potassium intake can alleviate some of that loss.

Potassium controls muscle heat and nerve conduction and like sodium is available in most fruits and vegetables such as bananas, oranges, cantaloupe, broccoli, peas, beans, tomatoes, spinach and potatoes. Unlike the trusty sodium, there is no built in system to warn you of a low potassium level. Every time your muscles heat up, they release potassium into the circulation system. This dilates the blood vessels, increases blood flow and takes heat away from the muscles: Alas, some potassium gets excreted via sweat and urine. Fail to replace the potassium, and you'll feel tired, weak and irritable. In fact, your potassium level can go down gradually over the course of a series of harsh sessions or races, and be a contributing factor to overtraining syndrome. Keep your potassium intake up so that any overtraining you feel is from tired muscle fibers instead of a potassium shortage.

Iodine maintains the thyroid glands ability to function. It's also needed for cell metabolism and the synthesis of vitamin A, protein, thyroxine and cholesterol. Sources include veggies, especially if grown near the ocean, dairy product, iodized salt, and sea food, with fish liver and fish liver oils being the best supplier.

Selenium is another trace element that acts as an antioxidant and is needed for energy release, fighting infections and heart muscle function. Sources include organ meats, regular meat, cereal, oatmeal, milk, dairy products, fruit and nuts.

Include whole grains (see next paragraph), dark meats, legumes, mushrooms and a little cheese, and a variety of fruit and vegetables and you've got most nutrients covered.

To paraphrase Runner's World columnist Liz Applegate Ph.D. "there is a whole lot of difference between wheat bread and 100 percent whole-wheat bread." Wheat bread is made with refined but enriched flour, which has lost 25 vitamins and minerals in the refining process, and only 4 or 5 of them are put back in, (i.e., the flour is enriched). In whole-wheat bread products the germ remains, thus giving you more B6, Folic acid, chromium and zinc, which are needed for energy synthesis and healing.

Whole grains also give you more fiber to keep your cholesterol down. Whole-grain sources such as oatmeal, whole-wheat bread, millet or brown rice should be at least half of your 6 to 11 grain servings which the USDA Food Pyramid recommends. Think that green pasta is better for you. Check how much spinach or whole-grain wheat went into its manufacture!

Looking to cheat by eating less often thus consuming fewer calories! Try high beta-glucan containing fibers: Oatmeal and barley contain high amounts of beta-glucan, a soluble fiber which may reduce your appetite. The food may stay in your stomach longer, thus making you feel full. You can lose weight faster. It is probably more prudent to spread your calorie intake over four or five "meals," two of which will be healthful snacks.

Eat from the wide range of foods and you'll get enough antioxidants (Vitamins A, C, E and Beta-carotene) to seduce your free radicals, and sufficient B vitamins, iron and zinc for the metabolism of energy.

Eat an ounce of nuts a couple times a week for the omega-3 fatty acids and the protein, but don't take a second handful to make you fat. It's essential to consume some Omega-3 fat because the body does not make its own. Cold water fish like salmon (preferably not farmed), mackerel, tuna and cod, plus flaxseed or flaxseed oil, and nut butters from almonds and walnuts are good sources of omega-3 fatty acids.

Omega-3s decrease triglyceride levels and inflammation (in training muscles and other parts of your body) and increase your immunity, decreasing your heart attack risk, menstrual cramps, cancer, rheumatoid arthritis and improve skin conditions. You can get fish and flaxseed oil in capsule form, and 2 to 3 grams per day is all you need. You can add the oils or butters to your smoothie or use them in cooking.

Eat fish regularly and you're also more likely to lose weight. Fish is also packed with zinc, iron, copper and protein. You'll have less depression than non-fish eaters.

According to a 2,001 report by the U.S. Department of Agriculture, you can lose weight using any diet provided it contains a low enough number of calories. Duh! The report recommends that you consume those calories in a balanced fashion, rather than a fad fashion where one or two sources of energy predominate.

Follow the food pyramid: This author will not debate the new style pyramid. The old or new style pyramid will work if you consume low fat versions of each group and consume the appropriate number of calories for your needs.

<u>Eat breakfast,</u> or you've insulted your body, which will pay you back later by making you feel weak or forcing you to eat a ton of calories because you've starved it. Breakfast avoiders are 4 times more likely to get a cold to mess up their training.

Too busy for breakfast? My favorite energy bar has 290 calories, only 5 grams of fat yet it's tasty. It has a nice 37 grams of carbs and spoils me with a 20-gram dose of protein. Add a bagel and a piece of fruit and liquids while driving to my first event of the day and I've got fiber, carbs and (quite frankly) too much protein. My disorganization is usually due to hitting the snooze button. Smoothies are another way to consume breakfast. You don't have to use the advertised 12 ounce smoothie versions for anorexics. You can make 36 ounce 500 calorie runner's smoothies, which give an hour of pleasure. You don't have to spend 20 minutes at the dinner table to eat a balanced breakfast.

Not partial to non-fat milk before sprinting to work? Fortified orange juice packs just as much calcium.

Your primary dietary goal should be to take your caloric consumption in the healthiest way you find palatable. Save all your arteries – in the heart, brain, legs, kidneys and other vital organs by getting 60 percent of your energy from carbohydrates. Match each rapidly absorbed fruit serving with a slower absorbed complex carbohydrate plus vegetables.

Carbohydrates First (Gold Medal).

Carbos should provide 60 percent or more of your calories. If you exercise one to two hours a day, you'll need 4 grams of carbohydrate per pound of your body weight. That's five hundred grams for a 125 pound person, or a glorious 600 grams for a 150 pounder. Sound like over-eating? Many runners regularly consume over 4,000 calories a day. At 4 calories per gram, the 600 grams per day person gets 2,400 calories or a near perfect 60 percent of their 4,000 calories from carbohydrate.

High carbo eaters start races and training runs with more glycogen in their muscles, their blood glucose stays at decent levels much longer than low carb eaters. Low carb eaters are borderline hypoglycemic after a mere 30 minutes of running, and after a mere 60 minutes, if they were in hospital they would be given a bolus of Intravenous glucose as they are already below 50 mg per 100cc. Carbo eaters stay above 70 (i.e. normal) for 2.5 hours or more of running.

The U.S. Dept of Agricultures food pyramid has been out for some time, and the public is getting used to the goal of 6 to 11 servings of grain per day, preferably whole grain, which retains the bran, the germ and the endosperm to protect us from a host of circulation and bowel related diseases. The grain group includes all grain products: bread, cereal, rice and pasta. Note: potatoes are at the base of the food pyramid.

According to a study by the U.S. Dept of Agriculture, people who consume at least 55 percent of their calories from carbohydrate consumed the fewest total number of calories per day and got more nutrients. Carbo eaters took in 300 calories per day less than protein and fat pushers, saving enough calories to lose over 30 pounds per year.

Unfortunately, many people still mix in or place too much fat on their whole grain products. The result: they still consume too many calories per day on average, and gain weight.

Oatmeal pancakes are good for you if they are not saturated with the saturated fat from butter or the unsaturated fat from margarine. Moderate the use of syrups too, or the meal becomes very high calorie.

Whole grain bread toppings need just as much scrutiny as white bread toppings do. Got a whole grain roll to go with your chicken breast. Half a pat of butter should not spoil the bread's taste, but you don't deserve it if you're eating the chicken skin!

Grains are at the base of the food pyramid, but the fruits and vegetables should almost match them. They have volume so they fill you up; they are also packed with a ton of vitamins and phytochemicals to complement your grain sources. Eat enough vegetables, plus nuts and soy and you can lower your LDL or wicked cholesterol by 28 percent.

Don't be afraid of sugar because sugar is a form of carbohydrate. But you should keep your "ingestion" of the empty calories from added sugar, such as in soda, to a minimum. Focus on complex carbohydrates which are broken down into their con- stituent sugars by your body. We need simple and complex sugars.

Just before or after exercise, there are advantages to consuming the monosaccharides - glucose or dextrose, plus galactose and fructose because they're absorbed quickly and can be utilized straight away. (Fructose is somewhat slower. It may slosh around in your stomach if you take it on the run, but it is a steadier energy source.)

The snack an hour before exercise, or fifteen minutes after, should contain some disaccharides, which have two linked molecules and need dividing before they can be used. Sucrose (table sugar), lactose (milk) and maltose (from cereal) are still absorbed fast, but not until the link has been broken.

Moderate amounts of polysaccharides in the form of starch (cereals, breads, rice and potatoes) can be taken two hours before exercise. Too much and you will feel bloated. These cereals give you the steady supply of energy to fuel aerobic activity. Eat these complex carbohydrates or starches within 15 minutes after exercise to discourage you from consuming too much of the simple sugars, and to ensure a steady supply of glucose once the initial rush from the juice and fruit is over.

Muscles and the liver store 1 to 5 percent of our body weight as glycogen, waiting to be released into the bloodstream as glucose during exercise. Do enough long runs and eat copious amounts of carbohydrates while resting in that last week and you'll store almost sufficient glycogen to run a marathon. Almost enough glycogen is fine because fatty acids will supply the other 20 to 30 percent of energy.

If you eat a low carbo diet, you'll have lower glycogen stores. If you run low mileage with only a few long runs, you'll have very low glycogen stores. Consume good quantities of carbohydrate to ensure that your muscles get re-supplied with glycogen for your next run. Unusual fatigue, a slowing of running pace, and achy muscles are symptoms of insufficient carbohydrates. Of course, they're also symptoms of overtraining!

Fail to eat enough carbohydrates and your body will use protein from your muscles for fuel. Include quality protein sources with your carbohydrates to help with muscle repair, and to replace the slither of protein which you use for energy.

After your next 10K race or speed session, drink a pint of water, do a mile warmdown, then try:

*   8 ounces of juice with at least two more cups of water;
*   A banana and orange for the carbo boost and electrolytes;

* A bread or other wheat product (bagel, pasta, cereals);
* A small amount of animal, soy or legume protein;
* Low fat yogurt or low fat milk;
* Then, within two hours, go eat a real meal.

Get most of your carbohydrates from unrefined foods such as fruits, vegetables, beans and whole grains because the sugar is absorbed slower than from refined stuff like candy, crackers, chips and soda. Unprocessed foods also give you more of the vitamins which are essential for a healthy you.

A nice way to monitor your fruit and vegetable intake is to consume all the colors.

* Orange and yellow for the antioxidants, carotenoids (including beta carotene) and bioflavonoids.
* Green for iron and phytochemicals lutein and indoles.
* Red for the phytochemical lycopene.
* Blue and purple for antioxidants and anti-infective properties.
* White, tan and browns phytochemicals include onion and garlic's allicin.

The most important carbohydrate you eat daily is immediately after exercise. The _carbohydrate window_ lasts from 15 to 30 minutes after exercise when muscles eagerly restock their carbo or glycogen stores. Eat during this 15 to 30 minutes to recover faster from your run, decrease risk of a cold and to make tomorrow's session feel easier and more satisfying. There is also a protein window, so include 15 to 20 grams of protein for muscle recovery.

A regular size bagel has 200 calories, but a nice 40-gram hit of carbohydrate. Its 7 to 8 grams of protein also gets you half way to your post run protein needs. But tastier and low fat bagels like the Fruit bagel in this table are not difficult to find. Page 204 takes a look at a few more carbo options and are listed by carbohydrate grams order in preference to calorie count order.

Sixty-five percent of the people in the United States are overweight. Figure out which stresses in your life make you consume empty calories in liquids or food and you will have an easier time controlling your weight.

Champion carbo sources (in grams) include:

Food	Amount	Carbo	Protein	Fat	Total Calories
Baked potato	large	67	6	-	290
Fruit bagel	one	64	11	1.5	310
Oatmeal	cup	54	10	6	300
Raisins	half cup	53	2	0.3	200
Whole grain bread	4 slices	52	11	4.8	275
Fruit yogurt	cup	47	10	2.5	250
Rice (brown)	cup	45	5	1.8	215
Pretzels	2 ounces	45	5	2	215
Smoothie (see below)	16oz	43.1	15.2	1.1	232
Pancake or waffle - one		43	10	9	293
Pasta	2 ounces	41	7	1	200
Beans (baked)	cup	41	15	1	225
Wheat Chex	cup	40	5	1	180
Fig Bars	4	40	4	5	220
Flask of hot cocoa		Varies			
Corn	cup	32	4.5	1.5	150
Banana	medium	27	1	0.5	116

Note: The smoothie in this table is made with one cup of strawberries, one orange and a low-fat yogurt. You can go above 50 grams of carbo by using bananas instead of the strawberries.

The pancake / waffle mix was made with one egg white, 4 ounces of non-fat milk and a store bought pancake mix (which is where all the fat comes from). The 43 grams of carbo represents one large pancake, not the two which can be cooked from this mixture. Add fruit to personal taste and you'll have much more carbo and a multitude of vitamins. Most runners will eat at least two hotcakes, and even at 53 grams of carb per serving, they'll probably use more than one serving of syrup.

If you cook the pancakes before running, you can microwave them a couple minutes after your run, and thus stay out of the cookie jar. Use self-raising flour or a lower fat pancake mix and you'll solve the fat content problem. However, if you use syrup and eat a piece of fruit, you'll get only 13 to 15 percent fat calories.

Syrup, honey or barbecue sauce are also useful to stay away from fat toppings on your baked potato.

A flask (or thermos) of cocoa works well on cold days when you return to your car instead of your home. It's ready for you and you can look forward to it during your run. It's available if a companion or you under-dress for that days conditions, and you get chilled. A pint of non-fat or soy milk, plus cocoa to taste, plus a banana for solid food gives you nearly 50 grams of carbo and 18 grams of protein to start your re-charging while warming your belly. Dry cloths and the car's heater will keep hypothermia at bay if you drink cool liquids while driving home, but the warm drink improves your mood and your core temperature.

The items in this carbohydrate table are all low fat foods. Oatmeal's 18 percent fat calories will come down below 10 percent for the meal with the addition of non-fat milk, a piece of fruit and some sugary flavoring on top of the oatmeal. Its only companion at 18 percent fat calories is the fig newtons, which is a pleasure snack, far superior to cookies, so we'll leave it at that. Whole wheat bread has healthful fat in its wheat germ; this author has no qualms about its 15.7 percent fat calories.

These food numbers do not include their traditional toppings or accoutrements such as milk on cereals. You can spoil the nutritional value of almost any of the above by using regular milk on or to make your cereals, by putting high fat spreads on breads, potato or pasta. Or you can heighten their perfection by using non-fat milk plus fruit on cereals, jelly on breads, low-fat meats and vegetables in breads or with your pasta or potatoes.

The glycemic index is a tool used to describe how fast a
source of sugar is absorbed into the bloodstream. The baseline uses glucose as 100. High numbers mean the sugar is absorbed fast.

Under 55 is classified as low glycemic;

55 to 69 is medium;

70 or higher is high glycemic.

Post exercise, eat foods with high numbers first, and add in foods with a lower index until you reach your real meal. Some researchers use white bread as the baseline for glycemic index numbers so published numbers can vary.

In a quirk of nature, overripe fruit has a higher glycemic index than under-ripe fruit. The sugar in overripe fruit is absorbed faster, and may score 30 points higher on the index. Your body won't need to do as much digesting.

If you want fast sugar absorption the general rules are:

A. The smaller the individual item of food, e.g. small shaped pasta versus large spaghetti.

B. The longer you cook the food.

C. The riper the food is...

The higher the glycemic index will be for that food.

Thus, spaghetti cooked for five minutes scores a slowly absorbed 38, at 15 minutes it's still only 44, but at 20 minutes it's a medium absorbed 61 (and probably mushy).

You can manipulate the glycemic index of a meal by adding protein. Low fat yogurt (31) and soy milk (43) have close to half the glycemic index of cheerios (74), cornflakes (92) or bagels (72). Use skim milk (32) on most cereals to bring down the index of that meal. Combine a protein with a carb source, and meals should come out close to oatmeal's 58 or cheese pizza's 60. Baked beans and green peas (48) are also great combo foods offering carbs and protein, and occupy the middle ground for absorption speed.

Add peanuts (14), boiled soybeans (23), kidney beans or lentils (28), broccoli (under 20), apples (40) or tomatoes (23) to your banana (51), watermelon (72), baked potato (78) or pretzels (83) to feel full longer. Fructose scores 21, demonstrating how slowly this typical sports drink additive reaches your muscles.

Watermelon should be looked at from the perspective of its glycemic load, which factors in the impact of the carbohydrate in one serving of a food. A watermelon serving has only 6 grams of carbohydrate available, or 24 calories. Its glycemic load is a mere 4, which is very low. The modest glycemic index (47) of cooked carrots has so few calories that the glycemic load is 3. Anything in single figures has a low glycemic load. Above 20 is high load.

Back to the glycemic index.

To decrease your insulin reaction: replace,

Canned peaches (60)	*with a raw peach at* (42)
Cranberry cocktail (68)	*use Actual cranberry juice* (56)
Orange juice (52)	*with an Orange* (42)
Corn Chex (83)	*with Bran Chex* (58)
Cup of sports drink (89)	*with tomato juice*
Bagel at 72 with a	*bran or blueberry muffin at* 60 & 59

The second group produces less of a spike in your blood sugar.
   750 plus foods are listed at
   diabetes.about.com/library/mendosagi/ngilists.htm!
A few people do have an insulin reaction to simple or high glycemic foods used as a pre-run snack, making them uncoordinated mentally and physically. Decrease this by:

*   Consuming low glycemic carbos, most of which contain a bit of protein or fat.
*   Adding a complex food like non-fat milk to either low or high glycemic foods.
*   Taking in 50 to 60 grams of carbo per hour during the run, including the first hour, and from glucose polymers.

A recent energy bar advertisement calls its sports bar a Low Glycemic Index Bar and it has the ratio of 50:25:25, which means you need only one piece of fruit, plus liquid to make it a balanced snack before or after exercise!

   No doubt the energy bar contained as much protein as a glass of milk, or perhaps the same as a bagel with a slice of low-fat ham. If you can't organize real food in a little cooler for post exercise recovery snacks, an energy bar plus water will do. However, read the nutritional contents plus the ingredients closely to see what you're getting.

   Another ad in the same magazine was for a muscle recovery bar which claims to be a "clinically tested dietary supplement". One would hope it was tested before being sold to the public, but what was the result of the testing?

Dumping is a physiological reaction to the consumption of too much simple or refined sugar. Symptoms include nausea and vomiting, sweating, faintness and palpitations, increased heartrate and hypotension. Simple sugars exiting the stomach too rapidly attract fluid into the upper intestine to absorb that sugar. If the blood is in your intestines, then it's not picking up and transporting oxygen to your muscles to help you run. Nor is the blood available to cool you off.

   Pre and post exercise, use complex carbs, plus a little protein and fat to ensure a slow emptying of the stomach.

Avoid those super drinks or power drinks which flood the market because their sugar solutions are too concentrated. Any drink with an action verb probably has too much sugar.

The worst offenders are goos (gels or Gu) with the quick fix of sugar for long runs. The 80 to 100 calories will only give you a mile of energy, yet you have several thousand already in your fat stores. The goop will raise your heartrate by 20 per minute, which should be sufficient for you to realize it's bad for you.

If you use a gel, fluid <u>races</u> from your blood vessels, dumping itself in your intestines, so you're less able to lose heat; the heart works harder due to your bloods increased viscosity; you've given yourself an instant dehydration affect. But you get a buzz. You get a psychological boost. Unless you also consume several cups of water, the goop will have deleterious effects on your performance.

Protein Second (Silver Medal)

Most of your protein need has been provided in the pasta, bread and legumes (beans, peas and nuts) already. You'll only need a small amount of other protein at each meal to "meat" your needs: 2 to 3 ounces per meal is sufficient.

One magazine included an article on protein needs, and said that in old age, we need up to 50 percent more protein than in our young days: namely, 81 grams per day. Like nearly every article on the subject, it then gave three sources to easily accumulate those 81 grams of protein: a cup of beans, a glass of milk, and a tuna steak. Sound quality protein sources I'd have to agree, with variety, taste and key minerals too.

Endurance athletes also need 50 percent more than the RDA for protein, but *the average diet already contains 50-75 % above the protein RDA*. Even a heavy trainer only needs half a gram of protein per pound of body weight...75 grams for the typical 150 pound runner. Some sources say that men need 0.6 grams per pound, which would take the 150 pound runner up to 90 grams.

Take another look at the carbohydrate table on page 204 and you'll notice the huge amount of protein that many of your carbos provide. Low-fat dairy and the meats of animal do provide concentrated sources of protein, but you need very few bovine products to reach your 75 to 90 grams of protein, and you certainly don't need protein supplements.

A mixture of protein sources (legumes + grains) will provide all 9 of the essential amino acids, or the 9 which our bodies cannot manufacture from the other 11 amino acids. The burrito with rice and beans is a good match, though you don't have to eat the rice and beans at the same sitting. You don't need high priced amino acid pills.

Lets take a look at what appears to be a purely carbohydrate meal which is eaten 40 minutes after a 20 mile run. Baked beans on a toasted large bagel, followed by fig newtons (see page 204), plus strawberries, provide 155 grams of carbohydrate to recharge the muscles, a ton of fiber to keep you active, and a whopping 30 grams of protein. Yet you have not eaten a single item for its protein. The prudent runner will have had a fruit juice and perhaps a fruit yogurt and a quart or more of water just after the run for an initial 76 gram carbo rejuvenation along with another 10 grams of protein.

Protein should provide only 15 to 20 percent of your calories. The low fat dairy product at breakfast will contribute to your protein and your calcium needs; a different animal source containing iron should be eaten at lunch and dinner. A half cup of cooked lentils and kidney and many other beans contain 7 plus grams of protein, 20 percent of your iron and potassium needs, and huge amounts of Folate which is crucial for production of red blood cells. Peas provide 4 grams of quality protein. A cup of pasta provides 7 grams of protein; those bagels you munch on, yet another six to ten grams...that's before you add the cream cheese! Oh yes, many cream cheeses have minimal protein but plenty of fat. Read the nutrition info.

Being endurance exercisers, we don't eat just one portion of these carbohydrates, which happen to also be good sources of protein. As most vegetarians will tell you, it's possible to get all your protein needs without entering into the meat and dairy section of the food pyramid.

Consume two to four servings of vegetables, plus your main carbohydrate sources in excess of 7 servings for most athletes, plus two small servings of animal protein, and it's difficult for western society people to be protein deficient. You don't need extra protein to build bigger muscles. Your body will use protein to build muscle only if you exercise those muscles sufficiently to stimulate them to be bigger and stronger. More protein does not make you stronger. Only a well balanced system of training will make you stronger.

Any extra protein at 4 calories per gram is burned as fuel or converted to fat.

Good protein sources include low oil fish and tofu, plus chicken to provide over 20 grams of protein in just three ounces. Fish, chicken, red meats and lentils are good sources of zinc and iron to decrease your injury risk, and to improve your healing capacity.

You should consume quality iron sources like beans, plus vitamin B12 every day. 92 % of vegans are deficient in vitamin B12, which is essential for the body to absorb iron. Animal food sources or supplements are needed for Vitamin B12.

Include a little protein in your healthful snacks and with each meal and you will not be weak from protein shortage.

Need lots of expensive protein for the Iron? Probably not. Drink or eat a good vitamin C source like oranges or its juice or tomato juice to make sure the iron in your vegetables, cereals and breads is properly absorbed; tomato juice has the bonus of containing 15 percent of your daily iron needs per serving: Then you will not need to eat steak just for its iron!

Protein or fat food sources eaten at the same meal with carbohydrates help to even out the absorption of sugar into your bloodstream, decreasing the peaks and troughs to your blood sugar. So does the protein in beans!

Restrict meat and its saturated fat. Yves Veggie Cuisine Hot Dogs, Lightlife Smart Bacon (4 pieces) and Gardenburger Chik'n Grill all provide over 12 grams of protein and zero fat in 90 to 100 calories with good taste. Tofu is another fine option to get the benefits from soy, and is also low calorie.

If you fail to consume the minimal amounts of protein prior to marathons and long runs, your feeling of fatigue could increase. A little bit of protein in your bloodstream before you start your runs, plus some easily absorbed amino acids during your run can either decrease the rate at which you burn your glycogen, or decrease your feeling of fatigue...provided you've done a realistic amount of training.

If you fail to do enough long runs to educate your body to build up its glycogen stores, your muscles will burn some of its protein. Smell of ammonia annoying you? You could be burning protein for fuel due to lack of carbohydrate. Eat more carbohydrate plus a little protein. This will save your muscle protein. Breath smelling nasty? You could be burning excessive amounts of fat due to low carbo and high protein intake. Ketosis, or the use of body fats for fuel also dehydrates you. High protein diets strain the kidneys and cause dehydration.

Protein is needed to repair muscle and other tissue, for all cells in fact, and for making enzymes which act as the catalyst for body actions. Protein also helps to keep your immune system in order. However, don't waste your money or your liver and kidneys by overdosing on protein.

Consuming some of your protein soon after weight training instead of waiting for two hours will help you to increase muscle mass. The same is true for carbohydrate and liquids. Don't starve yourself of any vital nutrient post exercise. The sooner you eat or drink your healthy snack and then a meal, the sooner your muscles will recover. The same rule applies after cardiovascular exercise.

Restricting your main meals to 1,000 calories also decreases your blood sugar swings. Consume balanced 200 to 500 calorie snacks between meals or an hour or two pre exercise and again soon after exercise to help your body cope and to recover.

Fat by default (don't give it a bronze medal).

Fat will provide the remaining 15 to 20 percent of your calories. You should never eat a food for its fat because you get plenty of fat elsewhere. Fat is stupid. Hold on runners, the author means that fat is dense…it contains lots of calories for its mass. One gram of fat has 9 calories, or over twice as much as carbohydrates or protein. Keep fat consumption low. Consume bulky foods which have a low calorie density for their volume such as apples and potatoes, instead of stupid foods like nuts, oils and creams (cream of soup, peanut butter, butter, margarine, salad dressing and mayonnaise).

Use mono-unsaturated fats (olive oil, avocados, peanuts) in preference to saturated fats (meats, dairy fats, coconut and palm oil). Keep trans fats (margarine, crackers, cookies and chips and other processed foods) to a minimum because they raise heart disease risk. Put another way:

* Eat small amounts of nuts instead of chips as a snack;

* Use avocado on bread instead of butter or margarine;
* You'll consume fewer calories and better fat if you use olive oil instead of butter on bread.
* Use olive or canola oil for your cooking or use a spray;
* Use flaxseed oil, olive oil or seasonings instead of those thick, unhealthful fatty salad dressings.

Most meat contains more fat calories than protein calories. Nuts are even worse. Yet in moderation, lean meats with the fat shaved off and nuts are good for you.

The dressings used on an otherwise healthful 400-calorie salad, often double the caloric value of your meal. Use low fat dressings, and please, if you must use them, keep the regular dressing at the side of the salad. Look at how viscous they are; imagine THAT trying to flow through your narrowing arteries. (Note: it doesn't reach the arteries in that form.)

Fast Food Chains hit the Salad Trail in 2,003

	Salad's Calories	Dressing's Calories
Jack in Box Chicken Club	290	**320**
McDonald's Chicken Caesar	210	**190**
Wendy's Mandarin Chicken	150	**250**

Most food chains offer 3 or 4 salad options; most food chains also do a baked potato with broccoli. You can eat without dressings, sour cream or butter! Note: Most of these chains also have a 40 calorie dressing pack, but you'll have to ask for it.

Minimal fat consumption will give a feeling of fullness after eating; it slows the transit of food through the intestines, while meeting your requirement for the fat soluble Vitamins, which were covered on pages 193 to 195. Whole-grain products also contain small amounts of essential fats.

We know that women with less body fat have lowered risks for many types of cancer. Exercisers, who potentially have a low body fat percentage, plus rapid bowel transit time compared to the sedentary, will have still lower cancer risk.

Rarely say never.

However, never eat a fatty food for its fat. Never place a fatty substance on a food when a near zero fat substance will work. Barbecue sauce is better than mayo.

* Like avocado? Fine. It's better for you than butter.
* Like nuts? Good. Eat a few for the protein, omega-3s and vitamin E, but don't eat them primarily to get their huge fat content.
* Partial to steak or eggs? Eat small amounts of meat with the fat trimmed of, including the chicken skin, but eat meat rarely; restrict yourself to 3 ounces twice a day. Keep egg yolk consumption to a minimum.
* Brownies your weakness? Celebrate, because chocolate is good for you. But, when making brownies, substitute non-fat milk for half of the oil, and use canola oil; use two egg whites instead of one whole egg. The batch of brownies which was 200 calories each with 40 percent of calories from fat, plus the saturated fat and cholesterol form the egg yolk, goes down a mere 20 calories to 180 calories per serving, but with a much more respectable 32 percent of calories from "healthier" fat. In fact, this brownie contains less fat than the so-called balanced energy or sports bars. Eat this brownie with a cup of non-fat milk, and you'll total 11 grams of protein and 40 grams of carbo in your 270 calories and a net 21 percent fat calorie snack. (Numbers based on adapting a double chocolate brownie mix with tons of chocolate chips in it!)
* One of the most balanced sports bars gets only 13.7 percent of its 290 calories from fat. A rocky road sports bar from Promax packs a whopping 20 grams of protein, which even if you're a vegan is more than you need from a sports bar. Though most is simple sugar, the 44 grams of carbohydrate is its saving grace. Eat a piece of fruit and down some water and your initial post exercise recharging, or your snack at any time is complete.

Special "so-called" Diets:

"The Zone" fad does raise an important point. This fad recommends only 40 percent of calories from carbohydrates, leaving 30 percent from protein to overburden the kidneys and the liver, which either excrete it or convert it to sugar; the remaining 30 percent is from artery-clogging fat.

One of the arguments for the 40: 30: 30 diet is that we burn more fat calories sitting down than we burn carbos. We only burn more fat by percentage while sitting; we <u>burn very few calories</u>.

Their argument is only true because we're able to take in sufficient oxygen to burn an inefficient fuel...fat. When we start exercising however, the efficient fuel, sugar, provides most of our energy needs.

Unless of course you consume too few carbohydrates. The body will then have no choice about which fuel to burn for energy. The body doesn't become more efficient at burning fat and protein while you walk or run: it has no choice about its energy source because it's being carbohydrate starved.

The second argument for 40:30:30 says carbohydrate intake makes the body respond by producing too much blood sugar. What actually happens is the body absorbs the sugar from the consumed food, then efficiently stores it ready for use. If you consume most of your carbs as simple sugars, with negligible fat and protein at a meal, your blood sugar will peak a bit, and then trough as the pancreas (secreting insulin) tries to correct your cruelty. The sleepy feeling is not from low blood sugar because it will still be in the normal range. The post-meal sleepy feeling is from the blood supply being diverted to your intestines, combined with the lassitude that occurs about an hour after returning to mundane tasks.

Eat complex carbs with a little protein and fat to slow the entire meals intestinal transit time and food absorption, including sugar absorption, will be steady.

Another Myth. As the Dept of Agriculture report said, a high carbohydrate diet does not make you fat. Consuming more calories than you burn or inactivity makes you fat.

Fat is a much less efficient fuel source than carbohydrates. It takes 10 percent more oxygen to run each mile if the energy source is fat in the form of fatty acids. You will have no choice but to run slower for a given effort or heartrate. Claiming that fat is the most efficient fuel is like saying crude oil is the best fuel for your car or to wash your face.

The zone and South Beach fads give the inactive 80 percent of the U.S. population an excuse to eat too much fat and protein.

Unfortunately, several energy bars belong to the zone camp. No surprise that the best tasting meat is usually high in fat. The same is true of energy bars. They contain so much fat, in fact, that you may as well eat chocolate, plus a multi-vitamin after a training run. However, some calories from protein helps to keep your blood osmolarity up, and to give a ready supply of amino acids for immediate repair work.

There's a simple way to correct the low amount of carbos in some energy bars, and the overdose of protein and fat. We can dilute the protein and fat by eating two pieces of fruit. The complex carbos, fiber, plus the nutrients from the bar will then be a fairly balanced recovery snack.

The 50:25:25 energy bar mentioned earlier needs only one piece of fruit to make it a balanced snack. Or eat a whole wheat bagel with fat-free cream cheese and a piece of fruit.

By the way, University of Connecticut researchers showed that cyclists on the high protein Atkins diet had significantly less endurance and muscle power than high carbohydrate eating cyclists. Don't try to run a marathon in the first two weeks of the South Beach Diet either.

Another reason to curtail Fats.

Want to cheat your body? Want to consume the same number of calories per year but lose weight? You can, and in a healthy way.

1,000 calories consumed as fat require only 30 of *your* calories to digest, absorb and to convert it to human body fat.

1,000 carbohydrate calories take a whopping 230 calories for the conversion process.

If your current diet contains the U.S. average of 38 percent fat calories, and you consume 3,000 calories per day, you get 1,140 calories per day from fat.

Reduce your fat calorie percentage to 25, and it will be 750 from fat. Every day, 390 fewer calories will be from fat, an amazing 142,350 fewer fat calories per year. For every 1,000 of these calories you'll use 200 more to convert the carbohydrate to fat storage compared to the minimal energy used to store fat sources as your own body fat. You will burn up to 28,470 more calories per year just by changing what you eat, yet you're consuming the same number of calories.

At 3,500 calories per pound, the 28,000 calories gets eight pounds from your girth each year to improve your running.

You also make huge health gains from the other factors of a lower fat intake:

*   Your arteries clog up slower;
*   Your cholesterol and triglycerides being lower;
*   Your energy level rising;
*   Due to consuming less fat per year while eating more total food with more carbohydrates.

Fat Potions.

Don't take anti-fat absorption pills that will give you fecal leakage, plus other side effects.

Don't think you're doing the body a favor by eating fat products which cannot be absorbed because the bloating and diarrhea are unfair exchanges for cheating the intestines.

Don't take metabolism stimulation pills either.

None of these will make your heart stronger, your circulation better, or raise your self-esteem.

Exercise does all three, and more.

Exercise raises your metabolism, burns excess fat, cures bloating, and suppresses appetite. Eating healthful food has no side effects and requires no prescriptions.

You're as likely to see a pharmaceutical company spending millions to encourage healthful eating as you are to see a tobacco company voluntarily encourage healthy breathing. Make lifestyle changes for a healthy life: don't sell your self-esteem to a pill.

So, people exercising more than three hours a week such as when training a marathon or 5Ks, should get

most of their extra energy needs from complex carbs. Remember: most complex carbs include a ton of protein.

The real problem for many people adding extra food is what they put on the carbohydrates. Bacon bits and butter is a poor choice on potatoes; barbecue sauce or salsa is better. Two ounces of shrimp with its mere 60 calories is better than eight ounces of hamburger for your extra pasta meal. Beware of store bought pasta sauce and dilute its fat with a tin of tomatoes, or make your sauce from scratch. Each meal needs a mixture of protein and carbos: The protein for muscle repair and to steady the foods absorption and carbos for re-fueling. Fat will be present by default.

While there is no evidence that vitamin or mineral supplements improve athletic performance, most nutritionists recommend a daily multivitamin with iron. Use the cheapest available; there's no such thing as a super vitamin pill. Get several types for your medicine cabinet. The days you missed fruit, take an anti-oxidant pill with Vitamins A, C and E. The days you eat fast food, down a multivitamin. No meat or beans today? Take an iron pill with calcium free orange juice.

Endurance athletes like marathon runners will not benefit from creatine supplements. Aerobic prowess is determined by nature and a long series of graduated training sessions.

How many servings from each section of the food pyramid? Try 12 of grain, 9 of vegetables and fruit; add your low-fat protein sources and you should be in homeostasis. Sadly, according to a recent survey, 20-year-olds consume only one or two servings of fruits and vegetables per day.

Start your day with 6 ounces of fruit juice, eat an apple mid-morning, drink a 12 ounce can of V8 with lunch, and eat a quarter cup of dried fruit mid-afternoon and you've got five servings down. Just look for a leafy green item, some type of beans and another piece of fruit at lunch and dinner and you're home free.

What you eat in the weeks leading into your race could dictate whether you have all manner of nutritional ailments. The last weeks eating will determine your race day energy.

Carbohydrate loading used to be associated with a depletion phase. You ran fairly long 7 days pre-marathon, then you shunned carbos from day 7 to 4 days pre-race. Four days pre-marathon you also did a short speed session at 5K pace to use the very last of your muscle's glycogen stores. You then loaded up your muscles and liver with glycogen by eating all the carbs you could handle, which also meant low fat and low protein for the last three days. The problem was that many people were fatigued from

the long run too close to the marathon, plus they felt lethargic during the first phase without carbos: the incentive for these inconveniences was that you got your muscles to store extra glycogen pre-race.

The kinder way to load is to ignore the first phase. Although you'll be running 12 to 14 miles one week pre-race, it is not a true depletion run, and will not fatigue you. You'll then eat normally for the next three days, but because you're resting up, your calorie intake should be a bit less than usual.

The last 4 days: If you're used to eating 60 percent of your calories from carbos, and you increase it to 70 percent for the last four days, your glycogen stores can go up 41 percent; the length of time you can exercise at 85 % VO2 max by 45 percent...if you're male. Females get no increase in glycogen, though performance does increase by 5 percent as they use more lipids. During moderately paced running, women get 40 percent of their energy from fat, while men get 30 percent from fat. Women therefore need less glycogen to run a good marathon.

Slower marathon runners get less benefit from carbo loading because you are exercising at a lower percentage of maximum effort and able to burn more fat in the krebs cycle.

If you follow the marathon schedules in this book, you'll do 18 to 20 miles 14 days pre-race. Your "almost a depletion run" 7 days pre race is a mere 10 to 13 miles, which is a very easy run for you. Remember to slightly decrease your overall calorie intake because you're resting up and doing only minimal exercise this week. Cruise through your midweek speed session to finish your depletion phase, and then eat the slightly higher percentage of carbos for the last few days.

Cycling a three hour race? You could do a short session at 5K intensity, finishing with a 30 second sprint a mere 36 hours before the race, and recover because there was no ground impact, plus stimulate the release of glycogen rebuilding enzymes which encourage your high carbo diet to go into glycogen stores instead of fat stores. But you're running the marathon, so provided you've done 4 to 5 mile sessions of speed running at these paces, use:

* 2 to 3 one mile reps at threshold pace 5 days pre-race.
* 1 to 2 miles of 400 meter reps at 5K pace 3 days pre-race.
* And carbo-load with complex carbs and fruit.

Marathon Race or Training Run Early?

While it is prudent to eat before long runs and early start marathons, it's not vital. You should have sufficient energy stores in your muscles already from three to four days of carbo-loading if it's marathon day (and from resting up). On race day, a carbo snack while you prepare and get to the start will keep your glycogen stores high. Make sure you drink several pints in the last two hours because your kidneys will not get rid of it pre-race. Never get separated from your 5 percent sugar liquids before big events: you may have to wait for hours so stay off your feet.

Just your normal long run? You ate a high carbo dinner didn't you? Took in 400 to 600 grams of carbohydrate during the 12 hours after yesterdays Interval session didn't you? You have enough energy stored to cruise 20 miles at easy pace.

Any weakness you may feel is the fatigue from yesterdays run, combined with that empty feeling due to lack of breakfast (it's mostly psychological), and slight dehydration.

The solution is simple (pun intended). Drink several pints of liquid while dressing and getting to the start of the run. Include half a pint of non-fat milk for its protein and sugar, and a pint of half strength cranberry, apple or grape juice for their vitamins, electrolytes and sugar or a sports drink if you only want sugar, no vitamins and fewer electrolytes. Drink lots of water too. A bagel or sports bar goes down easily and will keep your speed in check for the first half an hour of your run. Because you're training at a minute per mile slower than marathon pace, you're using more fat during training runs. Try runs with and without a snack and notice any difference.

If you can get up 2 or 3 hours pre-run or race to make toast, have cereal, and down some fruit or a can of boost or ensure, your intestines will be digesting this food for the first several hours of your run. You'll get a nice steady supply of energy. You'll also have more time to hydrate for your run. You can also shower (to warm and relax your muscles) and stretch prior to starting your long run or race. However, apart from a healthful 300 calorie snack, you should not *have* to eat before a 20 or a 26.2 mile run. However, fasting decreases your glycogen reserve, so at least eat a snack to top up your liver and muscles.

Other training runs.

Use the same snacking rules for lunch time runs. More than four hours since breakfast? Take a small snack an hour before the run. Yes people, one hour. Unless you are striding out long repeats at 2 mile to 5K paces, you can handle this small snack being in your stomach. Anyway, a banana and non-fat milk does not take long to exit your stomach. This snack is mainly a psychological boost, plus the liquid to help you feel energized. You'll probably need to pre-pack your healthful lunch for after the run. It's the most important meal of the day on lunch time running days.

The same rules apply for an evening run. Snack one to three hours pre-run. A sports drink is a poor snack choice. Sure it provides sugar, but it contains minimal electrolytes compared to tomato juice, rarely any vitamins, zero fiber and no protein. Sports drinks are nearly as nutritionally empty as soda. A better snack would be a low fat but high carb sports bar, 8 ounces of juice, plus 24 ounces of water; or drink a smoothie before your run. Start your runs well hydrated.

Tomato juice or V8 are good pre-run and post run snacks, providing the same number of calories as most sports drinks, but much more potassium and sodium, while also covering part of your vegetable needs for the day.

Research shows that people who use a sports drink during exercise have better sprinting ability at the end of a 40 to 60 minute session. However, you should not be sprinting the last 400 meter repeat. You should run your last repeat at the same pace as your first 19 reps, which will usually be 5K to 3K race pace. The place to run a great time in the marathon is by maintaining a stunning pace, or speeding up by 5 seconds per mile for miles 18 to 26, not by sprinting the last 385 yards.

Rehydrate and recarb in a timely manner. Include fruit for the antioxidant, anti-sore muscle factor and a little protein such as a serving of non-fat milk from cows or soy for muscle repair. Include calories in your liquid sometimes, such as just before, during and just after exercise. But for most of the day, drink non-calorie liquids, or flavor your ice water with one-quarter strength juice to encourage you to drink enough.

CHAPTER TEN

RESTING to RACE the MARATHON

After doing a series of Intervals at VO2 Max, Anaerobic Threshold Running, Hills & Strength Training, Base Mileage & Fartlek running, plus races at 5K to the half-marathon, you're ready to rest up for your first or your best marathon.

The goals of marathon training include:

* Getting you to the start line without injuries;
* Without hurting you mentally;
* And with the ability to run the <u>entire</u> distance using a high percentage of your VO2 maximum, and close to your anaerobic threshold.

You can't run when you're injured, so you've built up mileage and intensity slowly, and also at the slowest speed to give your various systems full stimulation. Those modest paced speed sessions did not overload your mind either, because you made the sessions more demanding in a graduated fashion. Dozens of long runs combined with "slightly demanding" sessions stimulated your anaerobic threshold and running economy to improve: you're now able to run mile after mile at close to your oxygen debt threshold.

While rest is vital when peaking for a marathon, you also need to run some short but good quality speed sessions to keep your legs energized as they freshen up.

The serious runner who follows this program for the first time can decrease mileage by 20 percent per week for four weeks, while running a few VO2 max sessions with medium reps at 5K pace combined with long reps at 10K pace.

The moderate to severe intensity runners, or people going through this program a second time may linger here for 10 weeks, honing their ability to run repeats closer to 2 mile race pace, combined with very long reps at 10K and 15K pace. Their mileage decrease should wait until the last few weeks.

Whichever group you belong to, these sessions will maintain your VO2 max ability while you learn to relax at modest speed and make additional muscle strength gains. Then you will do the remainder of your marathon taper.

According to a review of dozens of studies on tapering in *Medicine & Science in Sports & Exercise* the average improvement by marathoners who tapered was 3 %, which takes a 4 hour 7 minute marathon runner down to 3:59:36!

These key sessions combining long reps at 10K to 5K paces can feel hard. You need the experience from prior chapters of interval training before you run these final 4 to 10 sessions leading into your marathon.

You've raced at least 10 times by now. You've had a chance to experiment with modest paced starts when you speed up for the second half for negative splits. You've probably flirted with disaster by starting too fast, resulting in positive splits! You should know about the importance of even paced racing and even paced interval training.

This chapter will help you through the last few speed sessions toward your marathon, and introduce a new session to improve your marathon performance and enjoyment.

Combining Chapters 6 and 7.

Alternate these two sessions and you'll maintain the benefits from Chapters 6 & 7. Do each session twice.

* 2,000 meters at 10K pace; then 6 x 600 meters at 5K pace; then 2,000 at 10K race pace.

* One Mile at 8K or 5 mile race pace (about 5 seconds per mile faster than 10K pace); then 4 x 800 meters at 5K pace; then one mile at 8K pace.

According to the late Harry Wilson, one of the top British coaches of the 20th century, "During the last few sessions as you approach big races, you're not trying to run faster than before. Instead, you're trying to match your previous time, but in a more relaxed way. At the end of the session you should feel, Hey, if I'd wanted to, I could run faster."

Don't run faster; you don't need to. You're already giving your oxygen uptake system its maximum stimulation, and keeping your heart in its training zone for a huge percentage of the training. Save your muscle fibers for the marathon.

Practice running these reps with good form, and keep the running as effortless as possible. You know that you can run the session because you've done it before; think about completing the session in greater comfort than previously.

According to Wilson, "It's not just how high you raise the heartrate in interval sessions, but also how long you can maintain it at a steady high level." A key component of these peaking sessions is to run long reps at 5 mile to 10K pace.

Pay attention to your body. Top runners are said to be disciplined thinkers: they think positive thoughts while training. They associate with the discomforts of fast running by thinking how much good the last two laps of a 2,000 meter repeat is for them as they focus on running form and legspeed. This helps them and can help you to stay relaxed and enjoy the difficult sections of your training. Think about your running form, your breathing and the feel of the track, grass or trails as you float along at 5K to 10K pace.

Feel like slowing down because it's hard work to keep your pace? Have fun and relax during the most difficult laps of long repeats by thinking about your running form and the relaxation of all your muscles, about your position in relation to the ground and then ease your way through the second half of each repetition. Think of yourself as powerful and energetic during interval or other speed training, and the training will feel easier. Imagine strong, graceful animals...including your favorite marathon runners.

Fresh Legs.

You should run the interval sessions in this chapter with fresh legs, after an easy run or rest day. Wear the lightweight shoes which you intend to use for your marathon. Lightweight shoes put you in the mood to run fast. These four sessions of intervals, plus two runs at anaerobic threshold, and a fifteen mile run will break your new shoes in nicely. They will still have less than 50 miles on them come marathon day.

Do warmup and stretch the calf muscles and Achilles tendons before these sessions. Warm muscles are more efficient and less likely to strain. Your speed running can then be done with minimal injury risk from the lower heel possessed by many lightweight shoes.

Start these interval sessions at modest pace. For the short reps, use the middle lanes. Use the inside lanes for your long reps. Any runner moving faster than you must go around you.

Even in this peaking phase, you retain some sessions from each of the first four phases. Run hilly fartlek and anaerobic threshold to maintain your earlier fitness gains.

Most of the schedules in this book have you run the same mileage most weeks, but with an easy week once a month for a practice race. Some runners like to include a higher mileage phase of 4 to 6 weeks, which ends 4 weeks pre-marathon.

If you choose this route, restrict yourself to a 15 percent mileage increase to keep your injury risk modest. The simple way to overload your muscles is to add an easy 5 mile run with 16 x 100 meter striders, add 2 miles at threshold pace, and a mile or two to your long run for these 4 to 6 weeks.

Don't Reduce Mileage too Soon.

Unless you run more than 60 miles per week, you should avoid reducing your mileage until three weeks before your marathon. Reduce training volume too early and the size of your mitochondria, your blood volume and your muscle enzyme activity will decrease...compromising your marathon race. Don't lose months of strength and endurance training or de-train by cutting your running back too early.

You've rested every 4 to 5 weeks for a practice race, so your body should have had 12 chances to adapt to your training this year. For the marathon you'll rest enough to allow your body to completely recover and to adapt from your months and months of graduated training.

Add an edge with Differentials.

If you're staying in this section for more than 6 weeks, you could try a new session. The differential splits an interval into two parts. Run the first part at 10K pace to take the stuffing out of your legs: Then, accelerate pace by three seconds per 400 meters to about 5K race pace. For example:

4 x 1,600 in 6 minutes with a one lap jog could change to 2 laps at 90 seconds, and the last two laps at 87 seconds; take a 2 lap jog between reps. The final time of 5:54 will boost your confidence, while also boosting your VO2 maximum.

Predicting marathon times.

A strange thing happens to half marathon runners moving up to the marathon. Tables of actual performances show people slowing much more than you'd expect them to slow down. This is due to the high number of under trained runners.

Run 60 to 70 minutes for the half, and you can double your personal record for the half marathon and add eight to ten minutes to predict your marathon time. The 70 minute half marathon runner is at 5.20 per mile. The extra ten minutes allow him to slow down by 23 seconds per mile to achieve the rather nice two and a half hour marathon. If we give this runner a slightly more generous one-twelfth of his running pace at the half-marathon, which happens to be 5 seconds per mile of his half marathon pace, he or she should slow by:

5 minutes and 20 seconds per mile is actually 5.33 minutes (20/60 = 0.33)

5.33 minutes x 5 seconds, which is: 27 seconds per mile to give a 5.47 per mile marathon. Total time 2:31:31.

This is a slightly weaker goal. It is imminently achievable by all 70 minute half marathon runners who do sufficient mileage and a sufficient number of appropriate paced sessions of speed running.

For every minute per mile which you run the half-marathon at, you should slow by only five seconds per mile for the full marathon. That is, your running speed should slow by about one twelfth or 8.34 percent.

Of course, many minimal mileage people come on-line beyond a 75 minute half, which stretches the amount which the average person does slow by. The 80 minute 'half' person typically needs an extra 20 minutes; the 90 minute halfers' need an extra half an hour. These numbers are out of context to the percentage you'd expect them to slow down.

Just because the average person slows this much, doesn't mean you need too. Gear your mileage up, so you only slow down by one twelfth of your half marathon pace at the full distance. The keys of course are your two long runs most weeks, which will help you to achieve the 1/12th goal. But gear your quality mileage up also. Anaerobic threshold and 5K to 10K pace running will work your body systems while making you an efficient runner.

The 80 minute half marathon person runs 6:06 miles; he or she should slow by 5 secs x 6.1 minutes, or say 31 seconds per mile. Pace will be 6:37 per mile, which is a 2:51:45 marathon, or 8 minutes faster than the average person according to most published tables.

The 90 minute half-marathon runner is doing 6:51 per mile or 6.87 minutes. The average marathon performance of that runner is a convenient three and a half hours. If training diligently, he or she should actually slow by:

6.87 x 5 seconds = 34 seconds per mile

6:51 + 34 = 7:25 per mile and gives a 3:14:19 marathon, or over 15 minutes faster than the average person.

As I've suggested before, most runners should do several half-marathons prior to a marathon. If raced well, half-marathons form the basis for a fast marathon. Four to 8 weeks before your goal marathon, rest up to race a half.

You should also practice half marathon pace and anaerobic threshold running routinely in all phases of training. Do long fartlek in Phase One and formal threshold training later on, including 5 to 6 mile runs at half marathon pace and long repeats with minimal rest periods as shown in Chapter Five.

Several years ago, Runner's World printed a formula for predicting marathon times based on short races. Including:

Best current half marathon x 2.078 = Marathon time

80   x   2.078   = 166.24 minutes or 2:46:15

90   x   2.078   = 187.02 minutes or 3:07

I think these are unrealistic marathon goals and set you up to fail. An 80 minute half marathon runner has only six and a quarter minutes to play with, or about 15 seconds per mile slower than half marathon pace. Most 100 miles per week, 61 minute half marathon runners cannot achieve this goal.

Replace 2.078 with 2.15 and the 90 minute "half" runner gets a goal of 193.5 minutes, 3:13:30, which is 31 seconds per mile slower than half marathon pace. That is slightly more demanding than my 5 second per minute or one twelfth rule, but more realistic than a 3:07 marathon target.

The 2.078 goal may be realistic if you've only done half marathons as harsh training runs, have minimal racing experience, and did minimal speed running. Own those three short-comings and your half marathon PR could be weak. However, if you've raced to your potential at the shorter distances, try your first couple of marathons at the 5 percent slowing rule or by using 2.15 as your multiplier.

Other marathon predictions are based on shorter distance personal records, but will be unreliable if you avoid the long runs. Got a great personal best at the 10K and doing balanced marathon training? Manfred Steffny's "10K time multiplied by 4.66" may work for you. A 40 minute 10K runner (6:27 per mile) gets 186.4 minutes or a target of 3:06:24, which is 7:07 per mile. You'll slow down by 40 seconds per mile. A 50 minute 10K person is predicted to slow by 52 seconds per mile.

Road Racing and Training Magazine shows a nice formula by Paul Slovic which actually takes into account your recent training. Marathon time (M) should equal:
$$M = (T \times 2.98) + 46.6 - (W \times 0.04) - (L \times 1.3)$$
T is your best 10 mile race (to which I would add in the last 6 months and when you're fit).
W is your total mileage for the 8 weeks leading into the marathon.
L is the longest run in those 8 weeks.
The 40 miles per week, moderately intense runner in Chapter Eleven, with a gradual 4 week taper does 284 miles in the last 8 weeks and has a long run of 22 miles. A 65 minute 10 miler gets: $M = (65 \times 2.98) + 46.6 - (284 \times 0.04) - (22 \times 1.3)$
$M = 193.7 + 46.6 - (11.36 \text{ and } 28.6)$
$M = 193.7 + 46.6 - 39.96$
$M = 193.7 + 6.64$
$M = 200.34$ or a 3:20 marathon which is 7:39 per mile. Pretty weak if you can run 6:30 pace for 10 miles.

The only change using this formula for the 50 miles per week people in Chapter Fourteen is the number of miles in the last 8 weeks, which total about 370. Therefore:
$M = (65 \times 2.98) + 46.6 - (370 \times 0.04) - (22 \times 1.3)$
$M = 193.7 + 46.6 - (14.8 \text{ and } 28.6)$
$M = 196.9$ or about 3 minutes faster with the extra 10 miles per week.

60 miles per week people run about 424 miles and get a target of 194.74 minutes. Lest you've missed the point, because you're stronger, Slovic should give you a faster

marathon than the person who does 40 miles per week and is usually at your shoulder in a 10 mile race.

The fun part of this formula is that you can manipulate your training to sabotage your marathon. If you run 30 miles, two weeks before the marathon, the last section will be 30 x 1.3 for a massive 39 instead of 28.4, or over 10 minutes faster, yet your legs will actually be whooped on marathon day, so don't expect to run faster than you would with a 22 being your longest run.

If you don't taper you'll also get a higher number in the end block. 50 mile per week people are down to 25 to 30 total miles in the final week. Stay at 50s for the entire 8 weeks and that section is 400 miles for 400 x 0.04, or a score of 16, suggesting your marathon would be another 1.2 minutes faster. However, you would start the marathon un-rested with fatigue from a 20 mile run 7 days prior and from 5 miles of intervals two days before the race, which is far from the best way to prepare for a marathon.

The formula does not take into account speed running at half marathon to 5K pace or hill repeats which give you a much faster running speed. While your 10 mile time will benefit from speed running, if you fail to run moderately fast for 20 to 25 percent of your mileage during the final 8 weeks of marathon training, you will not stimulate your cardiovascular system and speed endurance, and it will be hard to run at relatively close to 10 mile race pace.

While the 2.98 and 46.6 are relevant numbers for many people, lets play with the following eight adjustments to Slovic's formula.

1. Use the total mileage in the 16 weeks before the final two weeks and multiply by 0.02 instead of 0.04. This allows a decent taper to half of your mileage in the last week, and takes into account your mileage 4 months pre-marathon, by which time you should have reached your peak mileage.

2. It would be tempting to give a 2 to 5 minute faster marathon to those who taper by 40 percent of their mileage.

However, this has already been taken into account with item one. Do add 2 minutes to your marathon if you don't decrease your mileage by 25 percent in the penultimate week. Add another 2 minutes if not decreasing all sessions by 40 percent in the final 7 days.

3. Use the *average* length of your 6 longest runs in the 16 weeks pre-taper x 1.4. No long runs in the last 20 days will be counted as one of the 6 longest for this calculation. Add two minutes to your marathon time if you run more than a 20 miler in the last 20 days. Add another minute to your marathon time if you run more than an 18 miler in the last 13 days. Add an additional two minutes to your marathon time if you raced a marathon in the last 20 weeks: it will not count as one of your long runs either.

4. Do at least 80 percent of each long run at one minute per mile slower than marathon pace? Decrease your marathon time by one minute because you've saved your legs for quality running. Run a couple miles at close to marathon pace during long runs? Take another 10 seconds off of your marathon for each of the first 6 sessions.

5. Run 10 percent of your weekly mileage at anaerobic threshold pace? If you do this session, your 10 mile time should be a fair reflection of your aerobic fitness. However, you can still take 0.1 minute off of your marathon time for each of the first 10 sessions during the 20 weeks pre-marathon. Add back one minute for any full session you do in the last 14 days, but take off another 0.2 minutes if you do close to half of your normal session in the last 14 days.

6. Done 10 minutes of hill repeats or hilly fartlek at 5K intensity in the 5 months pre-marathon? Claim another 0.1 minute off your marathon for each of the first 12 sessions.

7. Done 10 percent of your weekly mileage in one session of short reps at 5K to 2-mile pace? Claim 0.05 minutes for up to 6 sessions in the last 20 weeks. Done 8 percent of weekly mileage in one session of long reps at 5K to 10K paces? Claim 0.15 minutes for up to 8 sessions in the last 20 weeks.

8. Run a half marathon in the 6 months before your marathon? Take one minute off your marathon target time. Raced at 10K or 10 miles? Claim another half a minute for each of the first three. Add back one minute to your marathon for each race more than 5 in the 5 months at 10K to 20 miles pre-marathon. Raced more than 4 times at 5K in the 5 months pre-marathon? Add back one minute per additional 5K race.

Using the 40 miles per week, moderate intensity schedule (page 255) we'll get the following scores and bonuses.
1. Week 44 is the beginning of the taper but only by a couple of miles. Week 40 was a minimal resting up for a 10K also, so the 16 weeks gives about 628 miles instead of the maximum 640 which could be claimed. This section is 628 x 0.02 for 16.56. The original version was 11.36 so our bonus is 5.20 minutes faster for the marathon due to 16 weeks of decent mileage, and factoring out the taper.
2. No faux pas for us. We've rested up nicely.
3. There are 4 runs of 20 miles, one of 22 and the 18 in week 42 will give an average of 20 miles for the six longest. 20 x 1.4 gives 28, which is point six of a minute worse than basing the calculation on the single longest run of 22. Those of you who rotate 18, 20 and 22s during Phase Four would score an average of 21.34 miles for your six longest runs, which gives 29.9 minutes for this section, or 1.3 minutes faster than the one run of 22 calculation. See how easy it is to manipulate a faster goal time?
4. Of course you ran at the right pace, which is 60 to 70 percent of your maximum heartrate. You also did a pair of miles at marathon pace in your 12s and 15s (9 times in the last 20 weeks, but only the first 6 count, though actually it's the last six times you do this session which are most important). Score 2 minutes off your marathon time.
5. You qualify with only 7 sessions in 20 weeks because half of the threshold section was more than 20 weeks ago.

Score 0.7 minutes, plus an additional 0.2 minutes for the half
session in week 46 to make 0.9 minutes off of your time.

    6. You've got exactly 12 sessions, so score the maximum
of 1.2 minutes off your marathon.

    7. You have 14 VO2 interval sessions, and if you're here
for the second time, at least 5 of them should be long repeats.
Take 6 x 0.05 plus 5 x 0.15 for a score of 1.05 minutes.

    8. Oops. Your author only scheduled three races for you
to score 1.5 minutes. The author does expect you to race an
additional two or three times at the 5K though, which gives
one race per month from week 20. Most of you will race a
few times in the first 20 weeks for social reasons, and place
the hill session midweek. You make no time gains for your
marathon goal with 5K races late in the program because they
replace Interval sessions.

What is the marathon goal time for a 65 minute 10 mile racer
using the above adaptations?

Pure Slovic at 40 miles per week:		200.34
1. Mileage bonus (minutes)	5.20	
2. Resting up. No bonus, no foul	0	
3. Long runs (penalty)	(0.6)	
4. Correct speed & mile reps	2.0	
5. Anaerobic threshold sessions	0.9	
6. Hill repeats	1.2	
7. Intervals at 5K to 10K pace	1.05	
8. Races	1.5	
	<u>11.05</u>	
	189.29 minutes	

This is a 3:09:18 marathon at 7:13 per mile, allowing the
person a 43 second per mile differential compared to a 10
mile race. Note that Steffny's 4.66 x 10K pace was only a 40
seconds per mile slowdown...compared to 10K racing speed.

    You can use the 8 above adjustments for any of the
marathon prediction formulae and adjust them to your needs.
The longer the race for your starting point, the more accurate

your goal will be, especially if you're on modest mileage. The 80 miles per week 35 minute 10K runner can probably use the 10K as a starting point with few fears. The 40 miles per week runner should probably rely on the half marathon to find his or her target at the marathon.

Page 381 gives 5 common goal times with speeds at which to run your marathon. Work out your own goals using several formulae, based on your actual PRs instead of using the one closest to yours in a table.

While a half marathon race would be nice preparation about 8 to 12 weeks before your marathon, if you happen to have a half-marathon in your home town two weeks before your marathon, you can still take part. Simply use it as a hard training run with the last 8 miles at marathon pace and you've given yourself a dress rehearsal for marathon day. Include a 3 mile warm up and a 2 mile cooldown and you've got the 18 miles which are ideal two weeks pre-race.

Your last 5 Weeks & Pre-Marathon Race.

Five weeks pre-marathon, do your longest run, about 2 miles more than usual...a 22 is ideal. After two easy days, run a pleasant fartlek session at a range of intensities. Three easy days later, on legs which still feel some of the fatigue from the 22, race a half-marathon.

As you've already got an excellent personal record at this distance, do not try for a PR. You need to save something for your marathon. Run the first five to seven miles at 10 seconds per mile slower than PR pace for the half-marathon: You will still be running about 5-10 seconds faster than marathon pace! For the remainder of the race, run closer to your half marathon PR pace while passing many runners. With a three mile warmup and cooldown, you'll get a 19 mile session.

Three to four days later you should be able to run 5K pace for your short intervals. No heroics now. Two mile pace would be too demanding and counter productive. Besides, at

234 Best Marathons by David Holt

the weekend you will run long reps at 10K pace. It will be your big session. After 4 miles of 10K pace repeats at the weekend, sneak in a few 400s at 5K pace, but only for 20 percent of the total intervals.

Two weeks before your marathon do a 10K race, but please, no PR aspirations. Most of the 13 days leading into your marathon, that is, after your 10K race, will be easy runs of three to four miles...provided it's half or less of your normal day. The 40 mile a week person will only run on half of these rest days.

You'll do a nice speed session the weekend before the marathon, but the remaining six days will be restive. The closest thing to a challenge will be restraining yourself to 15K pace for 2 times one mile on marathon day minus three.

The last couple of weeks are simple: Run enough quality miles to stay fast, with sufficient mileage to maintain strength, while getting the rest that is essential to freshen up your muscles. The rest allows your muscles to make their final adaptation to all of your training. In the last week, your muscles also get charged up with glycogen and fatty acids for your race.

The last 36 days to your marathon Race.

Day 36...Speed session: long reps at 15K pace, save a bit for:

Day 35...Longest run in buildup, about 22 miles but slowly. You do not need to rest up for this run. You'll do your usual 4 to 6 miles of quality running a mere 24 hours before.

Day 34   Recovery run or cross train.

33   a nice 7 to 8 mile run at easy to steady pace.

32   Fartlek - including a few hill strides, long efforts at 15K pace and short efforts at 5K pace. Four miles at speed.

31   7 to 8 mile run at easy to steady pace.

30   Easy 4-5 miles to give you a 50 mile week.

Day 29   Half-marathon race. Pace it per page 233.

28   easy run

27   easy run or cross train

26   Tues: 6 x 400; 10 x 300; 6 x 400 relax at 5K pace.

Fail to restrain yourself in the half-marathon, and you'll fail to achieve this crucial economic running practice at close to VO2 maximum with fatigued legs from the weekend.

25 & 24   Short easy runs

23   Friday: 2 x one mile at 10K pace, then

    3 x 600 at 5K pace, then

    2 x one mile at 10K pace.

See Day 26 comment. Cruise and relax through these interval sessions. You've probably run these reps faster while training for 10Ks. Practice restraint at speed on a Friday.

22   easy 5 miles or cross train.

Day 21   18-20 miles – A rare treat because you'll have a rest day between speed and the long run, so if this feels like agony, you're running it too fast.

20   3 miles at anaerobic threshold. Relaxed cruising on tired legs from yesterday.

19   Short easy run.

18   4 to 5 miles of fartlek

17 & 16   short easy runs

15   10K to 10 mile race. Run about 10 seconds per mile slower than PR pace for at least the first half of the race.

Day 14   Easy five miles.

13   easy run or cross train

12   The last long run. As 1972 Olympic Gold Medalist Frank Shorter has said, training in the last two weeks will not help you in your marathon race. You are now beginning to rest up more significantly. Run 15 to 18 miles with 2 to 3 miles at marathon pace starting at mile 12. I know it's the middle of the work week for most readers, but take a half day off from work to easily fit in this crucial run. The alternative is to add a 7 mile warm up for your 10 mile race on Day 15. Or worse yet, run long the day after your long race. Heed Rob

236 Best Marathons by David Holt

de Castella's advice and "roll through" this run. Save the real racing for your marathon.

11   easy run

10   Include 15 to 20 times a relaxed 100 meters or very short session of fartlek running.

9   easy run

8   Long reps at 10K pace, plus shorter ones at 5K pace. Three times one mile and two times 800 meters work well. 2K, 4 x 600, 2K is just as good. Stay relaxed. Do one to two miles less than usual.

Day 7   10 miles easy.

6   easy run or rest (and rest in all spheres of your life)

5   Include 10 striders of 100 meters at 5K pace

4   easy 4 mile run or rest

3   Two times one mile at 15K to half-marathon pace

2   easy 2 mile run

1   Rest

Zero hour: Marathon race. Start at an easy pace. As Boston Billy (Bill) Rogers said. The first few miles are vital. Run too hard and you'll slow. Run even pace and stay hydrated. The slower pace will allow you to burn more fatty acids, thus preserving much of your glycogen for later.

Bill Rogers won the Boston and New York marathons 4 times. Years of long runs combined with track sessions such as quarter miles at 30 to 40 seconds per mile faster than marathon pace, and sometimes at 2 mile race pace, plus mile repeats at only 15 seconds per mile faster than marathon pace prepared him for the marathon.

Check your pace judgment and running form during the short speed sessions of the last few weeks. Your goal is to improve fitness by resting your muscles. Training hard here will not help you in this marathon.

Running your perfect marathon requires practice with short races, the use of all the types of training outlined in prior chapters, plus rest.

Peaking is best done with a combination of reduced overall mileage, while maintaining the key long run, and a graduated reduction in the amount of speed running.

Reduce mileage by 15 to 20 percent for three to four weeks, finishing with about 40 percent of your regular miles. An 80 mile a week person could run 65, 55 and 40.

Your muscles took months to adapt to marathon training: They'll need a month to fully utilize the rest during this peaking phase. You are learning how to relax at 10K to marathon pace.

Marathon: Running or Racing.

To run an enjoyable marathon you need great aerobic base. You need regular long runs and lots of 40 to 60 minute runs each week, and two gentle sessions at speed to build aerobic base and running economy.

To run faster marathons you need the strength and endurance from resistance training and threshold pace running to push your anaerobic threshold back, allowing you to run faster before reaching the oxygen debt which forces you to slow down.

To race a marathon you also need to run pure speedwork at 10,000 meter to 2 mile race pace. You need just as much speed and VO2 max stimulation and economical running practice as an Olympic 5,000 meter runner.

Marathon runners are not born. Nor are pronghorns born able to run at 60 miles per hour. In the first year of their life they hide from predators while gaining strength. Then their well trained large hearts, plus their naturally big windpipes allow them to race away from predators. Stay away from the marathon for the first few years of your running; train diligently and you'll avoid the pains and pitfalls of the novice marathoner.

While there's no single session to take your marathon record down, resting up, combined with the speed sessions in this and prior chapters should help you to race faster.

While resting, don't make these mistakes.

Don't spend hours walking round the exposition, or standing around at the pasta party.

<u>Don't sneak in a hard workout</u> because you're feeling fresh. You're supposed be running half of your normal speed session, and your legs should feel rested. You could easily run that last session of mile repeats 8 days pre-marathon, at 5K pace or faster, but it will make your muscles sore if done too close to your race. The final week, cruise the miles at threshold pace for relaxation and pace judgment. It's supposed to be a restive training run. Keep it restive, not cardiac arrestive. Warmdown properly, including a quarter mile of walking afterwards.

<u>Do research the race course.</u> Watch a video of the previous years race, and ensure that the course is the same. Review the course map with elevation changes. Drive the course. If you live within two hours of the course, take a field trip about 3 to 5 weeks pre-marathon and run the last 16 miles of the course, including the last 10 miles at close to marathon pace. Or practice on similar terrain closer to home.

<u>Get to the race on time</u>. Make travel plans well in advance and allow extra hours for the journey and for picking up race numbers (usually the day before the race). This saves your adrenaline for race day as you leisurely walk from the hotel to the start, (with a few pints of liquid to consume while you wait) or find your parking space after a short drive. Then void your reservoirs of excess content and find a quite place.

<u>Don't Change Eating Habits.</u> In the last 3 weeks you do not need extra protein to repair your muscles because you already get close to 100 grams in your western diet, which is way too much anyway. You do not need extra fat either, for a

back-up energy source as one magazine called it, because you already have enough fat for several marathons. But you do need to decrease your total calorie intake the last 3 weeks as you burn less energy with training. Keep the fruits and veggies for vitamins and antioxidants. The last 3 days will be mainly complex carbohydrates.

Include salt to help your body retain liquid and to keep your sodium levels up. A breakfast of oatmeal, whole wheat toast and banana or orange should ensure a bowel movement before the race starts. Use the same combination of food as before your 20 mile runs in training.

<u>Don't warm up very much.</u> A 5K race needs a two to three mile warm up. Unless all your miles will be under 6 minutes, a marathoner needs minimal running as warm up: probably less than half a mile, plus a bit of walking and 10 to 15 minutes of gentle stretching while staying warm. The last part of the warm up is getting to your start position, which at major events means walking.

Don't stand around. Do sit or lie down and relax.

While a long running warm up does decrease lactic acid build up, it's negated if you stand around for longer than a few minutes at the start. Avoid lactic acid build up by running the first mile ten seconds slower than your expected average race pace. Run the second mile at the same pace! Then gradually increase to your goal pace, but don't try to catch up your 20 second deficit. It's the best deficit you ever achieved.

The adrenaline surge at the start with thousands of runners and your rested legs are a disaster waiting to happen. Fast starts lead to painful finishes. Your practice races should have taught you self-control, but you still may feel as if you are running 7 minute miles, but actually be running at 6.30 pace. Run the first mile at 7.30 effort and see where you stand. Hopefully, you're now perfectly warmed up and will gradually ease up toward race pace.

<u>The marathon is not 26.2 miles,</u> it's four five mile tempo runs, with each 5 miles a bit faster than the previous 5.

You complete the day with a 10K...with a 5 second per mile cushion compared to the pace of your fastest 5 miles that morning. Note: The tempo pace on marathon day is 20 to 30 seconds per mile slower than your tempo training runs.

Got a studly 3 hour time target for a 6:52 per mile average? Run each 5 miles in 34:30, 34:15, 34, and 33:45 minutes. This gives you a 6.50 average pace so far, and a glorious 43:30 to run the last 10K, or 7 minute miles. Maintain the 6:45 pace from your 33:45 fourth 5 miles and you'll be one and a half minutes under three hours! Prefer two 10 milers followed by a 10K, go ahead.

Whichever way you break down the race, you should not be hurting at half way. You're cruising slower than in threshold sessions and you've rested up by tapering for 2 to 3 weeks. Save your mental and physical energy for the grafting which takes place in the last 10K of the marathon.

Feel so good in the first five miles of the race so that you're tempted to speed up? Don't. Changing your pace plan usually leads to problems. You should be feeling fresh, so conserve energy and enjoy the first half of the race. If you still feel great at 22 miles, you can finish at 6:40 pace. If you want to walk like a cripple afterwards, try 6:30 pace.

<u>Try nothing new on race weekend,</u> unless you've tested it (which means it's no longer new). Leave it at home, in the store, or on the roadside. No new socks or other clothing, shoes, food or drink. Been saving that 6th pair of lightweight trainers you bought two years ago? Had 500 miles from each of the first 5 pairs, including two speed sessions a week? You still need two or three speed sessions and a long run in your last pair before you race in them.

<u>Don't over or under dress.</u> Experience counts. Singlet or wicking shirt? Long sleeves, or even long johns (running tights of course)? The best running performances usually come at 40 to 50 Fahrenheit, windless and with slight cloud cover...while wearing singlet and shorts and pacing the race perfectly. You can easily discard a hat or gloves.

Windy, cold days will mean more clothing is needed. Wind on a hot day means you may be able to race faster than your adjusted time target based on temperature alone!

Be realistic in the heat. Fit and full of fluid? Paced the first 5 miles perfectly? Used to training in the heat. Maybe you'll race very close to your best on hot days? Maybe you'll wilt a bit less than most. Most runners will slow by 10 to 30 seconds per mile in hot or humid conditions. Get both, and you should run the first half at more modest pace.

Based on Jack Daniels' table on page 191 of his *Running Formula*, you should expect to slow down by about 1.5 percent for each 10 degree F increase in temp. Boston 85 instead of 55, (which it was in 2,004): The 3 hour marathon runner should start out at (180 x 3) 1.5 % or 31 seconds per mile slower. The new goal is 3:08:06.

The more conservative you are in the first 5 miles, the more likely you are to have a pleasant marathon experience.

Dictate your own pace. Take charge of your race. If you are running even pace (after that slightly slower first mile), by the third mile you'll have steady company. If you're straining to stay with a group of runners, or the group is running 5 seconds per mile faster than your pace plan (which should still feel easy because it's slower than half-marathon pace) *you have to let the group go*. Some of them will come back to you. There are other runners behind you wanting to keep you company, or wanting to stay 10 meters behind you.

Running in a group can waste your energy. So:
* Minimize the talking. Just enough to help you relax through those first 10 to 15 miles.
* Make no sudden changes in pace or running line.
* But, run the most direct route possible without stepping in front of others. Run close to the left curb on left turns.
* Run behind the person whose form and stride length is closest to yours. It will help you to relax.

* If the wind is from the front and left, your place is toward the back and the right of your group. Cruise slightly less to the right when running sweeping left turns. Wind from behind? Have a rest at the back and get pushed along.
* Run to the side if it's more relaxing, but don't get too close to them. They may change direction suddenly.
* Prepare for water stations by moving to the appropriate side of the road. Back off on pace to make an extra foot or two of space to ensure the cup holder can see you, or to get a clean grab line at the table.

Group running can give you 6.50 pace at 7.00 minute effort. It can also give you 6.40 effort at 6.50 pace if you:

* Talk excessively or constantly lead the group;
* Change pace frequently;
* Race to catch up after liquid stops;
* Use different running form to what you've practiced.

When running in a group, you still have to run your own race.

Changing pace by a few seconds per mile can alleviate stiffness from running mile after mile on a flat course.

Keeping the group together is the main goal at the marathon. No surges. Don't accelerate through corners to try and get a 3 meter gap, but do run with an economic cadence at all times.

<u>Drink liquids with energy in it.</u> Four 8 ounce cups of sports drink per hour will give you the 200 calories per hour which can improve your marathon. Prefer apple juice? At 15 calories per ounce you only need 13 ounces per hour for 200 calories. You'll need water too of course. One third strength juices are excellent rehydraters.

Drink before you feel the need to drink. Your thirst center is a sloth, and will not tell you that your body has turned into a dry sponge until it's too late. Drink before you are thirsty, at the early liquid stations, but don't overhydrate. Of course, drinking during the marathon is almost pointless if you started off dehydrated! Drink 2 pints or more two hours pre-race and continue with liquids which have up to 5 percent sugar right up to the start time. Including a little salt in your liquids improves your fluid retention. Coffee or tea is fine before any run because its diuretic signal is switched off once you begin exercising. Use non-fat milk of course, and see Chapter Two.

<u>Dropping out is always an option.</u> Target pace of 8 minute miles maintained until 16 miles, but slowed to 8:45 pace by mile 19. Clearly you're hurting, and the remaining 7 miles will be purgatory, while putting you at risk for physical and mental trauma, further dehydration or exposure depending upon what caused your slowing. Tough runners will drop out at the 20 mile point after running easily to that point for the psychological boost. If a sag wagon or ride is available earlier, take it. Only mad dogs, authors and Englishmen would continue or walk the rest of the course. Drop out, then after a restive break of a few weeks on minimal mileage, plan on several 10Ks and a half-marathon and a more realistic marathon time goal in 6 months.

What to do after crossing the Finish Line

Stay on your feet and shuffle through to liquids and a few simple sugars, warm cloths if appropriate, walk another couple of hundred yards to decrease stiffness, to keep your muscles pumping the blood back to your heart and brain to avoid collapse and then pick up enough calories and liquid for your first significant snack.

Lie down to eat your snack, but expect to need help getting up afterwards. More liquids and electrolytes and a slow walk and shower should precede a balanced meal.

Over the next few days, don't overdo the stretching because your muscle fibers are fatigued and can easily tear. Many people get a cold or other infection just after the marathon, perhaps secondary to shaking so many hands on race day. Overtraining, which running a marathon qualifies as, decreases immune function, making you more susceptible to infections. It will not affect your training because you're not doing any, but continue to consume a healthful diet with plenty of antioxidants from fruit and vegetables.

Make plans for after your marathon.

You enjoyed numerous races leading up to your marathon, so place a low key 5K race in your diary for 5 to 6 weeks after the marathon to keep you motivated, healthy and happy.

* Motivated because after virtually zero running for the first week after the marathon, and another week without fast running, in the third week you can begin striders and very gentle fartlek sessions twice a week for the remaining 3 to 4 weeks leading into your 5K.

* Healthy because you only need to run 5 miles three or four days per week, and ten miles once a week to stay fit for your post marathon 5K.

* Happy because you can still run with your buddies, and you know that a few days after your 5K you can begin hill repeats, or anaerobic threshold running or interval training again to prepare for a race at 10K or your next marathon.

* Setting an enjoyable goal for a few weeks after your marathon decreases the post marathon blues which people who only train for one race suffer from. Plan on racing for a lifetime, and you'll defeat the post marathon depression.

How often should you race a marathon?

Twice a year is plenty. There are so many other races to do, and great cities with 10 mile races or half marathons, you shouldn't even consider more than two marathons. You can give yourself a nice 15 to 18 week buildup for each marathon while racing shorter distances every 3 to 5 weeks. You'll have over 20 weeks per year to play at the 5K to 10K or a chance to take those distances seriously.

Many of you will need a year or more to prepare for your first marathon. Provided you stay in shape while racing 10K to the half-marathon once a month, subsequent marathons will only need a 12 to 20 week buildup.

Chapter Eleven

17 to 46 week Training schedules for 40 miles per week runners.

Putting Chapters One to Ten into practice.

The next few pages are a summary of the types of training you'll need to run a great marathon. Get marathon ready in 17 weeks to 46 weeks (see the box on page 255) depending upon your experience. First time marathon runners will probably use the one speed session per week schedule. Most printed marathon training programs would get you to the marathon in 12 weeks to four months, and give you perhaps two 16 mile runs and one 18 mile run for your longest runs. They would give zero speed running despite the fact that low mileage and beginners reap the *greatest* benefits from running at speed.

The 4 month program (17 weeks) in this chapter contains 4 runs of 20 miles (in weeks 5, 9, 12 and 14). It also includes races in weeks 6, 10 and 14. You will need to be in pretty good shape at week one to be marathon ready in 17 weeks.

Setting up for your first marathon? In this schedule, you need to arrive as 40 mile per week runners, and first time marathoners will not even enter phase two with its hill training until they can handle eighteen mile runs alternating with a 14 mile run on the easy weekends. You will then complete a 20 mile run every third weekend as you work through hill training, anaerobic threshold at 15K pace and interval training at 5K pace for 6 to 10 weeks each. You'll accumulate 6 to 9 runs at 20 miles, plus a 22 mile run. You'll peak for the marathon by tapering over a 6 week period.

If you're running less than 40 miles per week, use Chapter Three's program to reach 40s, and then join us at your leisure.

Seventeen weeks, or 46 weeks, or anything in between? The choice is yours based on your experience and how many weak areas you have. 46 weeks seem like a lifetime? You work 40 years for your pension. You should be running after you retire. Get used to 10K and half-marathon races before you run a marathon.

People already running fairly fast two or three times per week will need much less than 46 weeks because they will come in with a greater foundation or base.

Phase One: Base Mileage.

Your true base will have been achieved with the three years or more which you ran while racing at 5K to the half-marathon and the 20 miles. The big question is, how long should your long run be when cruising through the fourth year of marathon training while running 40 miles per week?

The 40 percent rule for your longest run only gives you a 16 miler, not really enough for the marathon! At 40 miles per week, you'll need to run half of your weekly mileage in one run, once every 2 or 3 weeks. Run at only 60 percent of your maximum heartrate, or these runs will be too grueling.

This leaves you 20 to 24 miles which you can split between 3 additional runs. Fewer, but longer runs give you more endurance than many short runs. At least one run should be 4 miles of fartlek as described in Chapter Three.

Very experienced runners may need only 1 week in this fartlek phase, and be ready for a marathon in 17 weeks. If you're entering Year Four of marathon training (after a year each focusing on the 5K, 10K and half marathon) for the first time, you may need 4 to 6 weeks here while getting used to 20 miles on alternate weeks. Those of you coming in from recreational running will need at least 10 to 16 weeks of fartlek, and eventually hilly fartlek sessions while building toward 17 mile runs, before moving to Phase Two where you'll edge up to 20s; you'll take 50 to 60 weeks to be marathon ready. You will all rest up once every 3 to 4 weeks to race at 5K to the half-marathon, thus maintaining variety.

Phase Two: Hills and Strength.

The number of hill repeats or speed training days dictate how seriously you take your marathon running, or how rapidly your body recovers from training to allow you to run hard again.

Serious runners run fast once a week to enhance running form and stimulate oxygen uptake systems as described in prior chapters. They can alternate hill repeats with their fartlek session each week, giving one hill session every two weeks or once every 8 runs. As you may recall from Chapter Three, beginners can actually include hill repeats from week one of marathon training. Start with two repeats of 60 to 90 seconds at 5K intensity up a 3 percent grade. Add one repeat every 2 to 4 weeks while also searching for slightly steeper hills and you'll get an entire year of progression.

Moderately intense runners enjoy two speed sessions per week. You'll get one session each of hills and fartlek every week.

The highest intensity runners will train fast three times a week, and add the hill session every week to their two fartlek sessions.

All of you should take care of your Achilles during hill training, and alternate long repeats one week with steeper, but shorter hills the next. You've done hills many times before, but you still need to increase the number of repeats sensibly, and run no faster than 2 mile race effort. No collapsing at the top of each repeat!

The long runs remain the cornerstone of your aerobic endurance and teach or perhaps force you to run economically for mile after mile. You'll include one or two times a mile repeat at marathon pace about four miles from the end of long runs. Strength training should be progressing nicely on two of those non-running days.

Provided you've been here before, and routinely run hills at all stages of your training, 4 weeks should suffice to achieve the 17 week marathon plan. Achieving the full rewards from hill training and mileage can take half a year of regular hill repeats! Ten weeks, with 10 hill sessions should give you 90 percent of this years potential.

Phase Three: Anaerobic Threshold Running.

15K pace running is another key to your marathon strength endurance. 15K pace is easier to run than 10K pace, yet it's more beneficial because:

* It stimulates your anaerobic threshold to rise, allowing you to maintain high race paces for longer. Forces you:
* To run economically and concentrate on running form.
* Leaves your legs rested for other speed training.

The serious marathon trainer who runs fast once a week will replace the hills or fartlek with one quality threshold pace session per week for 6 weeks. Or they could alternate a hilly fartlek session with threshold pace for 8 to 10 weeks.

Our moderately intense hero who runs fast twice a week will alternate fartlek with hills on Day Four, and run threshold pace on Day One.

Our highest intensity heroines will run one session every week of fartlek, hills and threshold pace while maintaining the ever present long run.

For all of you, injury prevention guidelines allow 10 percent of your mileage to be 15K pace, or four miles. See pages 101 to 120 for numerous options such as 4 x one mile and 2 x two miles. Start at 80 percent of max HR and increase pace to 85 or 90 percent. Start these sessions at half-marathon pace; end up at 15K pace. That's about 30 to 40 seconds per mile faster than projected marathon pace!

No races at 10K or 10 miles locally which fit into your marathon preparation? You can double your anaerobic session once a month instead of racing. Eight times one mile at 10 mile pace with a one minute rest is much easier than a 10 mile race provided you rest up for it. However, most areas have a race at 10K to the half-marathon every 3 to 8 weeks, so enjoy a race every month or so.

Going longer than 6 weeks without a race of more than 5K? Do the big threshold pace session instead of yet another 5K race. It is 20 percent of your weekly mileage, but that's much less than a half-marathon race would be!

Most runners should also run a 5K race once a month for the joy of it, cruising at high speed with no expectation of personal records because you did not rest up for the race.

* Socialization with numerous runners.
* A pleasant break from hill or threshold training sessions.

During your 20 mile runs, increase pace toward 70 percent of maximum HR for the second <u>half</u> of each run.

Phase Four: VO2 Maximum Training.

Two mile race pace, 5K pace and 10K pace training adds power to your legs and improves the amount of oxygen your lungs and heart and other systems can process, and therefore your speed potential.

As always, you have several options.

Serious marathon trainers will replace the threshold pace running, which had been a hill session, which had been a fartlek session, with the VO2 pace Intervals.

The moderately hard trainer can rotate hills, hilly fartlek with threshold running on Day Four, while running a series of VO2 max Intervals on Day One for 6 to 12 weeks.

The highest intensity 40 mile per week person can also do the VO2 sessions on Day One, but will also run two quality sessions on Days 4 and 6 such as:

Week One: Hills followed by threshold.

Week Two: Threshold followed by fartlek.

Week Three: Fartlek followed by hills.

The fourth week's one midweek quality run of hilly fartlek includes a few long reps at threshold pace to rest you up for a long race at the weekend. Don't rest up for 5K races because they substitute for your interval sessions once a month.

Keep doing 6,000 meters of intervals at 5K pace until you have no serious muscle aches afterwards. You'll probably need to run each full session three times for your muscles to fully adapt, and to teach yourself to relax and run economically. The long run is unchanged during Phase Four.

Phase Five: Marathon Peaking.

Rest and longer reps at 2 mile to 10K paces give extra pep to your legs while maximizing your running economy.

The serious trainer replaces the short Intervals with half miles and 1,200 meter repeats at 5K pace and may add 2Ks at 10K race pace. Three sessions of each should suffice.

The moderately intense runner reduces the midweek session of threshold or fartlek to 2.5 to 3 miles of speed running in order to be fresher for the Day One long repeats.

Highest intensity runners can run three miles of short Intervals at 5K pace for relaxation midweek, followed by a shorter session of hills or threshold running 2 days later. These highly experienced runners may run mile repeats at close to 3K race pace on two of the six weekends leading into the marathon; they may also be content with the 800s and 1,200s at 3K pace. 5K pace is fast enough for the marathon, though 2-mile repeats at 10K pace are well worthwhile too.

All of you can reduce the two midweek runs by one mile for the first two weeks, by two miles for the next two weeks, and by three for the penultimate two weeks. This takes your mileage down to 34ish.

Your long runs over the last six weeks will be 15, 18, 22, 15, 18 and then a 12 the weekend before the race. You will have run over a dozen 20s to prepare for that 22. It is four weeks pre-marathon, so you have plenty of time to recover. Your body also has plenty of time to make its physiological adaptations inspired by that run! Don't run the final 12 miler any faster than your usual long run pace: you're supposed to be resting up. Choose a flat course instead of a hilly course.

The last week will include 2 x one mile at half marathon pace. You'll also do a five mile run to give you 22 miles for the week. If preceded by low 30 mile weeks and decreasing length of long runs you'll be nicely rested for the marathon.

Training table abbreviations:

E = Easy runs...at 60-70 percent of maximum heartrate.
F = Fartlek
H = Hill repeats
HF = Hilly fartlek...a bit less vigorous than the hill session.
A = Anaerobic threshold pace running...15K speed.
V = VO2 maximum pace intervals...2 mile to 5K speed.

All types of quality running requires a warm-up and cooldown of two to three miles each side of the speed running. As you will be doing four miles at speed (or 2 miles for hill training), speed days give you 8 miles of running.

The drawback to using training phases is that you can lose the benefit from one type of training while perfecting the next type. Example: no more hills are scheduled after week 19. You can maintain your leg strength and knee lift by doing hilly fartlek, and by running one in three of your threshold sessions up a gentle hill of 2 to 4 percent grade. During the VO2 maximum phase, include a few hilly fartlek sessions with half of it being long efforts at threshold intensity.

<u>Serious Runners</u> move their legs fast once a week, but should also run two times one mile at marathon pace during each 15 mile run. Don't do the long repeats at VO2 maximum or 5K pace the first time through. Instead, spend the six week taper with 600s and 400s, learning the art of fast running while using very little energy. First timers may need more than 10 weeks in Phase One, and combine it with the hill phase just like in Chapter Three. You will of course be cross-training on days 3 and 5 until week 44.

Typically	Day One Sat	Two Sunday	Four Tues	Six Thur
Weeks 1,3,5, 7 & 9	8E	14	8E	4F

On even number weeks add to the long run, aiming for 18 miles by week 10.

	Day One	Two	Four	Six
Weeks 11, 14, 17	8E	15	8E	2H
Weeks 12, 15, 18	8E	17	8E	2H
Weeks 13, 16, 19	7E	20	6E	2HF
Week 20	Race 10K	12	6E	4HF
Weeks 21, 24, 27	8E	15	8E	4HF
Weeks 22, 25, 28	8E	17	7E	4A
Weeks 23, 26, 29	7E	20	6E	4A
Week 30	7E	12	2HF	6E
Week 31	Race 10 miles	8E	10E	4HF
Weeks 32, 35, 38	8E	17	7E	4V
Weeks 33, 36, 39	7E	20	6E	4V
Weeks 34, 37	8E	15	8E	4HF
Week 40	7E	12	2HF	6E

Practice long repeats at 5K to 10K race pace for six weeks.

	Day One	Two	Four	Six
Week 41	Race 10K	15	8E	4V
Week 42	8E	18	7E	4V
Week 43	7E	22	6E	4HF
Week 44	8E	15	7E	4V
Week 45	6E	18	6E	3V
Week 46	4E	12	4E	2A

Then race your marathon.

17 week schedule.

Want a shorter marathon training schedule. Spending 2 to 3 weeks in each phase gets you to the marathon start line in about 4 months. You still get four 20 mile runs with this schedule, plus a 22. You could cruise a half-marathon or 10 mile race instead of the 15 or 17 once or twice during the buildup, but don't do so in the last 4 weeks. Otherwise, stick with 10K races. Note: You are not after personal records during these shorter races.

	Day One *Saturday*	Two *Sun*	Four *Tues*	Six *Thur*
Week 1	8E	14	8E	4F
Week 2	6E	18	6E	4F
Week 3	8E	15	8E	2H
Week 4	7E	20	8E	2H
Week 5	8E	17	3HF	6E
Week 6	Race 10K	15	6E	4HF
Week 7	8E	17	8E	4HF
Week 8	7E	20	7E	4A
Week 9	8E	12	4A	6E
Week 10	Race 10K	15	6E	4HF
Week 11	7E	20	8E	4HF
Week 12	8E	17	8E	4V
Week 13	7E	22	6E	3V
Week 14	Race 10K	12	6E	4HF
Week 15	E8	20	7E	4V
Week 16	7E	18	6E	3V
Week 17	6E	12	5E	3A

And run a very nice marathon.

You'll also cross train twice a week with weights and 30 minutes of aerobic exercise. Cut it by 40 percent for weeks 14 and 15 and do none in the last 2 weeks.

Moderate Intensity Runners move their legs fast
twice a week, and should also run two times one mile at
marathon pace during 15 to 18 mile runs. You can spend the
final 6 weeks running long repeats at close to VO2 maximum
the first time through this schedule. See Chapters 10 & 12. Do
keep speed running relaxed at all times. Stretch, cross train
and weight train to maintain muscle balance.

You're very experienced runners, so you could decrease
the fartlek and anaerobic sections to four and six weeks. The
fartlek section is generally the recovery from your previous
marathon. If so, 12s would be sufficient for your long runs.
You've had at least two weeks of very low mileage after your
marathon before commencing the fartlek phase!

Strength is vital for marathon success. Reducing the hill
phase would be short sighted. Run plenty of hills and
continue to weight train during your VO2 max phases.

Because you run fast twice a week, you'll typically run
quality on Saturday followed by a long run on Sunday.
Consider a slightly shorter session the Saturdays before your
twenty. Run as little as 3 miles at threshold or VO2 max. The
weekends that you run a fifteen, make the speed session the
key session: run closer to five miles at speed. You run 5K to
15K paces to make you efficient at speed. You don't always
have to do 4 miles of repeats.

The occasional heart attack or death during a marathon gets
enormous press coverage. While running 40 to 60 miles per
week does not give you total immunity from cardiac
problems, you are much less likely than our typical citizen to
have, let alone die from heart disease.

Got chest pain during or after the race? Stop and call 911.
Your creatine kinase-MB will be positive after a marathon, so
your cardiologist will have to rely on your cardiac troponins
to diagnose your cardiac muscle damage.

See chapter 2 & 8s hydration tips to decrease your risk.

Two speedy days per week…moderately intense marathon training, at 40 miles per week.

Probably on	Day One Sat	Two Sunday	Four Tues	Six Thur
Weeks 1, 3, 5, 7 & 9	4F	15	4F	8E
Weeks 2, 4, 6, 8 &10	4HF	18	4F	6E
Weeks 11, 14, 17	2H	15	4F	8E
Weeks 12, 15, 18	2H	17	4F	8E
Weeks 13, 16, 19	2H	20	3HF	7E
Week 20	3HF	12	3F	5E
Week 21	Race 10K	12	4F	3HF
Weeks 24, 27	4A	15	4F	8E
Weeks 22, 25, 28	4A	17	2H	7E
Weeks 23, 26, 29	4A	20	3HF	6E
Week 30	4A	12	3HF	5E
Week 31	Race 10 miles	8	3HF	3HF
Weeks 32, 35, 38	3V	17	2H	7E
Weeks 33, 36, 39	4V	20	4A	6E
Weeks 34, 37	4V	15	4HF	8E
Week 40	3V	12	3A	5E
Week 41	Race 10K	14	4HF	8E

Then practice long repeats at 5K to 10K paces for six weeks, but include the 22 mile run half-way through.

Week 42	4V	18	2H	7E
Week 43	3V	22	3HF	6E
Week 44	4V	15	4A	7E
Week 45	4V	18	3HF	6E
Week 46	3V	12	2V	2A

And race your marathon.

The programs in this book are not 46 week programs for a marathon. They are typically 10 week programs for a 10K, then 10 weeks for a 10 mile race, then (e.g. weeks 30 to 46 above) a mere 17 weeks to prepare for your marathon. Plus you can race at 5K in the 5th of each 10 weeks.

Here is your 17 week option.

Repeat any 2 to 3 week phase if it is your weakness, or if you have 20 or 23 weeks before your marathon.

Probably	Sat	Sunday	Tues	Thur
Week 1	4F	15	4F	8E
Week 2	4HF	12	4F	6E
Week 3	2H	15	4F	8E
Week 4	2H	17	4F	8E
Week 5	2H	20	3HF	7E
Week 6	4F	12	3HF	5E
Week 7	Race 10K	15	4F	8E
Week 8	4A	17	2H	7E
Week 9	4A	20	3HF	6E
Week 10	4A	12	3HF	5E
Wk 11	Race 10 miles	8	12E	4HF
Week 12	4V	20	2H	7E
Week 13	4V or 5K	15	4A	6E
Week 14	4V	22	4A	5E
Week 15	Race 10K	15	4HF	8E
Week 16	4V	18	3HF	6E
Week 17	3V	12	2V	2A

Then race your marathon.

Peaking for your race requires a combination of reduced mileage and a reduction of your other training to allow your muscles to adapt from prior weeks training. Usually lift 50 pounds for 16 repeats on 12 different exercise machines? Decrease to 40 pounds for 12 repeats the penultimate two weeks, but continue to put your muscles through their range of motion. Biking 25 miles at 20 miles per hour (75 minutes) slow down and ride for 50 minutes. Do no cross training in the last 10 days prior to your marathon.

Highest Intensity Runners shift rapidly for part of nearly every run and 2 miles at marathon pace is still useful during your 15 to 18 mile runs.

	Probably Day	Sat One	Sunday Three	Tues Five	Thur Seven
Weeks 1 & 3		4F	15	4F	4HF
Weeks 2 & 4		4F	18	4F	4HF
Weeks 5, 8, 11		2H	15	4F	4HF
Weeks 6, 9, 12		2H	17	4F	4HF
Weeks 7, 10, 13		2H	20	3F	4A
Week 14		3HF	12	3A	2F
Week 15		Race 10K	15	4F	2H
Weeks 16 & 19		4A	17	2H	4HF
Weeks 17 & 20		4A	20	3HF	2H
Week 18		4A	18	2H	4A
Week 21		3HF	12	3A	2F
Week 22		Race 10 miles	7E	10E	3HF
Weeks 23 & 26		4V	17	2H	4A
Weeks 24 & 27		3V	20	3HF	4A
Week 25		4V	15	3H	3A
Week 28		3V	12	3A	1F
Week 29		Race 10K	12	3F	4HF
Week 30		4V	15	2H	4V
Week 31		4V	18	2H	4A
Week 32		4V	22	3HF	4A
Week 33		4V	15	4V	1.5H
Week 34		3V	18	3HF	3A
Week 35		3V	12	2V	2A

Race your marathon.

Weeks 30 and 33 have two sessions working on VO2 max. Midweek is usually short repeats at 3K pace. The weekend should be long repeats at 5K to 10K pace. You can shorten the schedule to 17 weeks by doing only three weeks in each phase. You can also increase the average length of your long run by alternating 18s with 20s for most of your build up.

CHAPTER TWELVE

Take it up

ONE MORE NOTCH

Some readers of this book have been waiting 11 chapters to move up to the next level, having experienced several marathons while training with short Intervals at 5K pace and long Intervals at 10K pace. After a couple of marathons you can all graduate to severe intensity marathon training by using a series of long repeats at 5K to 2 mile pace.

Prudent use of the sessions in this chapter will help you to run at a faster even pace and help you to personal records.

Remember from Chapter Six that physiologists agree the percentages at the higher level of VO2 max (100 - 95 %) should be done for 3 to 5 minutes' duration, repeated many times in one session: once you've run several marathons, it will be time to take another look at long VO2 max repeats.

Some of these sessions will improve your sprinting ability by bringing in the last of your fast twitch muscle fibers. The goal, however, is to improve your average marathon pace, not your end sprint. Exceptional sprinters at the end of a marathon probably did not run hard enough in the rest of the race. Don't save much for that last 387 yards.

Many runners slow down in the last 10 miles of the marathon. Chapter Ten showed several ways to predict your marathon time, from which you can compute average pace. We then manipulated some of those predictions to allow for your mileage and quality training. Any runner can sabotage a marathon by starting off too fast, or by running the first 10 miles more than 10 seconds slower than average goal pace.

The sessions in this chapter improve your maximum running capacity and can improve your maximum running speed over two to three miles: You will then run at marathon pace using a lower percentage of your capacity, allowing you to maintain a solid pace to the end.

As you've raced several marathons by now, you should know about even paced racing. You know your split times at key points such as 5 miles, and your running speed to achieve these times during your marathon.

You've developed the patience to cruise easily during the first miles of your marathon on rested muscles. Don't push the pace to get ahead of an even pace schedule. Don't race your companions in the early miles. Help each other to save energy with a steady pace and then speed up gradually by five seconds per mile for the second 13 miles or the last 10 miles.

Run Faster Marathons.

Running longer repeats at 2 mile pace to 5K pace enable you to tolerate higher levels of lactic acid in your body, and make you buffer wastes still better than before your first few marathons. You'll also feel more relaxed at high speed.

1983 Marathon World Championship Gold Medalist and former world record holder Grete Waitz was very keen on long intervals. Two days after her 20 mile run she would typically run 6 x 1,000 meters at close to 3K race pace (2-mile pace), or 5 x one mile with a lap recovery or 5 x 2,000 meters.

Try those three sessions or the two on page 260 to take your marathon training to a new level.

* Five times 1,000 meters at your 2 mile pace with 3 to 4 minutes rest is a good substitute for a 3,000 meter or two mile race: You also get more than 2 miles of training!
* Four times one mile at 5K race pace with similar rest does wonders for those of you who rarely race at 5K.

Both sessions, especially if combined with local low-key 5,000 meter and 10K races are great preparation for faster or for more comfortable marathons. These are the same sessions which you might have been aspiring to do at the end of Chapter Seven. Note that rest periods should gradually be reduced toward one minute for both sessions.

Most runners in the big marathons don't compete in track races. Long repeats at high VO2 maximum effort give middle of the pack marathon runners the same advantages which former track runners have. Top notch marathoners typically run 5,000 meter races, 10K and half-marathons while preparing for marathons, and often designate a 3 to 4 month period each year to work specifically on their 5K running. With the above two sessions, so can you.

You need to commence these sessions about six months prior to your marathon, and maintain a long run on alternate weekends for strength as you perfect your running economy. Pick two 5Ks and a 10K race about three months before your next marathon, and then 6 months before the marathon, use your own variation of these sessions every 7 to 10 days.

* 6 x 800 meters at 3K or 2 mile pace;
* 4 x 1,200 at one second per lap slower than 3K pace;
* 6 x 800 meters at 2 mile pace;
* 4 x one mile at 5K pace;
* 5 x 1,000 meters at 2 mile pace;
* 4 x one mile at 5K pace;
* 5 x 1,200 at one second per lap slower than 3K pace;
* 5 x 1,000 at 2 mile pace;
* Race 5,000 meters, or run 4 x one mile at 5K pace;
* 4 x 1,000 at two mile pace;

* Then: Run 5K to 10K races every other week for about 2 months. Run long repeats on the other weekends.

Progression for 800s. Note the transition from 800s to 1,000s at 2 mile race pace for the fifth session. Running the extra 200 meters is tough, so think about your running form in the second lap and retain energy for the last 200 meters while maintaining even pace. The first time you run at 3K pace you can alternate 1,000s with 800s, or do three reps of 1,000 and finish with two of 800 meters, and then a 400.

Progression for 1,200s. The sessions of 1,200s simply requires an extra repetition; run two 600s in the middle of the session the first time if you feel the need.

Progression for miles or 1,600s. The mile repeats should be your easiest session. You don't have to make any changes except to gradually reduce your rest period, and relax at 5K pace. You could also take the training up a notch by running one second per lap faster than 5K pace.

High mileage runners will usually do more than 4 repeats, and seasoned runners can run 2,000 meters to get even more of the session at 5K heartrate.

Hint: don't run the intervals which you find are the easiest very often because you're already competent at running them. Run the distances and paces which you found most difficult. Work on and teach yourself to run relaxed at your weak spot.

No weak spot? Try one mile at 5K pace; 1,200 meters a bit faster; 1,000 at 2 mile pace; and finish with a mile or 1,600 meters at 5K pace to finish. High mileage people will do a couple more repeats.

Only run these long reps at 5K to 2 mile pace if you've already done the interval training from Chapters 6 and 7. Support each session of long reps with speed sessions of short reps at 2 mile to 5K paces. Run them as hill reps once every three weeks for knee lift and leg strength and to get away from the track. Run at 15K to half-marathon pace too.

Make Three Attempts at each session before progressing further.

According to coach Harry Wilson, "Athletes usually need three attempts at a session before they can progress further. The first is an introduction - the second time is coming to terms - the third time is being in charge of the session...that's the time to move forward."

To restate Chapter 10, "You're not trying to run faster than before - you are trying to match your previous time in a more relaxed way." Feel as if you could run the session faster.

Practice running the second and third session of mile reps with good form: keep the running as effortless as possible. You know that you can run the session because you've done it before, so think about completing the session in comfort.

As Harry Wilson suggests, run three sessions of miles and 1,000s to practice for the short races at 5K and 10K. You can also run the last session of miles and 1,000s at a slower pace as you approach your races. Run 4 times one mile at 5 mile race pace instead of 5K pace the week before a 10K; run 1,000s 5 seconds per mile faster than 5K pace instead of at 2 mile pace the week before a 5K race. This makes it even easier to relax rather than strain your way toward the race.

As with your training in Chapter 7, you'll run these Interval sessions on fresh pegs. Take a rest day or easy run the day before long reps at 2 mile to 5K paces. Provided you've used the long build-up which started with years of 10K and half-marathon training, short intervals and anaerobic threshold sessions can be run on tired legs if you wish!

After three to four months of long repeats, and short races, use a 12 to 17 week build up for your next marathon.

Maintain Mileage.

One facet of marathon training is to educate your muscles to run fast while slightly fatigued: your muscles will be very fatigued in the last 6 miles of your marathon! You need to maintain 100 percent of your hard earned endurance fitness and muscle strength while running about 10 sessions of long repeats. Don't lose your ability to run long while running these long reps. Alternate 18s with 14s during these three to four months and you'll be ready for 6 runs of 20 to 22 miles over your final 12 to 16 week marathon build-up.

Don't neglect strength training during this speed phase. One set of reps give you 75 percent of the benefits of three sets, so try a short weight training session once a week and one long session. Or do weights once every 5 days instead of twice a week to maintain your earlier strength gains.

Lower mileage runners should consider longer repetitions. As stated in Chapter 10, "It's not just how high you raise the heartrate, but also how long you can maintain it at a steady high level. The person who runs 4 one mile repeats at goal 5K pace, is more likely to race a 5K at that pace, than the person who runs 4 miles worth of 1,000 meter reps at 5K pace."

Long fast repetitions will take your heartrate to about 95 percent of maximum during 5K pace reps and up to 98 percent at 3K pace. Except for the first rep, you should reach your goal heartrate within the first 400 meters of each repeat. During your recovery, allow your HR to drop to 110-120, then immediately start the next repetition.

Heartrate Training Zone.

When running 400 meter repeats, a person with a maximum exercise HR of 175 may only reach his 5K HR of 166 for the last 40 to 50 meters of each Interval. Here's the HR splits for 100s during a 400 meters. 148, 159, 164, 167.

This athlete was actually running slightly faster than 5K pace, so gaining very good skills at economical running, yet his heart was only at 5K intensity for about 10 percent of his Interval training. What happens if our hero slows down to 5K pace, but runs 800s?

Distance	HR	HR
200	159	157
400	164	163
600	169	169
800	171	167
Finish time	2.50	2.53

Yes my friends, that 167 HR at the end of the second repeat was a reflection of our runner slowing down. Observe:

* Slightly lower HR at 400 meters secondary to slower running (compared to his earlier 400s).
* But he was only seconds away from hitting his 5K HR goal of 166 at the end of the first lap, and spent over 300 meters above 166 (40 percent of his Interval training).
* If he took shorter recoveries, he could reach his 166 HR goal earlier in each repeat, though this would make the session feel and be harder. Your goal should be to gradually reduce your rest periods.

What happens when he runs 3 x 1,600 meters at 5K pace with a 400 meter rest taking three minutes for the recovery?

At	Heartrate for		
	1st rep	2nd	3rd
200 m	154	154	159
400	162	164	162
600	163	166	164
800	164	169	165
1,200	166	169	167
1,600	169	168	166

He reaches his 10K HR goal of 161 well before the 400 meter point. If you run mile repeats at 5K pace, you'll probably get over 80 % of your Interval time at or above 10K heartrate intensity, or 92 % of max HR. 400s at 5K pace give you less than 30 percent of your time at 10K HR or higher.

But the main interest here is on 5K heartrate. During the first rep in this session, he took nearly 1,200 meters to reach his 5K heartrate (166 or more) with fresh legs. However, after a three minute rest, he took less than 600 meters to reach a HR of 166 and spent <u>64 percent of that rep at or above 166</u>. Compared to 40 percent during 800s at 5K pace.

Run mile repeats at 5K pace and you'll spend a huge percentage of training time at your 5K HR goals, and be forced to make improvements to your running efficiency to achieve these sessions.

The lower heartrate in the last rep is probably a reflection of our hamster concentrating on his running efficiency while dealing with his fatigue, and perhaps because he had sweated off some of his over-hydration, so he was at ideal running weight for this final 5:53 of running at 5K pace.

You'll spend an even greater percentage of your time at 5K HR if you add a fifth lap to get 2,000 meter repeats! The fifth lap can feel a little gruesome though, so try to run it with company.

Greater Marathon Speed.

Long repeats teach you economical running, but you can use seven other sessions to gain legspeed at any stage of training.

1. Stride and Coast.

Run striders of about 50 meters, but with a fast 50 meter jog recovery. Start with a mile and build to three miles as you get used to them, to give you 1.5 fast miles. This is similar to the fartlek in Chapter Three, or the bends and straights in preparation for interval training. Now, in addition to the efforts being fast, the rest period must be fast. Don't allow your muscles to recover completely. This session develops speed and helps to refine your change of pace ability for racing. It helps you to stay with a companion when he inadvertently speeds up at every mile checkpoint!

Run it as a stride...coast...stride. Don't ease to a jog at the end of each strider. Seven minute mile marathon runners should stride out at 6:30 pace, not sprint; ease back to coast at 7:30 pace. Time your mile splits, not your 50s! Average pace is marathon speed. You'll work more of your fast twitch muscle fibers than in steady runs at marathon pace.

The 'coasting' section during this session does not last many seconds, but nor does the fast part. The cumulative effect after a mile, or sixteen of these efforts is your goal.

You can break up a 3-mile session by running a lap of striding the straights and jogging the bends, alternating with a lap of the 50 meters striders. You can also do this session on grass or by alternating speeds at each lamppost.

2. Sprint Drills.

You've been working on running form for about five years by now: form hints are in Chapter Three. Now you can run some 150 meter striders working on a relaxed, fast running action. Speed up in five stages every ten meters; maintain at close to mile pace for 50 meters, then ease down over the last 50 meters. Run these drills on smooth grass if possible.

Lean forward only slightly while staying tall. Reduce wasted motion...keep your head still. Run off your whole forefoot and give a final push from the toes. Feel the surface, pull the surface back to you like an ostrich does and devour the ground. Push off from the toes with full leg extension at the hip and in the calf muscles.

Practice these strides as a separate session; later, do six acceleration runs at the end of a track session once a week.

3. Speed during the Long Run.

Bring in more of your fast twitch muscle fibers on one long run per month. About two miles from the end of say your first long run each month, change up to 15K race pace for half a mile, or run two times a quarter mile. Run this fast part relaxed, and then cruise in the last part of the run. You can substitute this half a mile for part of your 2 x one mile at marathon pace in your long run, or add to the mile reps.

4. Downhills.

Running up a slight hill costs almost twice as much energy as you gain coming down that hill. Practice both ways with relaxed form. Details on pages 97-100.

5. Wind.

You can do long reps with the wind to help your legspeed, or while resting up pre-race.

To improve legspeed, run the reps at what you consider to be your normal intensity...at long rep heartrate for those who use a monitor, while letting the wind push you to a faster pace. Stay relaxed though, or you will lose the benefit. Running with the wind can give you 2 mile (or faster) legspeed at 5K effort.

When resting up pre-race, you can run at your usual pace, but the effort will be much easier because you'll be pushed by the wind. Jog back into the wind at easy effort.

Not yet resting but looking for high heartrates and an intense session? Run repeats into the wind and you'll work hard while saving your legs due to your relatively slow speed and decreased ground impact forces.

6. Lactate Buffering.

You can break a session of short repeats into sets. Run 300s or 400s at 2 mile pace, but take short recoveries...thus giving your muscle cells greater stimulation.

Start with two 300s, and take a fast 100 recovery between the reps. This pair is a set. Run a lap of the track as extra rest prior to another set of 300s.

The first effort will seem easy; maintaining pace on the second and third 300 gets progressively harder.

For the best training effect, the last 300 should be as fast as the first. When you've done this session successfully a couple of times, you can try sets of three, four, and then five reps.

Five reps will simulate a mile race. Don't do more than three miles of these intervals in a session.

Due to the short recovery, your muscle lactate levels remain high. This increases your lactate tolerance...the amount of lactate your muscles can hold before forcing you to slow down. Increasing lactate holding capacity allows you to maintain high speeds longer.

Exercise physiologists call it increasing your 'buffering system' or 'buffering capacity.' Like running long reps at two mile pace, you breathe deeper, thus increasing the maximum quantity of oxygen your lungs can take in, and which your blood has the opportunity to absorb.

You will also get your heartrate in the training zone for a greater percentage of your training time with short rest intervals. Our hamster from a few pages ago finished with 3 x 300 meters and took the entire first 300 meter repeat to reach a HR of 164, but by taking only a 40 second rest between intervals, hit a HR of 162 to 164 at the 100 meter point in his next two 300s, thus staying in the training zone for two-thirds of those repeats.

7. True Drills:

Form drills include High knees, Heel flicks, Rapid feet (calf flicking with low knees) and High Skipping. When doing drills, you'll move slowly forward but with rapid leg movement for 15 to 30 seconds, and then walk a similar amount of time before repeating.

These drills, plus weight training, hill repeats and plyometrics could give you the strength to add 2 inches to your stride length for the entire marathon. If you maintain exactly the same leg speed as in previous races, you'll run 4 minutes and 20 seconds faster at the marathon.

Tucking in behind other runners for most of the race while wearing lighter shoes can each save you 5 seconds per mile in effort expended, allowing you to maintain pace at another 4 minutes faster for the marathon. Keep the drafting low stress by not getting too close and picking someone at the right pace and striding style to match your style.

Run the above drills and running efficiency enhancers after a restive day so that you can run them fast. Keep your steady runs easy to allow recovery between speed sessions.

<u>As you approach your marathon</u> you can decrease the pace of some sessions toward 10K pace. Or, instead of three times one mile at 2 mile pace, run a mile at 5K pace, then 3 to 4 times 800 meters at 2 mile pace, then a second mile at 5K pace. Stay relaxed.

Don't run your short reps faster than 2 mile pace. Cruise through these intervals, putting more effort into your form than the actual speed. You'll be fast because you are fit. Unless you work on running technique during these weeks, the training will wear you down rather than relaxing you for the next marathon.

<u>When peaking</u> for your marathon, the weekend long run will be at least 20 percent shorter than your typical long run, and be run 10 seconds per mile slower than usual, on an easier course, at a cooler time of day. You'll also run more of your long runs on asphalt instead of dirt to get your biomechanics perfect for race day.

You can still run quite fast in the last week before a marathon. You have just enough miles mid-week to run 4 times 800 meters at 5K pace and 2 days later run 4 times 400 meters at 2 mile pace. Or stick to threshold pace repeats in that last week with 2 x one mile.

Reasons for Slowing Down in the second half of a marathon include:

Starting off too fast for the conditions or your training. Next time, slow down your first 10 miles by 5 seconds per mile to see if you can maintain that pace. Run even pace or negative splits by setting out at realistic effort...always.

Best half-marathon 85 minutes and you're in shape to run 85 minutes this month? That's about 6.30 per mile pace. Slowing pace by one twelfth as shown in Chapter Ten will mean a 3:04:45 marathon. You need to hit halfway in your marathon at 92 to 93 minutes, not in 88 minutes. Run at 7:02 per mile, not the 6:42 which would get you to half-way in 88 minutes, or you'll probably be walking by twenty-two miles.

How can you become fast enough to break 3 hours for the marathon? Easy! Spend a year concentrating on 10K racing, then another year at the half-marathon to improve your Half to 82 minutes. Then follow a 40 week marathon program while maintaining 82 minute half-marathon capability.

Want to build the endurance to run that second half of your marathon 10 seconds per mile faster...to equal your first half?

Add one mile to your 4 key runs each week for a total of only 16 extra miles per month. But where?
* Longest run. Add one mile.
* Second longest run each week. Add one mile.
* Two speed sessions each week. Add one mile to your warmdown.

After two weeks, convert those warmdown miles to quality running at threshold or VO2 max pace at a quarter of a mile per week. 10 weeks to get an extra 2 miles of quality running.

Then, while maintaining these extra 4 miles per week:

Add 60 minutes of cross-training every week. 30 minutes of weights and 30 of aerobic cross-training. See Best Half-Marathons. Already doing three similar sessions? Do a 6 mile run each week instead of adding a 4th weight session. After two months:

Add 2 more running miles per week: One more mile to your longest run each week, unless it is already 22, in which case, add it to your second longest run. The remaining mile goes onto your anaerobic threshold session, to give you greater endurance at close to marathon pace.

Do 16 x 100 meter striders once a week within an easy run at barely faster than 5K pace. Pick those legs up a bit with faster turnover for 20-30 seconds.

Train at your new full intensity for 40 weeks while doing 4 to 12 week phases of fartlek, hills, threshold, VO2 max (including long intervals), then rest up for another marathon.

If you'd been a 50 mile per week runner with 3 cross-training sessions, you're now a 62 mile per week runner who:
* Averages two miles farther each weekend;
* Does one mile per week more at 5K intensity;
* Runs two miles more each week at threshold pace, and,
* You do an extra 6 mile run at easy pace.

Formerly at 50 miles per week with no cross-training? You're now at 56 miles each week with one cross-training session. Like the 62 miles per week person, you also.
* Run two miles farther each weekend;
* Do one mile per week more at 5K intensity;
* Run two miles more each week at threshold pace.

Take another look at this author's adaptation to Slovic's predictive time in Chapter Ten, and you'll find that you've improved your predicted marathon time substantially. Now all you have to do is rest up properly for your marathon. Run the first half of your next marathon at your usual pace and there's a good chance you'll maintain pace...provided you improved your half-marathon best by 2 to 3 minutes during this training period.

Khalid Khannouchi and his talented opposition gave a pacing clinic at the 2002 London Marathon, and helped Khannouchi to take 4 seconds off his own World Record, taking it down to 2:05:38. 24 of the miles were between 4:43 and 4:55. The other two were 4:39!

Khannouchi made a gap on runner-up to be, Paul Tergat (who ran a new record 2:04.55 at Berlin in 2,003) and Haile

Gebrselassie, during the relatively slow 25th mile. Attrition slows the runners-up more than the winner.

Your ability to maintain pace in the last 6 to 8 miles is the key to fast marathon times. Start off at realistic pace based on your half marathon times and with 20 runs of 18 miles or more in the last 30 weeks, with at least 5 of them being 20 to 22 miles, and you should maintain pace. If you try to get 2 minutes ahead of even pace schedule at 20 miles, you pre-destine yourself to slowing.

Khannouchi finishes some long runs at the track with 3 miles at marathon to 15 seconds per mile faster than marathon pace. This teaches him to relax at speed with fatigued muscles, just like you must at the end of your marathon.

Do run your 2 x one mile at marathon pace toward the end of half of your long runs, either on a good road surface or a user friendly track. Run an easy mile to finish.

Paula Radcliffe's 2,003 London world record of 2:15:25 was also set with negative splits, her second half marathon took a mere 67:23. Radcliffe's record is only 7.8 percent slower than the men's marathon record, whereas the current 5K and 10K world records are 14.3 and 11.9 percent slower than the men's records. As a European Gold medalist at one event and Commonwealth Gold medalist at the other, Paula may revise those track numbers before she retires.

Reached a plateau? Enjoy the view before running back down the hill.

Running plateaus (long periods without improving) are usually due to doing the same training year after year, or because you've achieved your ultimate peak.

Do the many types of training out-lined in previous pages, improve your 5K and half-marathon times, and make some of your sessions more demanding or add a minimal amount of extra mileage to find the cure to plateaus. Some of you will need to reduce mileage to reach a higher level!

Chapter Thirteen

Average 40 miles per week.

This schedule is slightly different to Chapter 11's format, which is why it is separated by the chapter on long Intervals.

Consistency is the key to marathon training success. With this schedule, mileage varies from 37 to 45 for a total of 800 over the 20 weeks. You'll make subtle changes to your training from week to week and over the nearly 5 months to your race. The main difference to Chapter 11 is that the strength phase blurs into the speed phases, yet every type of training is included in the compacted 20 weeks.

There is one requirement for this schedule: You should have trained at 30 to 40 miles per week while racing 5K and 10Ks for at least 6 months. If not, then check the 10K or Half-marathon training advice in this author's other books, or use Chapter Three's schedule to get the fundamentals before embarking on this short-cut marathon program.

Like Chapters 11 and 14, this schedule focuses on strength followed by speed as you increase the length of your long run, but not in formal 10 week phases. Note that 6 of the 9 hill training sessions are in the first 10 weeks, yet strength is maintained because the ninth hill session is in week 17.

VO2 max training and 4 long runs (including week 16's race) dominate the last 10 weeks. Both will teach you to run economically. Except for the last week, a VO2 max session can be replaced by a 5K race; restrict yourself to two of them.

Fartlek training should be of high quality in the early weeks. In the second 10 weeks, fartlek running is used mainly as recovery from races and longer runs: run it less intensely.

The race in week 8 should probably be a 10K. You rest up for it. In week 13, a 15K to half-marathon race is ideal.

You do not rest up much for the week 16 race. A 30K or 20 mile race would be perfect. This is also the third of your 4 runs at 20 miles. It's a hard run. No race close by? Run 10 miles at half a minute per mile slower than marathon pace, then 8 miles at marathon pace.

800 miles to a good marathon.
You could add 2 miles to your Sunday and Thursday steady runs each week, plus a mile to one of your speed sessions each week to give yourself an average of 45 miles per week. But ditch the extra 3 miles for the last 4 weeks. You could also repeat a three week section several times to give yourself a 30 week preparation. The options are endless, so please adapt it to suit your needs.

Runners are apt to sprint up hills, run threshold at 10K pace by mistake, and do intervals at close to mile speed.

*   Hills hurting you? Run at 2 mile to 5K intensity for 60 to 90 seconds. Don't sprint.
*   Interval training feel hard? Slow down to 5K pace and it should feel relatively easy.
*   Hate threshold sessions because you hurt for ages? Slow down to 15K pace or half-marathon speed.

Ache for days after a 20 miler. You should have some fatigue, but make sure that you run them slow enough for cardiovascular stimulation, while pushing forward with your calf muscles: Run at 60 to 70 percent of max HR, or about one minute per mile slower your marathon pace.

Training table abbreviations:
E = Easy running at 60-70 percent of your max heartrate.

F = Fartlek or speedplay. See Chapter Three for details.

X = Cross training such as an hour of bicycle riding, a brisk walk, elliptical training, weight training, or 30 minutes of running in a swimming pool.

H = Hills. See Chapter Four.

A = Anaerobic threshold pace running from Chapter Five.

V = Interval training at VO2 maximum or 10K to two mile race pace. See Chapters 6, 7, 10 and 12.

As usual, all types of speed running require a warmup, stretching and a cooldown. For example, F4 means a 2 mile warmup, 4 miles of fartlek, followed by a two mile warmdown. Friday is always a rest day (R).

Day	Sat	Sun	M	Tu	W	Th	Weeks
Day #	1	2	3	4	5	6	Mileage
Week # 1	F4	E12	X	F4	E4	E8	40
Two	A4	E14	X	F4	X	E10	40
Three	H2	E13	X	F4	X	E10	38
Four	H2	E16	X	F4	X	E10	41
Five	A4	E15	X	H2	X	E10	40
Six	F4	E18	X	H2	X	E10	43
Seven	A4	E15	X	F3	X	E8	38
8	10K Race	E12	X	F4	X	E10	40
Nine	A4	E18	X	H2	X	E10	43
Ten	V4	E15	X	H2	X	E10	40
Wk 11	V4	E20	X	F4	X	E8	44
12	H2	E15	X	A4	X	E8	38
13	Race 15K	E8	X	F4	X	E10	39
14	V4	E20	X	H2	X	E10	45
15	A5	E15	X	V4	X	E8	40
16	Race 30K	X	E5	E8	X	F4	38
17	H2	E15	X	V4	X	E10	40
18	A4	E20	X	F4	X	E8	44
19	V4	E16	R	A4	X	E4	36
20	V3	E13	R	E3	A2	E3	30

Chapter Fourteen

Training schedules at 50 to 60 miles per week.

<u>50 mile per week runners</u> have many options for using their extra 10 miles compared to 40 miles per week runners: Add a mile or two to all four runs, plus run an extra four to five mile run to the complete the 50.

You can add your extra mile to the cooldown during quality days, or add that extra mile as speed running.

Running more than 20 miles in one run does little to improve your marathon...provided you run two marathons per year. Running closer to 20 miles on your shorter weekends will improve your potential. While rotating 15, 17 and 20s at 40 miles per week, you had an average long run of 17.3 miles. Alternating 18s with a 20 takes your average long run to 19 miles. 20 is still 40 percent of your weekly mileage, but it's easier to recover from if you keep it slow enough.

Adding to your 4 miles of fast running needs great care. Starting the first few repeats at appropriate pace is even more vital than in prior years. Add a quarter to half a mile every two weeks to reach your 5 mile speed running sessions. Two or three 5 mile sessions at the end of each 6 to 10 week phase should be enough the first time you train for a marathon at 50 miles per week.

The next time through this schedule, run the entire phase with 5 mile sessions, while increasing pace slightly from half-marathon to 15K in Phase Three's anaerobic threshold sessions, and from 5K to 2 mile race speed during most of Phase Four's VO2 max sessions and Peaking.

Hill training edges up to 2.5 miles of repeats, and you can do even more on the days that it's up a long gentle incline.

Half of your bonus 10 miles should probably be done on one of your rest days. Run just before your 30 minute weight training session as the warm-up, or 8 to 10 hours before it as a separate session if that works better for you.

Pages 246 to 251 gives a review of the Five Phases from Chapters 1 to 10, followed by the actual training schedules. The essential training elements are unchanged for you at 50 miles per week.

Phase One: Base Mileage while also doing fartlek running at 5K to 15K paces.

Alternating 18s and 20s leaves you 30 to 32 miles which you can split between 4 additional runs. Fewer, but longer runs add more endurance than many short runs. At least one run should be 5 miles of fartlek, see Chapter Three.

Phase Two: Hills and Strength.

At 50 miles per week, you'll probably be running fast on at least two days a week to stimulate oxygen uptake systems. Alternate hill repeats with fartlek sessions and add 16 times 100 meter striders on grass each week to maintain efficient running form.

You will increase pace toward 70 percent of maximum heartrate for the last 5 miles of each long run.

Phase Three: Anaerobic Threshold Running.

Half marathon to 15K pace running is another fundamental ingredient to your marathon endurance. Threshold pace is easier to maintain than 10K pace, yet it's more beneficial because you run economically and concentrate on running form, yet keep your legs rested for your other speed training.

Shortage of local races at 10K or 10 miles? As

shown in Chapter 11, you can double your anaerobic session once a month instead of racing. Ten times one mile at 10 mile pace with a one minute rest is a good substitute for a 10 mile race. Race at 5K once a month for fun, socialization and a pleasant break from hill or threshold pace training.

Phase Four: VO2 Maximum Training.

Two mile race pace, 5K and 10K pace training adds power to your legs, improves your biomechanics and the amount of oxygen you can process, and therefore your speed potential.

The VO2 Intervals will progress from four to five miles as described in Chapter Six and Seven.

You'll probably need to run each full session three times for your muscles to fully adapt, and to teach yourself to relax and run economically.

Phase Five: Marathon Peaking.

Rest and longer repeats at 2 mile to 10K race pace give extra pep to your legs and maximize your VO2 capacity and running economy. You will all decrease your cross training by 25 percent for the first three weeks, then by half for all but the last week, when you will do zero cross training.

Note: Don't run the final 13 miler any faster than your usual long run pace: you're supposed to be resting up! The last week will include 2 miles at 15K pace, and a five mile run to give you a 22 mile week. You'll be nicely rested for the marathon.

Training table abbreviations:

E = Easy runs...at 60-70 percent of maximum heartrate.
F = Fartlek
H = Hill repeats
HF = Hilly fartlek...less vigorous than the hill session.
A = Anaerobic threshold pace running...15K speed.
V = VO2 maximum pace intervals...2 mile to 10K speed.

Serious Runners should cruise two times one mile at marathon pace during each long run. Instead of doing long repeats at 5K pace the first time through, you could spend an extra six weeks with 600s and 400s. Learn to run fast while using very little energy. Run 16 times 100 meters once every week to practice running form.

Day	One	Two	Three	Four	Six
Probably on	*Sat*	*Sun*	*Mon*	*Tues*	*Thur*
Weeks 1, 3 & 5	10E	18	5E	8E	5F
Weeks 2, 4 & 6	10E	20	5E	6E	5F
Weeks 7, 9...15	10E	18	5E	8E	2.5H
Wks 8, 10, 12, 14,	10E	20	5E	8E	5HF
Week 16	Race 10K	13	3E	6E	2HF
Week 17	10E	13	5E	8E	5A
Weeks 18, 20 & 22	10E	20	5E	8E	5A
Weeks 19 & 21	10E	18	5E	8E	4HF
Weeks 23, 25, 27	10E	18	5E	8E	5HF
Weeks 24, 26, 28	10E	20	5E	8E	5V
Week 29	Race 10 mile	13	4E	3HF	5E
Week 30	8E	10	5E	8E	5V
Week 31	10E	20	5E	8E	5V
Week 32	9E	18	5E	8E	5V
Week 33	8E	22	3E	7E	5HF
Week 34	7E	16	3E	7E	4V
Week 35	6E	18	R	6E	3V
Week 36	13	4E	R	2A	4E

Then race your marathon.

As stated in Chapter 11, the drawback to using training phases is that you can lose the benefit from one type of training while perfecting the next type. Example: no more hills are scheduled after week 15, which is fine if you do quality fartlek sessions with many hills. You can also run one in three of your anaerobic threshold sessions up a gentle hill of 2 to 4 percent grade. During the VO2 maximum phase, include a few hilly fartlek sessions with half of it being long efforts at threshold intensity.

Although most Saturdays are 10 miles easy to give 28 to 30 miles for the weekend, it's inconceivable to this runner / author that 50 mile per week runners would only do one session of speed running per week. Saturday is your chance to run a few miles at close to marathon pace or Best Aerobic Effort (BAE). Restrict yourself to 2 miles early on and reach 5 miles at your BAE by week 17.

Here's a nice pair of pyramid sessions adapted from Chapter 11 of *10K & 5K Running, Training & Racing*. Any intensity runner can use these sessions. This one focuses on perfecting your anaerobic threshold. Take two minutes rest between speeds the first time you do this session, and reduce it to one minute over 4 to 6 sessions during the course of the year.
After a pleasant warm-up, run 2 x 1.5 miles at 15K pace;
then run three half miles at 10K pace;
finish with two quarters at 5K pace.

The second pyramid to focus on VO2 max training is:
Three times one mile at 5K pace; then
3 x 800 meters at close to 2 mile pace; then
6 x 400 meters at 2 mile pace.
Your recoveries need to be longer than the first pyramid session. Never done mile reps at 5K pace? Try 4 x 1,200 at 5K pace the first time.

Moderate Intensity Runners move their legs fast
twice a week. Like serious runners, you should run two times

one mile at marathon pace during long runs and run 16 times 100 meters once a week. You can spend the final 6 weeks running long repeats at close to VO2 maximum the first time through the schedule.

Strength is vital for marathon success. Cutting the hill section would be short sighted. Run plenty of hills and continue to weight train during your VO2 max phases to maintain muscle strength.

Consider 2 to 5 miles at BAE on most Thursdays.

Day	One	Two	Three	Four	Six
Probably on	*Sat*	*Sun*	*Mon*	*Tues*	*Thurs*
Weeks 1, 3,	5F	15	5E	5F	8E
Weeks 2, 4,	4HF	18	5E	4F	8E
Weeks 5, 7...13	2.5H	18	5E	5F	10E
Weeks 6, 8...14	2.5H	20	5E	5HF	10E
Week 15	Race 10K	13	3E	3HF	6E
Week 16	4A	12	5E	4F	8E
Weeks 17, 19, 21	5A	20	5E	2.5H	10E
Weeks 18, 20, 22	5A	18	5E	5HF	10E
Week 23	10 mile race	13	3E	3HF	6E
Week 24	4V	12	5E	4HF	8E
Weeks 25 & 28	5V	20	5E	2.5H	10E
Weeks 26 & 29	5V	19	5E	5A	10E
Weeks 27 & 30	5V	18	5E	5HF	10E
Week 31	Race 10K	13	3E	3A	5E

Then practice long repeats at 3K to 10K paces on Day 1 for six weeks. A 5K race is a nice break at week 35 or 36.

Week 32	4V	15	4E	4HF	8E
Week 33	5V	20	4E	2.5H	10E
Week 34	5V	18	4E	5A	10E
Week 35	5V	22	4E	3HF	10E
Week 36	4V	16	4E	2H	9E
Week 37	3V	18	3E	4A	8E
Week 38	13	3E	2V	3E	2A

Race your marathon.

Highest Intensity Runners shift their legs rapidly for part of nearly every run. Two miles of marathon pace practice is still useful during your long runs. You'll cross train of course, and run five miles on the most convenient day to you, and probably do your 16 x 100 meter striders that day. Your other days are something like this:

Days	One	Two	Four	Six
Weeks 1 & 2	5F	18	5F	5HF
Weeks 3, 5,7, 9	2.5H	20	5F	5HF
Weeks 4, 6, 8, 10	2.5H	18	5F	5HF
Week 11	Race 10K	13	3HF	2F
Week 12	4A	15	4F	2H
Weeks 13, 15, 17	5A	20	2.5H	5HF
Weeks 14, 16, 18	5A	18	5HF	2.5H
Week 19	Race 10 miles	13	3HF	2A
Week 20	4V	15	4F	2H
Weeks 21 & 24	5V	20	5HF	2.5H
Weeks 22 & 25	5V	19	2.5H	5A
Weeks 23 & 26	4V	18	5HF	5A
Week 27	Half marathon	10	3A	2F
Week 28	3V	5E	2F	3HF
Week 29	4V	18	2H	5V
Week 30	5V	20	5A	2H
Week 31	Race 10K	15	2H	4A
Week 32	5V	18	2H	5A
Week 33	5V	22	3HF	5A
Week 34	4V	15	5V	2H
Week 35	3V	18	3HF	3A
Week 36	13	4E	2V	2A

Race your marathon.

Note that weeks 29 and 34 contain two sessions working on VO2 maximum. The weekend session should be long repeats at 5K to 10K pace. Two or three 5K races at say weeks 24, 29 and 33 would be useful to break up the training, practice pace judgment with race day adrenaline surging through your veins, while running fast on tired legs because you only reduce mileage by a couple miles that week. For instance, doing 3 miles at threshold instead of 5 miles will freshen you up just a bit for a 5K race.

10 or 38 weeks, the choice is yours.

While you can adapt any 38 week program to an 8 to 20 week schedule, I'll make it easier for you with a 15 week schedule. This sample 15 week program is for moderately intense runners (two speed sessions per week). Just done a marathon or 20 mile race? Take 2 to 3 weeks of easy running and an occasional couple miles of fartlek, and do no runs over 12 miles while recuperating before starting this plan. Then:

Day	One	Two	Three	Four	Six
Week 1	5F	15	5E	5F	8E
Week 2	4HF	18	5E	4F	8E
Week 3	2.5H	20	5E	5F	10E
Week 4	2.5H	18	5E	5HF	10E
Week 5	5A	20	5E	2.5H	8E
Week 6	5A	15	5E	4F	7E
Wk 7	Race 10 miles	8	5E	4HF	7E
Week 8	4V	18	5E	10E	5HF
Week 9	5V	20	5E	2.5H	10E
Week 10	5V	18	5E	5A	10E
Week 11	5V	22	5E	4HF	7E
Week 12	Race 10K	13	5E	3A	10E
Week 13	5V	20	4E	4HF	8E
Week 14	4V	18	3E	4A	10E
Week 15	13	4E	2V	E4	2A

Race your marathon.

For the last few VO2 max sessions you'll be practicing long repeats at 5K to 10K paces on Day One. The 10K race in week 12 is on tired legs from the 22 miler. This is part of the plan so that you do not race too fast, and so that you run moderately fast with fatigued muscles.

And at 60 miles per week.

Running more mileage will improve your running economy, but will not make significant gains to your VO2 max. With better running economy, you should be able to out-race a person with the same VO2 max. However, if the high mileage is overtraining for you, injury or fatigue could mean the 50 mile per week, yet less efficient runner will beat you.

The 20 mile run is a convenient one-third of your mileage, but you still need to control your speed. You now have sufficient miles to run that long mid-week run...<u>with half of it at close to marathon pace.</u>

Most of you will do more than one speed session. A three to four mile session of hilly fartlek each week gives a great transition between the different intensities, especially as you have six miles to play with in your main speed session.

Potential 6 mile speed sessions include:

*   2 x 3 miles at half-marathon pace;
*   3 x 2 miles at 15K pace;
*   6 x one mile at 10K pace:
*   8 x 800 at 5K pace, followed by 6 x 500s;
*   10 x 600 at 5K pace followed by 300s at 2 mile pace.
*   And, hour long fartlek sessions when you wander and change pace for 200 to 1,000 meters, or 40 seconds to 4 minutes, depending on the system of counting you prefer.

60 miles per week allow you to:

*   Run even more 20s;
*   Run a 22 once every 6 weeks;
*   Include midweek fairly long runs of 12 to 13 miles;
*   Include more speed running in quality sessions.

The training is so much like the 50 miles per week runners that we only need to show the 15 week training table at moderate intensity. Day 3 and 5 short runs will be in conjunction with cross training. You can also shorten day 3 or 5s run to take Day Six's run closer to 15 miles some weeks, though only sub 4 hour marathon runners are likely too.

Lengthen this program by repeating weeks 3 & 4, or 5 to 8, or 8 to 11, depending on where your weakness is.

For most people, the rest day will be Friday. The Day one session will be at speed on fresh muscles on Saturday. Sunday is your long run on nicely fatigued muscles from Saturday.

Day	One	Two	Three	Four	Five	Six
Week 1	6F	15	8	6F	8	12
Week 2	5HF	18	8	6F	8	12
Week 3	3H	22	8	5F	13	8
Week 4	3H	18	8	6HF	12	8
Week 5	6A	20	8	6F	12	8
Week 6	6A	22	8	3H	13	8
Week 7	5A	17	6	5HF	8	6
Wk 8	Race 10 miles	5	8	4HF	8	12
Week 9	6V	22	8	3H	13	8
Week 10	6V	18	8	6A	13	8
Week 11	5V	22	6	5HF	10	6
Week 12	Race 10K	13	8	4A	12	8
Week 13	6V	20	7	5HF	10	7
Week 14	5V	18	6	5A	8	6
Week 15	4V	12	3	5E	2A	4

Race your marathon.

The 10 mile race at the end of Week Seven happens to follow three sessions at 15K race pace on the previous weekends. Running 25 percent of those 6 mile sessions at 10K pace would be useful. For example: Two mile reps with the last half mile of each one at 10K pace.

The 10K race follows three long sessions of shortish Intervals (Chapter Six) at 5K pace, but you'll probably run 20 to 30 percent of them at close to 2-mile pace. Your final three Interval sessions in weeks 12 to 14 will probably be at 5 mile pace, but may include mile repeats at 5K pace.

Finally. Reduce your cross training to help your marathon peak. Don't suddenly stop all cross training 4 weeks before your marathon. Ease off over three weeks.

You can also make prudent use of longer repeats during peaking. Used to 3 times 2 miles at 15K pace? Try two repeats of 2.5 miles.

Used to 6 times 1,200 meters at 5K pace...try 3 times 2,000 meters at 5K pace.

Like 10 x 600 at 3K pace, do 6 x 800 meters at 3K pace.

Those three original sessions were 6, 4.5 and 3.75 miles for a total of 14.25 at speed. The new sessions are 5, 3.75 and 3 miles for a total of 11.75 miles. You've saved your muscles two and a half miles of speed running, yet your heart has been stimulated for a higher percentage of its 11.75 miles.

During the last two weeks you can cut an additional mile off of each session to give yourself about nine miles of quality running over the last 10 to 14 days pre-race.

Example:
* Tempo: 2 at half-marathon pace, then 2 at 15K pace.
* 2K at 10K pace; 2 x 800 meters at 5K pace; 2K.
* 4 x 800 meters at 2 mile pace

Your final speed session will usually be 2 x one mile at half marathon pace to remind yourself exactly how running at 15 to 20 seconds faster than marathon pace feels.

Follow the basic and essential 4 sessions on Saturday, Sunday, Tuesday and Thursday with its 2 long runs and 2 quality sessions and you can add numerous 5 to 7 mile runs to reach 80 to 100 miles per week. Do what works for your body, your other activities and your marathon ambitions.

Chapter 15 has other options for greater than 60 miles per week, or for staying at 60 per week.

Chapter Fifteen

Balanced schedule

at 60 to 80 miles per week

This Chapter is adapted from Running Dialogue's Chapter 21.

As stated before, the marathon runner's main training goal should be to work on the endurance to complete 26.2 miles at close to half marathon speed. Most of you high mileage types will be coming from years of 10K and half-marathon running and can keep two speed sessions per week.

Moving up in distance? Simply increase the length of your long runs to 20 miles at the weekend and to 13 miles midweek. Add two miles to the Sunday run and one mile to the midweek run on alternate weeks. Run at 1½ and ½ a minute per mile slower than anticipated marathon pace.

The Sunday run might progress over the weeks as 15, 15, 10 mile race, 17, 17, half marathon race, 19, 19, 20 mile race, 17, 20, 17, 20, 13 followed by the Marathon race. Note the three races. Distance order is not important, but if the twenty mile race is early in the build up, it will need to be run slower than hoped-for marathon speed. A low key 10K or 10 mile race three weeks before the marathon with a long warm up to total the 17 miles will help to break up the last six weeks.

Cut down your training load starting 3 weeks

before the marathon. Reduce by 10 percent that week and by 20 to 30 percent for the next week. Cut the mileage in half for the last week. These actions allow the body to recover from the hard work of the build up. Do one gentle run in the final three days pre-race; resting and carbo loading gives the muscles an extra supply of energy to see them through the last few miles of the race.

Ignore the three or four speed sessions which some 100 mile weekers do. With your two quality sessions each week, you can still do all types of speedwork from hills to anaerobic threshold to Interval training.

The typical week will be:	miles
Day one... Interval sessions at 2 mile to 10K pace	10
Day two...longest run of week at one minute per mile slower than marathon pace	18-22
Day three...easy 3-7 miles	?
Day four... anaerobic threshold, with warmup etc.	8
Day five...easy 6	6
Day six...second longest run at half a minute per mile slower than marathon pace. Every third week, include up to six miles at marathon pace.	12-14
Day seven...easy 0-7	?
Total	60-80

A one percent decrease in the energy cost of running can save 2 minutes off a 3 hour marathon. Efficiency is economy, so practice striders twice a week in easy runs...and:

Every three weeks during marathon training, instead of doing a steady 15 to 20 miles, consider 20 to 30 x 400 meters at 10 seconds per mile faster than marathon pace with only a 15 seconds rest. An area of grass allowing straight 400s works well. If the area is big enough, vary which section you use for each strider. An accurate 400 is not needed. Don't try to run at 5K pace. 5K pace is for a different day. This day, practice the change of pace and running at barely faster than marathon pace for a total of 5 to 7 miles.

One or two percent grades are fine too because they give still more variety and you can practice your form on very gentle slopes. On a track, 30 x 300 with a fast 100 rest around the curve will save you 3,000 meters of bend running. Better yet, do 500s with 100 rests to decrease the number of reps needed to make your five to seven miles at speed.

Do four 100s with a few seconds coasting after every 8 to 10 reps to help break up the session.

This is high level aerobic training. Add the warmup and cooldown, and you'll easily get in 15 miles.

If you slow down in the last 8 miles of a marathon, studies show that your legspeed is likely to be unchanged, but your stride length shortens. Running long repeats at half-marathon pace, plus the above session will give you a good chance of maintaining stride length and hence racing speed. So will starting off at a realistic pace for the first ten miles!

Both of these **sessions** teach you running economy or efficiency, which **increases** the potential for good marathon times.

Do at least a **couple** of miles the day after your long run each week, or ride a gentle 10 to 20 miles, or take a walk. How much mileage you do beyond the four basic quality sessions is up to you. Exercise physiologists tell us there are minimal gains to be made beyond 80 miles a week.

Intend to progress beyond sixty miles?

If all sessions were increased by a couple miles, mileage could easily go up to seventy-five, but it would place great strain on the body. Twice a day training is another option. The body recovers quicker from two seven mile runs at a given pace than from one fourteen mile run at the same pace. Of course, the longer run does build greater endurance!

It may have taken several years to build up to your sixty miles of good quality running on a consistent basis. Most of these sessions will at some stage feel hard, but to add another mile would make it intolerable. However, by adding a gentle 20 minute run say eight hours after the long Sunday run, many runners feel looser and more relaxed the next day.

After a few weeks it can be increased to 30 and then 40 minutes. Then practice lifting the knees up for fifty meters at a time. In a few months you'll be doing a gentle fartlek session. Meanwhile, the other main sessions aren't feeling any harder and you'll run at the same paces as before. Provided you rest up for them, your improved endurance should show through in faster race times.

Then you can add a five miler once a week at pleasant pace; a few months later add another. For alternate additional short runs, include some strideouts: do about 8 pickups of 100 meters to make sure the hamstrings and fast twitch fibers get some work. Otherwise:

* Keep your feet close to the ground to minimize the shock from ground impact;
* Take short, fast strides to maintain legspeed;
* Be efficient and economical; don't let these short runs become junk miles;
* Watch for body changes and injuries.

Take care with your regular speedwork. If you're too tired to train at 15K pace on your designated day, make adjustments to your mileage. You should always be able to cruise long intervals at 15K intensity, though not necessarily at 15K pace! When you can no longer hold 15K intensity running for long repeats, you may need to decrease mileage by 10 percent to reach your ideal level (for this year).

If you're planning a higher mileage phase, get the support and encouragement from training with others twice a week. If the plan is 12 runs, get out 12 times. We often don't know how we will feel until a mile or two into a run. If you still decide on a rest day, run back and you've got 4 miles before hitting the shower. It often happens that the day you didn't feel like running at all will turn into a great run.

Some runners train 14 times a week. Most take a day or two of short and easy runs, but they're able to train at moderate to high intensity on the other five. The trick is to find your limit. Provided you still enjoy most of the training, and you remain fresh enough to run at the right pace in your speed session, go ahead and test your limits. Include fartlek, strides and weight training every week.

However much training you add, consider the possibility that rest might help you improve more than the extra training would. Some people need 100 miles per week to run their best marathons; some marathon runners compete better on only 50 miles: there are no definite rules on mileage. Enjoy your running and aim to reach a realistic target based on your ability.

Fuel is vital for the marathon. Your body is capable of increasing the size of its fuel lines. At marathon pace, blood levels of epinephrine and norepinephrine, which make carbs more available to muscles, is increased.

Longish tempo runs at marathon target pace teach your muscles to process those carbs, and prepare your muscles for the marathons' demands. See also carbo loading page 217 to delay your encounter with the wall.

Training table abbreviations:

E = Easy runs...at 60-70 percent of maximum heartrate.

F = Fartlek...5K to 15K pace

H = Hill repeats

A = Anaerobic threshold running...15K effort.

V = VO2 maximum pace intervals...2 mile to 5K speed. i.e., the 300s, 400s, 800s and the two sessions of 1,200s.

Mile repeats and 2Ks are done at 5 mile to 10K race pace. Very advanced runners may also run some of the 2 mile reps at 10K pace. Most of you will run them at 15K pace.

All types of quality running require a warm-up and cooldown of two to three miles each side of the speed running. As you will be doing five miles at speed (or 3 to 4 miles for hill training), most speed days are 9 to 10 miles.

One or two 6 to 8 mile runs will also be done on days three and five of each week to net you 60 to 80 miles per week.

	Day One	Two	Four	Six
Week 1	15 x 300 hill	15	5A	8E
Wk 2	6x1200 @ 5K	15	2x2mile@A	8E
Wk 3	Race 10 miles	6E	4x2K@A	10E
Wk 4	8 x 800 hill	17	5x1mile@10K	10E
Wk 5	20x300 hill	17	8x800@5K	8E
Wk 6	Race 13.1 miles	5E	4HF	12E
Wk 7	20x400@2mile	19	5A	13E
Wk 8	6x1200 @ 5K	19	3x2mile@A	10E
Wk 9	Race 20 miles	5E	4HF	13E
Wk 10	25x300@2mile	17	6A	13E
Wk 11	8x800 hill	20-22	6x1mile@10K	13E
Wk 12	20x400@2mile	17	6A	13E
Wk 13	15x300 hill	20	6x1200@5K	10E
Wk 14	6X800@2mile	15	4A	6E
Wk 15	3x2K@10K	13	10x100	2x1mile@A

And race your marathon.

Note that you repeat most sessions every 6 to 7 weeks.

You could insert an extra week before week 14. Some physiology experts recommend 4 weeks to recover from the last 20 mile run. You could also run a 22 during your build-up at week 13. Whether a 20 or a 22, consider inserting:

Week 13B   14x500@2mile   17   5x1mile@10K   10E

The 500s total half a mile less than the 20 x 400s, yet it gives you an additional 100 meters with your heart in the 5K intensity training zone of 95 percent max heartrate on <u>every</u> repeat. That gives you an extra 1,000 to 1,400 meters of quality training at goal heartrate despite running less.

If you do a 10K race instead of the 400s in week 12, you'll probably reduce mile reps on Tuesday of week 11 to 4 or 5 reps with the last 2 at 5K pace as a nice contrast to, and preparation for the 10K. Three days after the 10K you would reduce the session (6A) to 2 x 2 mile repeats at half marathon pace, to again give a greater contrast to the 10K pace of the weekend. In week 13, you could replace a couple of 1200s at 5K pace with 400s at 2 mile pace to practice relaxed 400s, that is: 2 x 1200; 6 x 400; 2 x 1200. The alternative weeks 11 to 13 would then be:

Week 11	*7x800 hill*	*20*	*4x1mile@5K*	*8E*
Week 12	*Race 10K*	*17*	*2x2mile@half*	*13E*
Week 13	*15x300 hill*	*20*	*4x1200@5K*	*10E*
			+6x400@3K	

For all of you, the 100s in week 15 should be at 5K pace for relaxation. You'll be doing 16 x 100 once or twice a week anyway, so this is nothing new. The 2 times one mile is at 15K to half marathon speed for pace judgment.

<u>**If you rested up properly for a 10K race,**</u> why would you need to rest for several weeks after the 10K?

The day after your race is the first day of your next month's marathon training or base build-up. You usually run half your normal mileage for the week leading into a serious 10K. Take one easy run and it's time to enjoy your fitness and freshness as you cruise along at 70 percent max heartrate for whatever mileage you like. Don't lose fitness with inactivity.

If the last race was a 10K, a 17 miler will do you good the next day. Only after races at the half-marathon to the marathon do you need substantial rest with say 5 miles on alternate days.

You don't rest up much for races in a marathon build-up, merely decreasing your Tuesday quality by a mile, cutting the Thursday run by a few miles, doing only one cross training session, and decreasing your Monday and Wednesday runs. Ah, I suppose you do rest up, and you'll see from the program that your legs are babied for a few days afterwards.

CHAPTER SIXTEEN

WALK & JOG THE MARATHON

Like Chapter Fifteen's program, this one is adapted from Chapter 21 of Running Dialogue.

This is not the Beginner Marathon program. The Beginner Marathon program is in Chapter Ten, and is run on 40 miles per week with one main speed session. This chapter is for those of you who wish to walk and jog the marathon on minimal mileage.
* Perhaps you have some physical ailment which prevents you from adding a mile per week to your current 15 miles per week of walking or running, and which would prevent you from reaching a steady 40 miles per week after six months. If so, please enjoy this walk / run program for the marathon. However, you will probably be better off sticking with the half-marathon.
* Perhaps you are very overweight. If so, stay with modest mileage and enjoy short races plus copious amounts of cross-training. Make subtle lifestyle changes as suggested in the

nutrition chapters. Then, as you get your weight under control, increase to 40 miles per week and do so with only one minute walk breaks every 10 minutes.

For the rest of you, here we go.

While the emphasis of this book has been to encourage you to get several years of running background before you attempt a marathon, provided you've already had six months of training and running 10Ks, most people can complete 26.2 miles.

It only takes 20 to 25 miles a week to be able to run-walk a marathon. It won't be fast, but it doesn't have to be ugly, and you can have fun. While I'm not keen on minimalist training, this section should help you to complete a marathon with only modest injury risk.

You will do most of the sessions which 40 mile per week runners do, but do them every two weeks, including hills, 5K pace and tempo runs.

Saturdays...Alternate long reps with a tempo run at anaerobic threshold. Keep doing 2 to 3 miles of running at 20 seconds per mile slower than your 10K race pace. You will then start Sunday runs with modest muscle fatigue.

As usual, the most important ingredient is your long run at close to marathon pace. How fast is marathon pace?

Multiply your current 10K race time by five and divide by 26.2 to get your running pace. Higher mileage people would use 4.66 times their 10K race time, but you won't have the endurance for that, plus you will be taking walk breaks. A 50 minute 10K runner (eight min miles) gets 250 minutes for the marathon, or about nine and a half minute miles.

Starting with your 40 minute run in week one, add five minutes, or half a mile on alternate weeks in your build-up until you get to 10 miles or 100 minutes of continuous running at marathon pace. Take a one minute fairly fast walk every 10 minutes if it suits you. If this run feels too hard, you're probably running too fast.

Walk breaks make it easier for you to add distance; walking 100 to 200 yards every mile sets you up to walk up to four miles of your marathon. You will then be able to handle 22 miles of running. Walking is also good cross training for runners at all levels. Wear a water bottle fanny pack so that you don't need to stop to drink very often. Refill the bottle as appropriate.

For even weeks, your long session is a run-walk starting with 60 minutes. Add ten minutes each time to give you three hours after the 24 weeks. The running should be at one half to one minute per mile slower than marathon target pace. Run fifteen minutes at this pace, then walk at relaxed tempo for five. Practice taking in liquids with a little carbohydrate. You can also run 5 minutes and walk one minute if it suits you better. Use whatever combination works for you.

Include walking sections early in the session and make them routine, to keep the body fatigue modest. You went through the walk for five minutes and run for one minute while building up to 10K races. Hopefully, by now you're at the run for 5 and walk for one minute prior to contemplating a marathon. Your second marathon could be on 10 minute runs and one minute walks.

Midweek quality is for variety and to stimulate economic running, and to allow you to train almost anywhere.

Once every 3 weeks do hill repeats, but slowly. They are described in Chapter Four. If you prefer, do reps through mud. Hill training is even more important for low mileage marathon runners: You need all the anatomical benefits which resistance training will give you. Six to eight long hill reps are better than short ones.

Every 3 weeks, run intervals on the track. Sorry, did I say this was a minimalist schedule! Read Chapter Six. Try these sessions: Six 400s; five 600s; eight 400s; four 800s; eight 400s; six 600s; 4 x 800; 6 x 400.

Run at 5K pace or up to 3 seconds per lap faster (VO2 max pace). Walk the recovery, taking the same length of time as your repeats for the rest. This is clearly a vital day's training; you've had three rest days...so make the most of it.

The third week can be a bit more relaxing with fartlek using 200 to 300 meter striders on trails and grass.

<u>Resting up</u>: The last walk-run 2 weeks prior to your marathon should be an hour less than your longest.

The last continuous long run should be 7 days before your marathon, and take a mere 60 to 70 minutes because you are resting up. Only 50 minutes of it should be at marathon pace.

Two times one mile at marathon pace should be the only speed session in the last seven days. Do it either three or four days prior to the marathon.

Everything is geared toward the long runs which build aerobic base to enable you to complete the marathon. Speed sessions give you the benefits of every type of training which international class runners use.

If you come to this program with 10K fitness, you'll be able to run-walk the marathon after six months. Hopefully, you'll do a few 10Ks and a half-marathon in the build-up. You can also stay at week 24-25's level for a couple of months while repeating it several times. Then:

* Do a little more on your easy days;
* Add another mile to your continuous runs every two weeks to reach 13 miles;
* Add another 15 minutes to your walk-runs every two weeks to reach 4 hours;
* Do an additional mile of speed on your quality days.

After your month of consolidation at week 25s level, it should take 8 weeks to reach the 30 mile per week level, and you should stay four weeks before resting up for a marathon. Your training schedule stretches from 26 weeks to about 46 weeks.

You will then be more likely to run most of the race at marathon target pace with minimal walks. Resting up may allow you to run for 30 minutes at a time with a five minute walk break, or 15 minutes with a one minute walk break. If

298 Best Marathons by David Holt

you sense you're approaching poop-doom, settle back to 20 or 15 and five minutes walk.

You should never try to something in a race unless you've practiced it in training. Unless you've run at least 18 miles non-stop on at least three occasions, don't attempt to run the marathon. Take at least a one minute walking break every mile. This will leave you only 24 miles to actually run because the walking will take care of the other 2.2 miles.

When changing to a walk, look behind first. Move to the side of the group or the side of the road so as not to impede or surprise the other runners. If your watch beeper tells you to walk at a narrow point or just before a corner, ease the pace through the "slow down zone" and begin walking just after the zone, when you're out of most peoples way.

Water stops too. Don't add to the congestion and hold up biped traffic by stopping. Pick up two cups and walk quickly through to drink it. Note: You'll probably drink one cup of sports drink and one or two of water.

Only replace the liquid which you've sweated out. Don't dilute your electrolytes with too much water or with too much sports drink.

Training table abbreviations:
40@M = number of minutes at marathon pace.
CI2 = 2 miles of Cruise Intervals (anaerobic threshold);
T2 = Tempo 2 miles.
H2 = 2 miles of hill training.
BAE = Best Aerobic Effort is about 40 seconds slower than 10K pace.
70 WR = alternate walking with running at 60 seconds per mile slower than marathon pace.
2F, 20x100 or 16x200 = Run these striders on soft surfaces and no faster than 5K pace.
6 x 400 = no faster than 5K pace.

Low mileage recreational marathon.

	Day One	Two	Four	Five	Six
Week 1	CI2	40@M	4WR	2F	4WR
Two	T2	60WR	3E	2H	4WR
Three	CI3	45@M	4WR	6 x 400	3E
Four	3BAE	70WR	4WR	3F	4WR
Five	T3	50@M	4WR	2H	3E
Six	CI3	80WR	4WR	5 x 600	3E
Seven	3BAE	55@M	4WR	3F	4WR
Eight	T3	90WR	4WR	16 x 200	3E
Nine	CI3	60@M	4WR	2H	3E
Ten	3BAE	100WR	4WR	8 x 400	3E
Eleven	T3	65@M	4WR	3F	4WR
Twelve	CI3	110WR	4WR	2H	3E
Thirteen	3BAE	70@M	4WR	4 x 800	3E
Fourteen	T3	120WR	4WR	3F	4E
Fifteen	CI3	75@M	4WR	16 x 200	4E
16	3BAE	130WR	4WR	2H	4E
17	T3	80@M	4WR	8 x 400	4WR
18	CI3	140WR	4WR	3F	4E
19	3BAE	85@M	4WR	2H	4E
20	T3	150WR	4WR	6 x 600	4WR
21	CI3	90@M	4WR	2H	4E
22	3BAE	160WR	4WR	4 x 800	4E
23	T3	95@M	4WR	3F	4WR
24	CI2	180WR	3WR	20 x 200	4E
25	T2	100@M	4WR	2H	3E
26	3BAE	120WR	3WR	6 x 400	3E
27	T2	50@M	3WR	CI2	2WR and

then run/walk the marathon.

Growing older is a delight and perhaps a privilege. We have experience, plus we get to stay fit because we exercise. But we do tend to lose strength and speed. Incorporate 30 minutes of weight training twice a week; add a little aerobic cross-training and you can slow the rate at which you lose strength.

Don't Run a Marathon Until You're Ready.

Be Macho. Be strong and save your body for another race. If you missed some vital training or you have a cold you should stay at home on the big marathon day. Instead of an injury from the big event, you can have a successful marathon later. It's not macho to run yourself into the ground.

The side effects of running a marathon with insufficient training.

According to Dr. Sonny Cobble, of The Orthopedic Hospital of Los Angeles, who assists the hospital supported 'leggers' running group, "absolute devastating fatigue, can result when attempting a marathon with insufficient training." Problems include, "blisters, chafing, knee discomfort, hypothermia, dehydration, fatigue and in one case a fractured femur."

Chronic Fatigue Syndrome with anemia and other side effects is a long term problem. Normally associated with overtraining - which running a marathon can achieve in just one run - this syndrome involves illness, stress and injury due to exhausting body reserves. A near constant feeling of weariness is often present, and lasts for weeks. You probably run slower at the shorter distances and you should not even contemplate another marathon.

*   Exercise physiologists tell us physiological adaptation relating to endurance and muscle strength takes at least 14 days to show up: fourteen days after the training! Therefore, the longest run must be at least 2 weeks before the marathon to give any benefit. According to most coaches, the longest training run for a marathon must be at least 20 miles. But it takes a good series of base runs to build up to the 20 miler.

Bone and connective tissue adaptation takes months rather than weeks. Assessment about marathon readiness should be based on the length of runners' longest run each week for at least the last 8 weeks ending two weeks before the marathon, and how well the body reacted to the longer runs.

* Provided you've done 20 percent of your weekly mileage as speed running at faster than marathon pace, your race day pace should be based on 30 to 60 seconds per mile faster than the speed of your easy long runs done in training. Other factors are the number of runs over 15 miles, the length of the four longest runs, and the quality of speed running. If you do negligible speedwork, half of your long runs should include a long section at marathon pace. See Chapter 10.

* Come to terms with not running the marathon. It's much better, healthier, and even acceptable to pass over the hyped-up event, in favor of a smaller event when your body is ready. Give your body the opportunity to perform to its potential, without the pain and medical bills of a serious injury. It's not heroic to run a marathon before your body is ready. Reduce the number of runners staggering across the finish line, and stop your fellow runners and TV viewers from thinking those who do so are brave, determined or courageous. They are silly people who should have caught the safety van to the finish or not started at all.

* For those of you with the wisdom to wait 2 to 3 months, build on your current fitness level. Repeat a 14 or 21 day schedule several times. Each time you go through the schedule, add two miles to the longest walk / run, (until it reaches 20), and a mile to the two most important speed sessions, (until you're doing 4 miles worth). Take part in several 10K, 10 mile and half-marathon races at monthly intervals, then go to the marathon start line with an excellent chance of success based on realistic time goals.

CHAPTER SEVENTEEN

Your Running Future

TRAINING TIPS TO DECREASE INJURY RISK

Staying well nourished, stretching every day, cross-training two times a week and only running five days a week at appropriate speeds and distances for you? Glance through this chapter as you prepare yourself mentally for your marathon.

Avoid injury by backing off when early signs of stress occur. When running is no longer a joy for 90 percent of the miles, the rest of your life is probably affected. Back off on training and enjoy your other pursuits.

Overtraining & Injury warning signs include

stress from too much running, or from work, money, family or house moving etc. Monitor for:
1. Dull aching pains in joints, tendons or muscles, and slower recovery from training sessions. Your endorphins may override the pain signals after a few miles, or the pain may get worse: Either way, find the cause.
2. Sore feet and lower leg muscles for many days at a time.
3. Pain at old injury sites? Take an extra day or two off and do your next quality run in water or do biking or elliptical training intervals to allow for healing.

4.   Stress or fatigue usually decreases your running speed for a given effort. See the Fitness Test below.
5.   Feeling tired, cranky or sleeping poorly.
6.   Many illnesses such as sore throats, colds or flu; or skin conditions, mouth ulcers or swollen lymph glands.
7.   Loss of weight or extreme thirst in the evenings.
8.   Decreased sex drive.
9.   Higher than usual resting heartrate in the morning. 10 % higher and it's time to cut training volume back by 20 %, and run 30 seconds per mile slower for this mileage.
10. Heartrate 20 % higher, or does not return to normal after a week of easier and less running? Add extra rest days.
11. Feel dead at the beginning, middle *and* end of several runs, and with unusual fatigue levels. Take a few days off. Stretch daily and slowly while taking your break.

Consistency is vital for marathon training. Don't make a sudden change because you feel no difference after just 3 sessions at anaerobic threshold or hill repeats. Do months of these types of training while patiently awaiting results and make no sudden changes.

Fitness Test for Overtraining.

One of the best ways to check for overtraining is with a regular, but easily achieved pace trial. This is not a time trial. This fitness test requires that you run at a set speed for a modest distance. Wear training shoes instead of racing shoes to remind yourself it's not a time trial. You'll record your heartrate and compare it with previous pace checks.

A two mile trial check at 10K pace allows you to do it every two to four weeks depending on what races you're doing during the marathon preparation. You don't have to use the same area every time. A road, a running track or a treadmill at one percent elevation can be used depending on the days temperature and wind. Look for:

One: Same heartrate as usual indicates all is well, which may include that your muscles can handle the extra 5 miles per week which you added five weeks ago, or that you've recovered from your half marathon of three weeks ago.

Two: Lower heartrate than usual means that you're either fitter or more relaxed at 10K pace. Expect your heartrate to go down over the first three fitness tests as you learn to relax at 10K pace. Check your speed every quarter of a mile or 400 meters, but your heartrate every 200 meters of the second mile to monitor your progress. Done three sessions at 5K pace since your last fitness check? If the sessions were short enough for your muscles and tendons, and if you've recovered, you may achieve a lower heartrate in this test.

Other indications that training is going well include feeling very relaxed and rested mere minutes after the fitness test, with a high desire to do some additional quality running. After the test you could do a half session of training with 800s at 5K pace, or half a dozen hill reps, or cruising mile reps at anaerobic threshold depending on your current needs.

Three: Heartrate higher. 16 x 400 meters last week may have been too much. How achy you feel in the hour to 96 hours after a session is one clue, but it may take the fitness test to confirm that you're overtrained. Too much mileage, long runs too fast and other stressors have the same effect.

If your fitness test shows a higher than normal heartrate, you'll cooldown and begin a rest phase of from a few days to several weeks.

The second kind of Fitness Test which you can alternate with the above test is your running speed at a permanent heartrate. You will need to choose a heartrate which is relatively close to your favorite or best race distance. For instance, if your favorite event (despite training for a marathon) is the half marathon, and you know that your heartrate averaged 160 during your last half marathon, you'll run 20 to 30 minutes with your monitor showing a steady 159 to 161 beats per minute. Adjust your pace to stay within one beat per minute and record your total distance.

Warm up for the fitness test and do your striders, but then take about one mile, or up to 8 minutes to reach your goal heartrate. To reach 160 faster requires you to start off really fast, and you'll find running the rest of the test difficult.

As with the first fitness test, the terrain must be comparable, yet treadmills and tracks mean that you can do your test in any city. A dirt track will make your average pace 4 to 8 seconds per mile slower than usual. Treadmills vary too, so if the speed at a heartrate of 160 nets you 15 seconds per mile faster than usual, chances are that it's the machine.

If you cover the same distance as usual in 20 minutes at a heartrate of 160, your training is fine. Covered more distance than usual? You're improving. Less distance suggests overtraining.

Reduce stress levels before an injury occurs by:

* Reducing mileage by 20 percent;
* Cut a mile or two off of most runs;
* Take an extra day off from running;
* Do 3 miles of long reps at 15K pace instead of 4 miles of long reps at 5K pace;
* Run 12 relaxed striders on grass instead of a hill session;
* Swap relaxed sessions of fartlek on grass for track reps.

Address the cause of your stress. Take control of the stressors you have control over and learn to live with, or get away from those that you don't have control over. If you need to, change jobs or your living situation. Inertia, or not taking action to get away from a stressor is more damaging to you than taking action to break the cycle of stress in your life.

When moving house and or jobs, take at least 6 weeks of easy runs, with 3 miles at 5K effort once a week. When settled, you can gradually return to your former running duration and intensity.

Repeatedly getting small injuries can be the result of overtraining. When you're fresh, the awkward foot placement which sends you off balance can usually be corrected over the next few strides. However, when you're muscles are fatigued from high mileage or excessive amounts of quality running, you're less able to make rapid adjustments to your stride: You're more likely to injure yourself.

Warn-out running shoes are a big contributor to injuries. See page 323. Do the last 100 miles for each pair on very soft terrain.

When you get injured, ease off or rest for a few days to allow the tear and muscle strain to heal. Don't train through the injury if it hurts because you will put more strain on the healthy muscles due to your running style compensating for the unfit area. If you train with the first injury that would have taken two or three days to heal, you can strain another area which takes weeks to heal.

Don't overstride.

Run with a stride length compatible with your body type, height, joint ranges, muscle flexibility, footgear and running surface. You must have control over unnecessary movements, and keep good leg speed for the whole marathon. Overstriding slaps you in the face.

Your feet should kiss the ground at impact, not hit the ground. Flow across the ground. Find a nice running groove while looking 50 or so yards ahead to remain upright, or with a minimal forward lean. Don't look at your feet or you'll miss 90 percent of the joy from running. You can also reduce your trauma from ground impact by cross training. Your goal will be to build endurance into your running muscles, including abs, back and shoulder muscles.

Long strides are inefficient. Your stride length should not put you at a stretch on each revolution of the legs or stride cycle. Adjust your stride length and leg speed according to the distance you're running. In a ten mile race, runners automatically (if after blowing up a few times), start at a slower speed than in a 5K or five mile race.

Poor planning & Self-inflicted Injuries

The warm up and warm down, including stretching and strides must be sufficient to prepare the body for its task, and to relax afterwards. They are of equal importance.

Liniments or creams massaged into the skin help to warm up the local area, which can be useful for old strains and aches, but not to 'hide' an injury when rest would be more appropriate. The major benefit of creams is self massage, and thus the tendency to get this muscle well warmed up before commencing the run. Warm up exercises are more time efficient because you'll get your whole body ready to run.

A 10 percent volume increase for two or three weeks may be okay, but consolidate for a few weeks at your new level while converting some of that increase into speed running before moving up again. Restrict your pace increase to 8 seconds per mile or 2 seconds per 400 meters.

Olympic medalists run at 5K to 3K race paces most weeks in winter. So should you. This helps to maintain good form, thus decreasing injury potential. Move gradually to track sessions during Phase Four of each marathon preparation while maintaining strength and endurance with long runs.

Not following any of the training programs in this book? Independence is good, but plan your schedule to put stress on a different aspect of running on consecutive days. You may be able to handle 16 efforts of 200 meters up a hill on a Monday, but don't repeat it on the next four days, and "kill" your Achilles in the process. Don't run six miles hard and repeat it either. Spread the training load.

Certain sessions require easy, restive runs for the day or many days after. The body takes at least a week to get over a 10-mile all out race, and 4 weeks to completely recover from a marathon. During this time, the body needs rest, easy runs, some gentle running at modest pace and gentle stretching.

Assess how much time you need to recover from a particular training session. You may need four easy days a week, which allows you to do three quality sessions. Or, you may need three easy days after every quality session...which probably means those quality sessions are too harsh for you.

Back to back moderately hard days (the second day gives your legs a feeling which is close to the mid and late race fatigue), followed by two easy days may work for you. Or they may be your undoing because it would be overtraining.

You would also run the second session before the worst of the natural swelling from the first session hits you. Your back-to-back days must complement each other. A hill session at 5K to 2-mile intensity, followed 23 hours later by 600 meter repeats at 5K pace will usually result in a poor second session. Match either of those two sessions with 2-mile reps at 15K pace on the second day and it's more likely to be a success because there is 35 seconds per mile difference for the second day. Three days later do your second session at 5K intensity and you'll have the appetite and legs to run 4 to 5 miles worth of reps.

You must vary your training:

Did you run fast yesterday? Run at 70 % of max HR today. Last speed session short hills three days ago? Run long repeats at 10K pace today, and 800s at 5K pace on the grass three days later. See the sessions on pages 139 and 155. Long run of 13 miles last week? Do 15 or 18 this week.

As you get fitter, increase the quantity of your quality running. Build from 8 toward 16 repeats at 5K pace, using 300 meters to 800 meters repeats. Build from 3 to 8 repeats at 15K pace using half miles to over a mile, or up to 4 miles as a continuous run. Then gradually reduce the recovery between all intervals toward one minute.

Soft or forgiving terrain is important for injury prevention. Treadmill running beds half inch or more give on each stride, plus the four rubber pads which support the typical running bed is clearly an advantage over asphalt with its camber. See Chapters Two and Four. However, grass and trails get you scenery and stimulation from the light to enhance your mood and your speed.

Training tips to avoid the overtraining woes.

Perhaps you skipped Chapter Four?

Do Strength before Speed.

Run hills or hilly courses or run in mud or sand before attempting the speed sessions of Phases Three to Five. Use jumping and bounding exercises too. It may take 12 to 20 weeks of regular resistance training before your muscles are ready for the stresses of speed running.

Make sure you start well hydrated, and do a 10 to 15 minute warmup before stretching. Start your speed running sessions with striders of 100 to 200 meters on grass at 5K pace. Nothing flashy or fast. Practice your running form.

In the hours leading into a speed session, psych yourself up a bit. Visualize your running form and your strength, then put it into practice while controlling the speed of your first few repeats. Run with people of similar abilities mostly. Note: You can run 800s at 2 mile intensity while companions are doing 2 miles at 15K pace; run the first and last 800 meters with them. You can train with someone who is more than 2 minutes faster than you are at the 5K.

Run long repeats at 15K race pace (about 15 seconds per mile slower than 10K pace) before doing serious speed training. Alternate sessions of mile repeats with continuous tempo runs of 20 to 25 minutes at 15K pace. See Chapter Five.

You'll then be ready for VO2 max training. For most runners, 5K pace is fast enough. Experienced runners may wish to run 10 to 12 seconds per mile faster, which is 2 mile race pace. This is only 3 seconds per 400 meters faster than 5K pace, but it's 100 percent of a persons VO2 max. Running any faster than 2 mile race pace is pointless and adds substantially to your injury risk, and you spend very little time at ideal training heartrate.

Practice landing gently on even grass at 5K pace before running at speed on the track. Do one mile of gentle striders at 5K pace before moving up to 300 meters then 400 meter repeats. Gradually build up the number of repeats toward 10 percent of your total weekly mileage.

Having a bad track session? Cut out a few reps if you need to. Next time, don't run it the day after a 20, start the session well hydrated, at appropriate running pace and after a warm up with stretching and striders and you'll have cured 90 percent of the causes of poor speed sessions. You get 90 percent of the benefits from the first two thirds of the session, so 10 instead of 15 reps is still a success.

Variety during track sessions:

Doing 12 times 400 meters to improve your running economy? Run the first one nice and relaxed at 5K pace; the next repeat one second faster; the next with shorter, but faster strides yet restraining yourself to 5K pace again; for the fourth one, do the first 200 meters at 5K pace, but increase legspeed to 2 mile pace for the last 200 meters; then run a 5K pace rep but with higher knees than normal; then one where the emphasis is on whipping your leg through faster, or make full use of the ankles by pushing off with the calf muscle properly to propel you forward rather than upwards.

Mess around to work on different aspects of running form, while only changing pace by about one second. Your form changes can be so subtle that few people watching would notice that you are varying your workout!

Protect the hamstrings & butt muscles.

Twice weekly striders and sprint drills help keep these muscles in shape and avoid the bun burn when you run eight times a gentle 150 meters at the end of your summer track sessions. If your main training session was at 10K pace, run your 150s at a relaxed 5K pace. Your goal is to practice good running form while tired, not to get ready for a mile race. If you had done your main session at 5K pace, your 150s could be at 2 mile pace. Run 8 minute miles for a 10K? Try these two sessions:

4 x one mile in 8 minutes with 2 to 5 minutes rest, then 8 x 200 meters in 58.5 seconds. (10K pace followed by 5K pace).

6 x half mile in 3.54, followed by 8 x 200 in 57.5 (5K pace followed by 2 mile pace).

Whether you run 200s or un-timed 150s depends on your pace confidence. If you can restrain your pace for the 150, then 150s are far enough to practice the skill of running fairly fast at the end of a session. If you have a tendency to run more than half a second faster than the above times for the 200s...stick with 200s or move up to 300s so that you are forced to restrain your pace.

Marathon runners should be no more injury prone than 10K runners. Make sure you run efficiently in the last few miles of your long runs. No overstriding.

Minor pace changes on long runs too.

Your body talks to you constantly, but just like your significant other's ramblings, you're not always listening. Sleep studies show that humans change position almost hourly, yet many runners do three to four hour runs using the same stride length and surface the entire way. Vary your pace by 10-15 seconds per mile on purpose instead of due to the fatigue of the constant pace. Run a few hundred yards on grass and dirt every mile or two. Stretch the shoulders and arms every 30 minutes when you take your big hydration stops. Running in the city? Loop through schools and parks to include a bit of grass running, and to drink at the water fountains.

Run fast during long runs.

Long runs require more of your muscle fibers to work because the first ones used become tired...the technical word is fatigued!

During long runs your fat metabolism improves, and if you get dehydrated, your heartrate increases. Over many months, your VO2 maximum increases and your endurance rises! Once your running muscles have got used to the demands asked of them and adapt to their task, you can boost the training benefits by:

* Varying the pace by 10 to 15 seconds per mile;
* Increasing effort up some hills to maintain running speed with good form, instead of slowing down. Let your heartrate go up 10 beats per minute.
* Running close to marathon race pace toward the end of the run, which will make you concentrate on running form, while bringing in the last of your muscle fibers.
* But do not push yourself to maximum effort during these speed sections. Remain well under control. No sprinting.

You're training for the marathon, so try two times one mile at marathon pace at mile 14 of an 18. Do these speed sections on the grass or a track, and then finish your long run with another two miles at 70 percent max HR.

Your main speed sessions come later in the week, so keep the fast sections of your long runs to 10 percent of your long run. In your main speed sessions you'll be running 10 to 40 seconds per mile faster than race pace.

Four Weeks of Race Recovery.

Do a seven mile run each weekend and some gentle striders during this extended recovery, and then ease into a 5K or 10K program at modest mileage for a race about 10 weeks after your marathon. Significant numbers of injuries occur shortly after a long race.

Training Diaries show patterns which can help you prevent a

potential injury or overtraining. Anything significant about your drinking or eating habits that day or running at higher intensity, whether on purpose or not...record it. How you felt during or 6 hours after the run if significant or running in new shoes or have a potential injury ache...record it. Heartrate 10 beats per minute higher than usual during a steady run at known speed? You have another sign of overtraining, though perhaps it was dehydration or a hot day. Later, you can highlight items in the diary for ease of reference. Most days you'll only write 10-12 words.

You are not perfect!

Aim for consistently good training runs, not perfect training sessions. Be prepared to change your run if conditions make change the right choice. Your training does need structure, but you don't have to run 8 times half a mile at the track on a cold gusty day just because it's week three of your cycle. Some days you will run like the aged old dog that you are. Take a shower. You can run like an old dog again in 23 hours. Learn to accept your bad days. Had three old dog days in a row? It's probably time for a rest day. It could also be time for some gentle speed running!

Be positive. Be the engine which *can* get up the hill, at appropriate speed and with good running form. Tell yourself you *can* run those 800s at 5K pace; the wind is *only* 15 miles an hour; it will be relaxing to run into the wind with a slight forward lean.

As mentioned before, associate or think about your state of fatigue, running pace and breathing. Relaxing at appropriate pace while staying hydrated helps you to cope with your exertion, so monitor your body and running form every mile and you will end up running faster races. Visualize yourself running with good form before you train.

Don't try for personal bests in every session.

Usually, running a little slower than your best for a particular session is best. If you take a couple of rest days you'll be able to run 16 times 400 meters at 2 mile race pace. Sandwich that track session between a 10 mile tempo run at marathon pace and a 20 mile run at one minute slower than marathon pace, and the 400s will need to be at a more realistic 5K pace.

Just done a personal best for a training session? You either:
* Had it coming because of a solid month or months of training;
* Put more effort than you normally do into that days run;
* Had more rest in the last 96 hours;
* Recently lost some puppy fat;
* Preceded your run with the best sex of your year, and your partner did 60 percent of the work;
* Ran your weakest route on a course which you've rarely tried to run fast on before.
* Had a training partner, and actually ran the first 2 repeats at the right pace instead of too fast.

Most of the above leave you very relaxed and ready to race. Perhaps you should save it for your races? However, good training sessions are needed to prepare for races. But don't repeat the session tomorrow. Instead, take a steady to easy training run because in two or three days you'll need another quality run to work at a different aspect of your running.

Be specific:

Once a week, do a training session that is very specific to your next goal race. Racing a half-marathon soon? Tempo runs of 4 miles at 5 seconds per mile faster than goal pace, and mile to 1.5 mile repeats at 10 to 15 seconds per mile faster than goal pace would be your key sessions to improve your anaerobic threshold.

You still need tempo running if you're racing 5Ks; you still need 5K pace sessions to race the half-marathon.

Next race disgusting hilly or pancake flat? Do key sessions on similar terrain, but do some training on completely different terrain for variety and to prevent over training a particular group of muscles.

While we cannot stop chronological aging, we can slow physiological aging. You can aim to race at the same age graded performance as you did at your peak. If you entered this sport late, you can also compare your current performances on the age graded tables to see how fast you could have been in your late 20s or early 30s, which is the peak for distance runners.

Once you've reached your actual peak, expect and accept a 5 percent decrease in your performance *times* per decade. Train for the same length of time, at the same relative intensity of previous years, and you should maintain the same age graded performance. See londonheathside.org.uk/wava.htm click on age-grading.

No mile should be a wasted mile.

Every mile has its purpose. An easy warm up mile sets up the rest of the run, reducing injury risk, while also working your muscles and adding to your endurance.

It's the easy 4 to 8 mile runs between harder sessions which gives you the endurance for those hard sessions, while also giving you recovery from the hard sessions. These runs must be easy enough to rest your legs; your speed sessions must be easy enough that it only takes three days to recover from them. Example: Did 15K pace intervals on Monday? You should be ready for hill repeats or VO2 max training by Thursday and you should be rested for a long run by Sunday.

Time to relax? Use Chapter Three's

Fartlek or Speedplay instead of Track Sessions.

Don't feel like the formality of a track session? Run 2 miles easy on the most enjoyable surface convenient to you, then pick up the pace for a few seconds. Run at 5K pace for 15 seconds, gliding along nice and relaxed with good running form. Be generous to your stressed out mind, and run easily for 45 seconds. Stride out again for 15 seconds. Then start another strider every minute, but run two each of 20, 25 and up to 40 seconds. By starting every minute, the 40 second efforts will give you a 20 second breather. Now you're training!

Still want an easy session...two each at 30 and 20 seconds gets you out with 16 repeats. Running *actual* 5K pace instead of sprinting? Used to three miles at speed in a session, and feel like doing a solid session? Run two efforts of 45 seconds, and then go back down the pyramid 5 seconds at a time gives you 26 repeats. The intensity is as high as you're willing to make it. Two-mile race pace is a thrill, or stay at 5K intensity.

The running environment for this run should be pleasant, and if you're lucky, inspiring. You can count footfalls instead of timing the repeats. Count just the left foot, or the right foot. Or you can count breathing cycles. Former Boston marathon winner, European and Commonwealth Champion Ron Hill would call this a number stride fartlek session. It can be done on roads, trails, huge grass areas and in deep sand or in dry and muddy river beds.

Want to give up halfway through your track session?

You probably need to adjust the session because you're:
* Not ready to run this particular session. Don't jump from 10 x 400 meters at 5K pace to 12 repeats at 2 mile race pace. Instead, reduce to 8 repeats the first time, running the first four at 5K pace, then two seconds per lap faster than 5K pace for each of the remaining four. Next time (about three weeks later

because you'll be rotating several sessions) try 3 at 5K pace to set you up for 6 reps at 2-mile pace (3 seconds faster for the 400 meters). Next time, try one rep at 5K pace, one at one second faster, before hitting 2-mile pace for the remaining 8 repeats. Gradually move up to 12 reps.

* Still want to give up? You started the session too fast, or with insufficient warm up, or neglected to include several striders before the first repeat. Run the first 100 meters of each rep at the right speed.
* Insufficient recovery between repeats. Heartrate should come down to 110 before your next effort.
* It's significantly hotter or colder than usual; you're over or under dressed.
* Wearing your slow shoes instead of your lightweights.
* You had a stress filled day or week.
* You are dehydrated, bloated or overtrained.

Completing two-thirds of a session will give you 90 percent of the training benefits. Continue your session to reach and run the 8th of 12 repeats, and if you still feel the need, warmdown and go home. Otherwise, make the adjustment. Change the pace, increase the rest, take sips of water, run 400s at 5K pace instead of 600s. Do whatever it takes to get your planned 3 or 4 miles of repeats.

Parts of some sessions have to hurt a bit. Avoid sudden changes and you'll know you can complete the session, and still run a 2 mile warmdown afterwards.

VO2 Max Does Decline.

Unfit people lose one percent of their oxygen uptake capacity and muscle strength each year. In steady training? You should only lose half of one percent each year. Staleness comes from doing the same thing week after week without goals. As you have a marathon planned in 10 months, with races at the half-marathon and several 10K and 5Ks too, you have many goals. Because you'll be using five training phases, you also vary your training. Still losing too much fitness or slowing down? Possible causes are:

1. You're about to get injured. Go back to page 302. You may need a few weeks of easy training to rest from a race or to heal an injury.

2. Circulation and other internal health problems such as anemia: Do an exercise stress test with a cardiologist who is used to testing fit people. Get a full physical too. Several diseases come on line in our 40s and 50s.

3. Running too fast. Running as fast as you did 6 years ago in training is probably over training now. If you did 10 miles at 7.30 per mile at age 46 because your 10Ks were at 6 minute pace, (37:17) you need to slow down by 10 to 15 seconds per mile at 51 (because your 10Ks are now 39 minutes). This years sessions will be taking more out of you if you continue to train at 7.30 pace, making you more fatigued.

4. Need some speed variety. Legspeed is one of the first things to go as we age. You can maintain most of it by running 8 to 16 times one hundred meters twice a week (in addition to your formal speed session). Running on grass works well. Practice good running form for the 100s and during all of your running. No need to do more than one mile at speed for these pick-ups, but do a few of them with high knees, a few with a bounding high and long (and inefficient stride) to gain strength. Do most of them with good form though. Don't run more than 10 seconds faster than 5K pace.

5. Don't forget your hill training. When running short hills, this author favors 10 minutes of hill repeats at 5K or up to 2 mile intensity. This could mean 10 repeats of 60 seconds, or 15 of 40 seconds. One in three hill sessions should really be up a longer, gentle hill. Five mile to 10K race intensity, with 15 to 20 minutes of up hill running works well (using repeats of 3 to 5 minutes).

6. VO2 max variety. Unless you can run about 8 times 800 meters at your expected 5K pace, with a one minute rest, you should not expect to be able to race a 5K at that pace. Run some 300s and 500s at 2 mile pace. Run some 1,200s and miles at 5K pace. You can rotate 4 to 6 different sessions.

Running magazines keep stressing that we need more rest days between hard sessions as we age. However, if you train at this years 5K pace you may still only need the one or two days rest you needed at age 36.

Do the same percentage of your training miles that you did at your peak. Did 6 miles at 5K pace when on 60 miles per week at age 30? Mileage now 45 per week at age 50? 4.5 miles at this years 5K pace is your session, but do mostly mile reps instead of 1,200s to get nearly as much training time at 5K heartrate level as you did 20 years ago.

Reduce the recovery when you run 800s (Chapter 7).

Continue to do a bit of running at 2 mile race pace for the joy of it by running say 3 x 300 or 2 x 400 meters at the end of your 800s. Stay relaxed though.

7. Don't forget anaerobic threshold training. Do long repeats at 30 to 40 seconds per mile slower than 5K pace. In general, start with two miles at 15K pace, and add a quarter mile each week for a second rep. After 8 weeks, run 2 times 2 miles one week, alternating with a 4 mile run at 15K pace. It takes another 6-10 weeks to show up as improved fitness with faster races.

8. Long runs should be over 15 miles consistently, but preferably be only *one third* of your weekly mileage. Consider putting your bike ride onto the end of your Sunday runs to build endurance, and rehydrate while exercising.

9. Don't let cross training dominate. Running requires specificity. These were covered in *Best Half Marathons.*

* Provided you're already doing hill repeats and bounding, weight training is the most important cross training. Do 2 sets for 90 percent of the gains of 3 sets. Then add:

* Pool running, which keeps you cool with no impact forces.

* Elliptical training, which requires that you stand up and weight bear. 20 minutes at 70 percent of your maximum heartrate after a 5 mile run will make the session equivalent to a 7 mile run.

* Cycling, which builds quadriceps and lengthens the hamstrings. Ride 20 miles twice a week, then save your legs for running.

10. Rest up before your major races. Three or four times a year, decrease all sessions by 20 percent in the penultimate week, and by 40 to 50 percent in the final week. This will be for your two marathons and for a couple of half marathons.

Once a month for the other 8 months of the year, rest up by 40 percent for one week to allow your training to take hold physiologically, and to do a 5K to 10 mile race.

<u>Here are 3 Golden Rules of Speed Training</u> from a national running magazine (*in italics*) followed by this authors' contrary view!

* *Follow speed training days with easy running.* Absolutely agree. 24 hours after your speed session, run your 18 to 20 miles at one minute per mile slower than marathon pace. A nice easy paced run as recovery from speed running.

* *Don't do speedwork until your muscles have zero aches.* Follow this rule and you'll never be able to do speed running because we always have some residual aches from our long Sunday runs. You can train at 15K pace on very tired legs; train at 5K pace on fairly tired muscles. Run an appropriate amount at each pace so that you can run an easy 10 miler between the speed sessions.

* *Don't do speed running if the weather turns hot, cold, windy or wet.* Rubbish. Oops, wrong country, I mean garbage. Run intervals into the wind and driving rain, but dress to remain warm though not toasty hot. You can work at 10K intensity into the wind while your legs are ambling along at half marathon pace. Jog 30 seconds if it's cold, and then cruise back with the wind, but at half marathon intensity for your heart, while at 10K pace for your legs.

  Two days later, if the weather is still nasty, you can wear two layers of clothing for 500 meter reps on grass or at the track. Run two straights into the wind, and one straight with the wind.

  Heat the problem? Find some shade. Take a few ounces of sports drink while walking recoveries in the shade. You don't have to use a track for speed running. Wooded trails save you from the sun and the wind.

  Treadmills save you from all the elements. Find a pay by the day club for emergencies. If your speed running is faster than the 10 miles per hour which is the typical machines maximum speed, raise the elevation. Each 1 % increase is worth 10 to 15 seconds per mile for most of us (see page 92).

Races are rarely cancelled due to inclement weather. Learn to run in all kinds of condition. Learn the joys of running in the rain, snow and 100 degrees Fahrenheit. See Chapter Two for safety tips in nasty conditions.

The relatively minor problems of the next few pages can lead to major connective tissue damage or muscle strains. Treat these problems as injuries because your running style may change to keep pressure off of the sensitive area.

Chapter Two suggested you carry a bottle of diluted fruit juice or sports drink to decrease injury risk from dehydration. Pack a small tube of petroleum jelly, some lip balm and a dollar fifty "First Aid To Go" mini first aid kit which has antiseptic wipes, antibiotic ointment, band-aids and a couple of pain pills and you'll be covered for most falls and blisters.

Athlete's foot is a fungal infection that is itchy and painful. Avoid it by drying your feet soon after running because the fungus loves warm, moist places. Use a fungicide such as Tinactin or Lamisil several times a day. Or try a 1:1 apple cider vinegar and water soak three times a week. Treat for another 10-14 days after the symptoms clear.

Black toenails are often from shoes with insufficient room in the toebox or from downhill running, which is when your toes get intimate with the end of your shoe. Buy a half size bigger next time. Use a sterile needle to drain the blood or blister which is often under the nail, or let the body reabsorb it. Antibacterial creams will decrease the risk of infection. The nail will fall off in a month or two. Keep your nails short (cut them strait across) to decrease this problem.

Blisters Repetitive friction causes the top layers of skin to separate, and then fluid comes in magically to decrease additional damage. When you get a blister, adjust the position of your sock or other annoying item, and run home because walking home takes at least 80 percent more strides to get you there!

After a shower, pop the blister with a sterile needle at the blisters edge, leaving the skin to protect the area; or you can leave the fluid in. Use antiseptic creams on raw or broken blisters.

Avoid blisters by building mileage up slowly; break in new shoes with a walk and a few short runs before using them for a long run. Throw out old socks. Buy plenty of wicking, synthetic material socks. Antiperspirant helps keep your feet dry. Use baby powder inside of your socks and pad problem areas with moleskin, band-aids or use stuff such as Blister Block or Second Skin.

If your smaller foot is significantly so, wearing a second, but thin sock that side may help.

For Bunions, a bony protuberance on the outside of the big toe, wear shoes which are wide in the forefoot. Pronation is a causative factor, and wearing pointed narrow shoes speeds their development. Use a spacer between the big and second toe. Doughnut pads can help. Don't wear pointed narrow shoes. Painful bunions may need surgery, especially if they restrict movement of your toes.

Calluses can be a later stage to blisters and should be welcomed as they protect you. Don't let them become too thick because the edges have a habit of blistering. File them after a shower, or use moisturizers. Use well-fitting shoes and thick socks.

Chafing is first cousin to blister, and is raw skin secondary to constant rubbing, especially of nipples, at bra lines, under the arms and the inner thigh. Prevent or decrease problems with ointments such as Vaseline, petroleum jelly, A & D cream, or Body Glide. Even when you wear soft, breathable clothing, an uneven seam can catch you out by mile 18. Don't let your shorts ride up into your groin. Avoid race day t-shirts for running because the pretty pictures will rub your nipples raw. If you smear some cream on your nipples, place a band-aid on top, running in appropriate thickness t-shirts is usually fine, but don't use the one which you got for entering today's race.

Hammertoes: claw like toes and the longer small toes may buckle under. Wear shoes which are long enough for running and for the rest of your life. Plenty of wiggle room and at least half an inch from the end of the longest toe to your shoe.

<u>Heel Pains</u> can simply mean too much slippage because your shoes are loose, but are also a warning sign for:
* Plantar Faciitis due to the fascia being pulled off its attachment to the heel bone.
* Achilles trouble from its insertion into the heel bone, or from an inflammation close to the insertion.
* Ankle ligaments and nerves being pressured or strained.

Refer to the relevant sections in Chapter 19 and see an expert it necessary.

<u>Ingrown toenails</u>: Signs are pain, swelling and redness. Use warm soaks to treat. Cut toenails straight across and wear shoes which are wide in the forefoot.

<u>Morton's foot</u> is not a disease, but it means your second toe is longer than the big toe, may make you more prone to black toenails, predisposes you to stress fractures of the second metatarsal, and makes you more likely to overpronate: so get your running shoes checked and keep plenty of space in the forefoot area or toebox, and half an inch at the end of your longest toe.

<u>Warts</u> are a viral infection and respond well to salicylic acid in liquid form.

The next 47 pages show numerous types of injury which will either prevent you from doing your planned marathon, or merely take you out of training for days to weeks and require that you adjust your training program such as spending two weeks less on 10K pace Intervals.

You don't have to run this marathon. Once you're over the initial injury, you can ease up to 40 miles per week for 3 to 6 months and then commence a 15 to 17 week marathon program.

You may enjoy your 3 to 6 months a bit more if you take an easy week with just three runs of 5 miles once a month for relaxation. You can also use the very easy week as a rest before a 10K, but cruise 3 one-mile reps at 5 mile pace and 5 x 800 meter reps at 5K pace at 7 and 4 days pre-race.

Chapter Eighteen

MUSCLE INJURIES

Never take pain pills before running. Never take anti-inflammatory painkillers so that you can train. Don't mask your pain. Do use ice or cold water on muscles and tendons after your longest or hardest sessions to speed your recovery.

Simple actions prevent many injuries. Getting sore Achilles tendons? Stretch the calf muscles regularly, decrease mileage and cut the tabs off the back of your shoes and you may be cured in a few weeks. It can take a bit more skill to recognize some problems.

Though you increased mileage and intensity gently to prepare for your marathon, because every runner has a different injury threshold, you're likely to encounter the frustrations from injuries from time to time. Exercise don't train is this books motto, which is an exaggeration of the train don't strain philosophy. When you've got used to 8 mile runs most days, the first 5 miles of each run is simply exercise when done at the right intensity. The next 2 miles are no faster, but feel a bit harder. These are your training miles. The last mile includes easing up: don't ever sprint the last 400 meters.

The same with speed running. The first mile of 5 times one mile at 5K pace is very pleasant. Take 60 second rests and you'll be cursing this author at the 800 meter point of your third repeat, and for all but the first 400 meters of the last repeat. Only half of your 5 miles will feel like training, and you should still not be straining because your "job" is to focus on relaxed running at 5K pace.

Provided you do your speed running at the appropriate pace, high mileage is the best predictor of injuries.

While each running ailment has its own causes, the injuries discussed here and in Chapter 19 can nearly all be caused by:

* Inappropriate running shoes which make your overpronation or over supination worse for you. Use appropriate shoes for your feet and running style, plus orthotics if needed to correct most of your problem.
* Running on hard or hilly surfaces;
* Not warming up properly;
* Not stretching enough, especially the calf muscles;
* Making sudden changes to your training, including:
* Increasing mileage too fast or simply doing too much;
* Adding speedwork too rapidly:
* Running your speedwork so fast that it becomes work.

Any of the above can cause early fatigue, which your body will compensate for by changing your running biomechanics, placing stress on muscles and joints. Sometimes you will come up lame or achy. Eventually, you'll injure yourself.

Minor aches can develop into significant injuries. Try to sense what your muscles are telling you using Chapter 17s tips and back off before an injury.

Lets look at the first item, <u>running shoes</u>, because there are three general ways in which we run. Have a podiatrist or an experienced runner watch your running form, or get yourself video taped. Experts in running shoe stores can be your specialist. Show them some of your old running shoes and have them watch you test run a few new pairs. Make sure that you also test a neutral shoe with no special devices even if you've got a history of over pronating.

You can also test yourself at home. Walk a few steps with bare feet and then place them about 3 inches apart. The normal feet possessed by about 50 percent of people will be directly below the knees. The big toes will point forward.

You're a <u>neutral runner</u>, and your feet should roll nicely or pronate about the right amount. You probably will not need an anti-pronation or anti-supination shoe, but you still have three choices based on measuring the length of your feet when sitting and standing.

324 Best Marathons by David Holt

* No change? Your feet are rigid and you'll probably get a good ride from cushioned shoes.
* Foot length increase by 3 millimeters or less makes you a normal, normal. (Normal pronation and normal flexibility.) Weird, but your shoe type is a stability shoe.
* Highly flexible feet increase in length by more than 3 millimeters and while stability shoes work for many, others appreciate a motion-control shoe.

The wet foot test is another predictor of your arches' habits. With wet feet, stand on a few sheets of newspaper, and then check your foots shape. If you see your entire arch in your footprint, you have a low flexible arch or flat foot, and as you'll see in the next paragraph, you'll probably overpronate. If you see almost nothing of the arch in your footprint, you're high arched and likely to underpronate. Have a footprint that is narrower in the middle of the foot than at the heel? You lucky and some would say normal people should have a neutral foot plant in running because you have medium arches.

One quarter of peoples' feet splay outward when standing (called duck feet by some). Arches usually collapse during impact shock, which can wreak havoc on your Achilles, shins, knees and hips. Your shoe type is clearly a stability or motion control for <u>overpronators,</u> and most of your mileage should probably be on board lasted or combination lasted shoes. There are racing shoes and performance trainers for overpronators. Orthotics allow many runners to use cushioned or regular running shoes.

<u>Wear anti-pronation</u> shoes if appropriate. Different pronators need different amounts of resistance on the inside to stop their feet from rolling over. Just because your pronating friend swears by his 'Ni-bok' 720s, doesn't mean they'll suit you. Based on advertisements you would think that 90 percent of runners overpronate, but you're only about 25 percent of the running population. If your shoes are bashed in on the inside after a hundred miles, you need a meatier anti-pronation device and or orthotics, but you can also work on running form a bit to roll through your stride more efficiently.

Roughly one quarter of peoples' feet splay inward which is pigeon toed. You have a tendency toward high arches and rigid feet which <u>underpronate</u> on each stride, decreasing your ability to absorb shock. You'll need extra cushioning and perhaps a single-density midsole. A curved last or a slip lasted base will assist your cushioning, making them soft and flexible which encourages you to pronate a bit. You may also be called <u>supinators</u> because you land on the inner part of the foot and then roll outwards, though many of you are partial to landing on the outer part of the foot (anywhere from heel to little toe) but not pronating or rolling over enough.

All runners should buy their shoes late in the day, when your feet have expanded to their largest point. Wear your normal running socks and your orthotics to test them. Get your feet measured. Your shoes will need to be about half an inch beyond your big toe when standing. Buy for the largest foot. If you need to, add padding or an extra sock to your small foot. Wear a size 9 running shoe? Some manufacturers may be a full size either way. Test them. You'll need a snug fit at the heel to prevent slipping on every stride, but the ball of your foot needs comfort too. After checking comfort with walking, run a few hundred yards to give the final test. Don't go shopping a few hours after your 20 mile run!

Your feet may roll at different rates, so the wonkiest foot needs correcting. Stop that one from wobbling on each stride, and the better foot's workload is also lessened. Heed the store-person's advice but give a nod to how each shoe feels to you. Arch supports or orthotics inside the shoe may also be needed.

If only your right foot overpronates, running with the traffic (the right side in the U.S.) will allow the camber to correct your body's fault. However, long term, it's better to get your footwear corrected by using orthotics so that you can run on a variety of flat surfaces, plus you won't have to trust drivers to avoid you.

In cold temps, polyurethane can become rigid, so consider gel, air or other cold resistant adaptations for your winter shoes.

Orthotics or a simple heel lift one side can also adjust your leg length differences, which reduces the strain on your longest leg. A shorter leg alters the alignment of the spine, increasing injuries such as sciatica and I-T band syndrome. It also decreases running efficiency.

Pelvis to foot x-rays are the most accurate way to measure leg lengths, however, most therapists can measure you adequately in their offices: They'll have you lie down, place your hips in alignment, perhaps raise your legs to 'shake them out,' then check for the position of the heels.

You can self check while standing. In the mirror, see how level the top of the pelvis is. If one side is lower you have your first hint. Place a magazine under the foot of the short leg. Add more magazines until the hips are level. Your spine may have curved over the years to help compensate for the difference.

If you've had unexplained problems with any of your leg joints or back, see a specialist. Try a heel insert for the short leg, and consider orthotics to avoid future injuries, while shaving minutes off of your marathon time.

Each foot has 26 bones and 20 muscles kept together by ligaments and tendons. Keep it supple and free of cramps with stretching; place it in comfortable shoes with at least a half inch of space at the end of the toes; tie the laces for a firm, but not a tight fit; correct any leg length differences and there's a good chance they won't frustrate your running ambitions.

The foot absorbs shock on every stride, adapting to the ground, relaxing and rolling inwards (pronating) during midstance or the support phase as some call it, and then becomes rigid again as it becomes a lever, with the strong calf muscles acting on them to spring or propel you forward.

Got a pain on the top of your foot? Are your feet high arched? Do you tend to have tight calves? These can cause your extensor tendons on the top of the foot to overwork. Pain can extend to the toe, especially at push-off. Loosen those laces, use a good warmup with stretching, and the first time you make a mistake, use ice.

Finding an Injury Expert.

Muscle and non-muscular injuries are frequently related to each other. Biomechanical imbalances, overuse and sudden changes in training cause most running injuries. See a sports specialist from any field that has an interest in and an understanding of the mechanics specific to running.

If the front office questionnaire includes a section for your typical training, and other hints suggesting athletes or runners are given individual attention, you could be at the right office.

Your mechanical problems are unique. Get yourself measured for leg length, muscle size or strength and flexibility. You should also be watched when running.

Your treatment should emphasize...Injury Prevention, Stretching, Strengthening, Special Treatments which need to be done by the specialist, and Rehabilitation. Retain control over your rehab decisions, just as you do with your running decisions.

Inform the specialist of other recent, even minor injuries which you have suffered. Give the person a chance to diagnose you properly.

Just like serious diseases, there are several stages to an injury.

Denial: Runners find it difficult to stop running. It's Wednesday, so it must be an 8 to 10 mile run, but the back of your right knee really hurts from the 800s that you did last night. After a 400 meter walk, you ease into a gentle run and the knee still hurts. If you walk back and shower and then ice the offensive body part, you've overcome denial and will not make the problem worse, but you may still have some problems with...

Anger with yourself for running one extra 800 or for doing them 4 seconds faster than usual on Tuesday, or perhaps it was only 3 days after a superb 10K race!

Acceptance: If your pain level is the same the next day, and you prevent yourself from trying to run, you're half way to the cure for your injury. But you're probably still not ready to see an expert. You do some research and find out about the popliteal muscle (or popliteus) which crosses the back of the knee and helps to flex the leg. You weight train at modest intensity, during which the only exercise that hurts is the first few inches of the hamstring curl. Hmm.

You still hurt on Friday, but you're positive the tendons of the large muscles are OK, and you call an injury expert, who based on your symptoms, suggests you:

328 Best Marathons by David Holt

1. Ice behind the knee for 10 to 15 minutes several times each day.
2. Take NSAIDs every 4 to 6 hours for a week because it takes several doses to get the full anti-inflammatory response from these medicines.
3. Use Epsom salt soaks. The magnesium relaxes muscles once its absorbed through the skin, soothes pain and helps your muscles to repair themselves.
4. Drop the saddle on your bike by one inch for a couple of weeks to reduce the strain behind the knee with less risk of hyperextending the knee.
5. Walk instead of run this weekend and take short steps.
6. If pain free at walking pace, you can re-commence running, but run slower than usual on Monday to test the knee and call back for an appointment if you have not managed 2 miles, but he asks that you do no more than 4 miles and use a short stride.
7. Says there is a good chance you'll be back to full sessions at threshold pace in three weeks, and can ease up to 5K pace after a couple more weeks.
8. Next time you're at 5K pace, increase the speed of your 800s by 2 seconds per mile, not by 2 seconds per 400 meters.

Running and other aerobic exercise produces a feeling of wellness and is an anti-depressant. Because you're a regular cross trainer you avoid feeling sorry for yourself.

You do show patience: You help out at the 5K race you'd been intending to do as a time-trial, and swap injury war stories with what seems like half of the runners, all of whom are racing this day. You know that you will be back in a few weeks, and take and enjoy the recommended walk with your spouse.

Note: Some injuries take months to heal - usually the ones that took months to show themselves. Find the cause while healing the current injury or you'll re-injure yourself.

Your injury rehabilitation commences the minute you get hurt. Early use of cooling measures...a pond can reduce the swelling while you wait for transport...will save you much distress. To prevent the problem getting worse, stop running.

MUSCLE PROBLEMS, treat with PRICE.

<u>Prevent or protect</u> your muscles from more damage with Rest, Ice, Compression and Elevation.

<u>Rest:</u> A slightly strained muscle responds well to running fewer miles at a slower pace than which you normally train.

When you injure yourself, and it's you who does the injuring, blood vessels at the injury site expand. The extra fluid or edema causes pain. Don't mask pain with Tylenol.

<u>Ice:</u> Blood is needed to bring in repair materials but too much inflammation constricts blood flow, and can interfere with healing: combat the swelling with ice. Use ice for 15 minutes each hour for two days.

Ice decreases inflammation, preventing many sore spots becoming injuries. Hosing your legs with cold water after a run has the same effect, and it can ease significant fatigue, plus it'll bring your body temperature down. You can use real ice to cool the inflamed area or use frozen peas or other vegetables or use gel packs, including Velcro wine chillers which can be fastened to your legs. Within minutes of taking off the ice pack, blood will rush to your injured area and bring in nutrients to help with healing.

Place a thin towel on the ice pack and you can lay your leg on the pack, allowing your weight to add pressure to the pack. Because heat brings in more blood and fluid, use warmth only after all the swelling has subsided, typically at least 48 hours. Lay warm packs on top of your legs and with a towel on top of the skin to decrease risk of burns from too much pressure.

<u>Compression bandage:</u> Use a wide crepe bandage in preference to a narrow one. Apply it in a series of figure of eight, working toward the heart, with each layer half over-lapping the previous layer. Ace bandages require less skill. Don't let either type become a tourniquet.

<u>Elevating</u> the achy limb for an hour at a time helps to decrease inflammation also, but your main partner is ice.

Still hurting after multiple ice applications and elevation? Take an appropriate dose of NSAIDs (non-steroidal anti-inflammatory drugs) to reduce the inflammatory response, but not on an empty stomach. Pure painkillers like Tylenol are better for some people.

Your decision depends on whether you'd like to risk your stomach (one to two hundred thousand hospitalizations a year are from NSAIDs use and ten percent result in death) or your liver.

NSAIDs can decrease your muscle inflammation and pain. Some inflammatory response is needed to bring in nutrients and get rid of damaged cells so don't overdo the pill popping. Don't turn off or mask the pain with pills so that you can run or you'll miss your body's warning to slow down or stop. Painkillers should not be taken before exercise to allow you to train harder. Use pain pills for short-term aches due to slips while running or mistakes in training. Don't use pills for a chronic problem. Find and cure the cause of the problem.

Take appropriate doses of analgesics. A few years ago, the NY City Marathon included an 8 Advil sample pack in its goodies bag. Hundreds of people took all 8 pills straight after the race and had stomach problems. While NSAIDs are decreasing the inflammatory response at your joints and muscles, they are also decreasing the lining of your stomach. Whether taking enteric coated pills or not, you're still increasing your ulcer risk. The newer Cox II inhibitors also cause stomach problems, have not been shown to be any better, and Vioxx was removed from the market in 2004 due to side effects on the heart.

Stay hydrated when on analgesics or the side effects are more likely due to higher drug concentrations in the blood.

Heavy exercise raises the level of free radicals, which can make your muscles sore. Finnish researchers showed that taking 2,000 milligrams of vitamin C before, during and after a 10K race speeds recovery. Vitamin E works too. Use this combination for 5 or 6 key sessions per month to avoid the side effects from too much vitamin intake.

As a rule, muscle strains at the back of the legs are from running too fast, or overstriding. Rest and slow down.

Cutting out speedwork for a few days of active rest, and putting your muscles through a comfortable range of motion will bring nutrients to the muscle and stimulate repair. You will also maintain fitness.

Massage can increase circulation, bringing nutrients and oxygen to cramping or damaged muscles to speed healing or at least make the ache more comfortable for you. Massage can reduce pain and stress levels, but try not to use it to enable you to get straight out to the track again and restrain the original torn muscle. Deep tissue massage, moving in the same direction as the muscle fibers can get rid of adhesions and give you back your range of motion.

Muscle tears are graded from first-degree strains with little muscle damage and no restriction in range of motion; to second-degree with more damage and swelling; to third-degree with complete rupture of the muscle unit and severely limited movement. Usually, the more it hurts, the greater is the area of muscle tissue strained. Third degree strains often need to be seen by an injury specialist, who will help you overcome the pain and the potential for lasting damage if not properly and patiently rehabbed. Specialists also have ultrasound treatments to increase the blood flow and to decrease the scare tissue.

A major muscle tear requires that you stop running for 7 to 10 days; minor tears, if not hurting when you run, heal with active rest. But, run 30 seconds per mile slower than usual;
* Avoid long runs...do two sevens instead of a 14;
* Avoid hills...you tend to run too fast down them.
* No speed running.
* Don't overstride.
* Run on soft, even surfaces while rehabbing.
The combination of easy running and RICE for the acute phase of about two days, then stretching to regain your range of motion should help your muscle recuperate.

Practice good running form before you do speed sessions again. Wear appropriate shoes. If you use lightweight racers for speed sessions, do copious stretching of the calf and Achilles to prepare them for the lower heel. Ease into the fast running after your warmup, stretching, drills and striders. Do fewer reps for the first couple of sessions back.

Be aware of burnout and overtraining syndromes such as DOMS (page 332). Once you've chosen the right shoe type for you, rotate several pairs. Use sorbothane inserts to absorb up to 96 percent of the shock from hitting the planets surface.

It may take several little injuries to find your training threshold this year, or this life, and to find an exercise, or shoe or training regime which enables you to overcome it. By training a little below this injury threshold limit, and investing time to correct a weakness, you can maintain improvement.

<u>Delayed Onset Muscle Soreness (DOMS)</u> is

the muscle aches and pains you feel after a particularly hard workout or race. DOMS typically peaks 48-72 hours after the session, but may last for several more days. DOMS is an overuse inflammation of the muscle tissue: The swelling reduces blood flow leading to muscle spasms. Exhausted and inflamed muscle fibers express themselves to you as pain and you'll suffer from many micro charley horse cramps due to your muscle tears.

Walking at the end of the original session (because you knew the session was harder than normal!), plus stretching and easy exercise for a few days should see you back to normal. Ice and cold water does wonders in the early phase.

Be careful about exercising these achy muscles because they are prone to straining. If your pain is severe, or throbbing, or lasts more than a few days, heed its warning before you permanently harm yourself. If running still hurts after several days, take a complete rest and go see a sports injury specialist.

Ignore training pains at your peril or you'll get what you deserve, which is a long break from running.

See Chapter Eight for hydration skills to decrease your risk of DOMS. Eat a balanced diet with loads of antioxidants such as in cranberries, blueberries, black beans and the citrus family and vegetables to help decrease muscle soreness. You can also decrease your risk of DOMS by not making sudden changes to your training.

Cramps toward the end of tough sessions or races are due to poor conditioning compared to what you're currently asking your body to do, which is the same as overexertion or fatigue. Poor nutrition and dehydration (see Chapter Two) can bring on these cramps and possibly DOMS after a relatively small increment in training pace or distance.

Raced a marathon to perfection? You deserve aches and, except for three to five miles at a leisurely pace every other day, you deserve several weeks off from running. Former marathon world record holder Ingred Kristiansen usually had to take the elevator after marathons because her legs hurt so much, and took a week off of running and then an easy week before gradually increasing mileage and intensity.

Completed five miles worth of 400 meter repeats at your 2 mile race pace? You probably overtrained. You should be running 15 miles the next day. For most runners, 16 times 400 at 5K pace would be ideal and not too strenuous the day before a 15. Don't whoop your legs so much on Saturday that you're unable to feel relaxed during your long Sunday run.

You should have moderate amounts of aches or fatigue from a previous days solid, yet not too demanding session. Engross the slight soreness which is the result of a sensible increase in training volume or intensity but be careful to what degree you ache.

It's okay to feel slight soreness for several days at a time. Slight soreness from your long run, heaped upon slight soreness from sensible speed running. Do many types of session because each session gives your body a different challenge and takes your muscles and joints toward overload, but not beyond overload.

Overuse injuries are from doing the same thing at the same pace day after day, from which you accumulate fatigue in a small range of motion. Run two of your days at a variety of paces slightly faster than marathon pace, and two days at significantly slower than marathon pace. Warm up and stretch before speed running to reduce injury risk and do striders to decrease the amount of lactic acid which you produce.

Do appropriate amounts of speed running at 5K and 15K paces, and you'll never need 3 days to recover from a speed session. Don't suddenly jump into 10 miles of 400 meter repeats because you read an inspiring article about Zatopek, or because a current world record holder does so. They took a decade or more to be able to run long sessions at 5K pace.

Rest days and the easy weeks allow your muscles to recover from moderately hard sessions: you should be stronger the next time you work through the schedule and you'll have fewer aches.

Don't repeat harsh training sessions which give you DOMS again. Do fewer repeats, at a slower pace next time. Some training must feel moderately harsh, but you should be able to run quite well the day after a quality speed session or long run. You should be able to train without recourse to analgesics.

Many schedules in this book are based on 4 runs per week. The worst training this author has seen this century was in the October 2,002 issue of a major running magazine which also had 4 running days per week but 4 key errors:

1. Only one long run during the entire marathon program;
2. No cross training;
3. No hill training; and
4. Speed running which was at 40 seconds per mile faster than their 5K pace, (which is faster than mile pace).

Number 4 would be fine if your goal is to race the mile or 800 meters, but fast sprints are useless for marathon runners. Restrict most speed running to 5K pace or 10 seconds per mile faster while running 800 to 1,600 meter repeats and you'll avoid running at mile race pace, which is the least useful speed for marathon runners to train at. See Chapter Six. You'll also need more than one 20 miler to run a decent marathon, and you need the strength from hill training and the strength and injury prevention from cross training.

To run or not to run.

If an injury hurts when you run, stop running. Some runners need to rest every injury. If running does not increase the pain, it is often OK to run through injuries. Remaining active will help it to heal. If the pain disappears during or after your warmup, or the pain is fairly minor, enjoy the moment and run less intensely than you do normally. Provided the pain does not make you change your running form, or put pressure on a related part of your body (hint: every part of your body is related to other parts), do some running.

However, lumps and bumps as one expert called them, visible swelling or warmth suggest no running. When reading the "Should you run" tips in this and the next chapter, consider them to be in addition to the above paragraphs.

Regular and slow stretching will decrease your risk of muscle cramps, as will plyometrics. Also:

* Do quality sessions at and faster than marathon pace, but don't add much each session. An increase of a quarter mile at speed

per week would take you from 5 miles at speed per week to 10 speedy miles in only 5 months.

* Expected race temp 90 degrees and humid, but you run mostly at 70 degrees. Check your sanity for choosing such race conditions, and then wear an extra long sleeve shirt for half of your training runs to prepare your body to sweat. Hydrate before the run, on the run and afterwards.

* When you get a cramp, stop. See the calf muscles spasm (charley horse section). Drink something with electrolytes in it. Walk or run slowly to bring blood to your muscles.

The most likely injury for beginner runners is:

SHIN SPLINTS - painful shins, also called
Medial tibial stress syndrome, which is simply an inflammation along the inner side of the shinbone.

A stress fracture pain is likely to be a continuous pain and restricted to one spot. Do not run, and see page 359.

However, if you have a more diffuse pain or tenderness in the lower third of the leg on the inside, or along the entire shin, and if stretching eases the pain, a fracture is less likely. Run on soft surfaces if the pain is not severe and read on.

With shin splints, pain is felt on extending the toes and weight bearing. It hurts if you press the area with your finger. Physiologically, it's an inflammation of the tendons OR muscle in this area. Pain gradually gets worse as you run, though for some shin splint types it eases when you're well warmed up, but resumes at the end of exercise. Other types ease shortly after stopping.

Causes include:
* Running with the weight too far forward;
* Striking the ground with the first third of the foot;
* Over-striding;
* Overpronation;
* Shoes too tight around the toes or inflexible shoes;
* Weak arches may be present;
* Short calf muscles which stress the shin structures;
* Calf muscles too much stronger than the shin muscle;
* Calves tighten and pull on the shin muscles;

* Beginner runners are very susceptible;
* Overtraining is its trademark; especially:
* Increasing mileage too quickly, running on hard surfaces & too much speedwork, too early, on hard surfaces.

<u>Prevention:</u> Flexible foreshoe—Wear a combination or slip lasted design in preference to heavy or stiff shoes. Replace shoes every 300 to 400 miles. Use a sorbothane heel lift to reduce jarring, along with arch supports or padding if necessary. Don't make a sudden increase in training or run too fast too soon. Balance your training. Run fewer miles and do them on softer surfaces. Include pool running, elliptical training and other cross training. Consume 1,200 mgs of calcium per day.

Concrete is 6 times harsher to your tissues than asphalt. Asphalt is three or more times harsher than packed dirt trails. Grass and muddy trails are still softer, and significantly decrease your risk of shin splints. Bring back road mileage a mile or two at a time as you ease back to full training. Use orthotics or anti-pronation shoes.

Stretch before running, and again after warming up. Made a training mistake and hurt your shins? Ice them, take some NSAIDs and don't do it again!

Shins always hurt after a track session? You probably need to slow down to 5K pace, or do shorter sessions with shorter strides, but you can also do your speed running on dirt, grass, sand, up hills, on a treadmill, or do pool running. Also, correct any other training errors. Do an appropriate amount of speed running and shift at a reasonable pace. Gradually work up to 10 percent of your weekly mileage in one session, and run no faster than 5K pace until you can do that 10 percent without severe aches and pains.

Do not forget your warmdown...perhaps the most under rated part of a training session. Running for two to three miles may sound gruesome if you've just done 20 times 400 meters at 5K pace. It *is* gruesome if you were not in good enough shape to run those intervals with a bit to spare! Easy running brings in blood with its nutrients and speeds the extraction of the waste products from fast running. Add a quarter mile of walking at the end and you'll also decrease your post exercise blood pooling which adds to muscle inflammation. Hose your legs with cold water, put your feet up for 20 minutes while you rehydrate and cool down, then take your shower and stretch gently.

The shin muscle works against the large calf muscles, is the last muscle to warm up and the first to cool down. Wearing long thick socks will help to avoid the chill when not running, and make it easier to warm up the muscle before you do run. You can also consider knee high hose which are adapted from:

A. Short stockings used by ladies wearing long skirts or pants.
B. Pressure "Ted hose" to prevent DVTs in hospitals and in people who are inactive or who stand for long periods.

These thin, pressure stockings are said to improve VO2 max by returning more of your blood to the heart. However, your calf muscles' contractions are already returning the blood, so the main incentive to wear this type of sock would be warmth, comfort and to copy the great Paula Radcliffe.

Do an exercise to build up the shin muscles. While sitting in a chair, draw large circles with your big toe, and then write the alphabet with your big toe. After a few weeks, add the paint pot exercise (sit on a table, hang a weight from your toes and pull your toes up i.e., flex your ankles for sets of 12). Or hook an elastic belt or similar item around your toes and push against it ten times, then pull it toward you 10 times.

Reduce your mileage to get over the shin splints.

Pain on the outside of the shin? Walk with your toes pointed in for one minute a day.

Pain on the inside? Walk with toes pointed out for one minute. Build up toward five minutes.

Then practice walking on your toes and on your heels with toes pointed in and out.

Treatment: Use ice and NSAIDs for the initial swelling. Take a couple of rest days and commence flexibility work: Stretch pre and post exercise. Lie on your back with one foot in the air. Place a towel around the sole of your foot, and pull with your left hand to bring the toes down and to the left, which will stretch the muscles on the right. Hold for 30 seconds and repeat to the right and then with the other leg.

Also, massage gently down the muscle to your pain tolerance, and then back off by 10 percent to avoid damage. Use ice alternating with moist heat, and then put the muscle through its full range of motion. When you've been pain free for several weeks, gradually increase mileage at 5 percent per week for three weeks, but then stay at that level for 5 weeks before increasing again.

Shin splints is mainly an injury of new runners and people who make sudden changes to their training. Find the cause of your pains and then deal with it patiently.

COMPARTMENT SYNDROME.

While there are numerous muscle compartments in the body, for runners, this malady usually relates to the anterior or front compartment of the lower leg, which is on the outer part of the leg, in front of the fibula. The inner part of the lower leg is dominated by the tibia bone. The compartment set up by these bones is surrounded by a tough sheath containing muscles, nerves and blood vessels.

Compartment syndrome is a muscle pain due to the muscles growing or in acute injuries and infections, expanding faster than the sheath surrounding them. It includes one form of shin splints, though it also affects the other smallish muscles of the lower leg. Your shin muscle will feel tight, numb (if nerves are involved) and you may have a sensation of pressure due to excess fluid or muscle development. The pain is on the outside of the leg, and unlike true shin splints, the pain comes on during exercise and lasts well beyond the finish of your session. Diagnosis is with a pressure check, though your specialist will usually rule out shin splints and stress fracture too.

Massage, ice and anti-inflammatories can help, but several months off of running may be required. Surgery (fasciotomy) may be required if the pains return, releasing pressure and allowing the muscle more room to expand. First though, reduce mileage to allow your muscles and the sheath surrounding them to adapt.

Like shin splints, compartment syndrome is attracted to people who make sudden mileage increases or suddenly introduce speed running. Stretch regularly and weight train using light weights for many repeats to decrease your risk.

Some muscles grow so much that they constrict the blood flow into the sheath, resulting in necrosis which is a medical emergency. However, emergencies are usually due to traumatic injuries such as whacking your shoulder, arms or legs during a fall, or losing a battle against another moving object.

CALF MUSCLE STRAINS.

Causes: Similar to Achilles tendonitis at page 354, but especially overload, too much track speed running in low heeled racing shoes, or a series of minor twists on rough trails. Early warning signs for calf strains include cramps and charley horse, so read that section too.

Many problems are resolved by using a heel lift in all shoes, plus regular stretching. Some experts say avoid walking barefoot; others say walking or running barefoot will stretch the calf to its ideal length.

The gastrocnemious responds well to ice, strains more when running up hills, and because the tendons of origin cross behind the knee joint, it requires a straight knee to fully stretch it. Because the soleus is under the gastroc, it's less amenable to ice therapy. The soleus works hard during downhill running, which is when you're likely to strain it. Because it originates below the knee, it can be stretched while the knee is bent.

Between the gastrocnemious and soleus is the plantaris muscle and all 3 combine to form the Achilles tendon.

Inflammation is decreased with a compression bandage if properly applied. An anti-embolitic stocking probably gives the safest amount of pressure. Elevate the leg to the level of your heart or slightly above.

After the initial 3 to 7 days or acute phase, both muscles are receptive to massage. Use fingers or finger shaped gismos or a roller to break up adhesions. Massage toward the heart and then do some cross-fiber massage.

Rehab: Stretch gently once you're pain free during walking. Raise your leg up while you're sat on the floor and rotate your foot clockwise for a minute and then reverse for one minute at your ankles' maximum range of motion.

When pain free, add weight training. Point your toes away from you and practice raising your body weight up by standing on your toes. Stand on both feet and support part of your weight with your arms for the first few sessions. Move up and down over 5 to 10 seconds for 6 to 10 repeats. Do a set three times a day.

Next, while standing with a hand support, rock back and forward from heel to toe for a minute and repeat after a rest.

Ready for harsher stuff? Stand on a step and allow your heels to drift down below the step before pushing up on your toes.

Small calf muscle strains heal well with active running, but keep to soft even surfaces. Use mental preparation when you head back to the trails. Expect and look forward to adjusting your stride. Be ready to take several short strides or relax at the knee to make those adjustments. See sprained ankle at page 357.

CHARLEY HORSE or SEVERE Muscle Cramp

is...An acute agonizing spasm caused by prolonged contraction at the muscle fiber level. The cramp can last for several minutes.

Causes include:

* Post exercise, often many hours post exercise, due to dehydration and possibly lingering pockets of lactic acid;
* Or small areas of muscle damage;
* After repetitive movement such as five miles on a treadmill at constant speed and the same elevation without changing cadence or running style;
* Exercising more than usual: Over-fatigued muscles;
* Or your greatest race ever:
* Sitting or lying in an awkward position, which compromises circulation;
* Excessive sweating or exercising with a fever or in hot conditions;
* Loss of sodium; insufficient intake of calcium; low potassium or magnesium;

Avoidance: Correct the above to decrease the potential for cramps.

Treatment: Many books say massage and stretching. However, if you massage a cramping muscle, you will certainly strain it; if you try to stretch a cramping muscle, you'll strain it some more.

Or try this: Place the cramping muscle in its shortest anatomical position. For the calf, this means bringing the foot back toward your butt, and letting the toes drop down. The calf is less likely to remain in spasm because you have told the stretch proprioceptors that the muscle is in its absolute resting position.

As the muscle relaxes, you can use gentle touch followed by gentler massage, a slow kneading to locate the sore spots. Then use ice alternating with low temperature moist heat to further relax the muscle and bring nutrients in, while flushing wastes out. Eat fruit that contains sodium and potassium to correct your electrolyte imbalance; take a tum or glass of non-fat milk for calcium; add an anti-inflammatory for pain. Replace lost fluids. Diazepam, diphenhydramine, Vitamin E, B complex vitamins and tonic water can decrease the frequency of Charlie horse cramps too. And avoid sudden changes to your training.

Stretch slowly before and after running. If the cramp was due to a muscle strain, you may need several rest or cross training days.

Except in the case of a minor spasm while exercising, delay long sessions of stretching until after the acute phase.

Popliteal muscle strains were discussed on page 327, so lets cruise up the leg to the:

HAMSTRINGS.

Hamstring strains are an injury of fast running. Hamstrings get tired and sore if you lift the foot behind you too far, or extend your stride too long. You don't need to kick your butt on every stride - leave that to sprinters. Long strides overextend the hamstring muscles, which is not a good idea at any time, but once you've fatigued the hamstrings they'll easily strain. Leaning forward when tired can lead to muscle strains at the back of the legs, the hamstrings and glutei's or gluteals. Chronic hamstring problems may originate from the back or from an unequal pelvis, so see an expert if the following tips don't help you.

Keep your stride short and keep your legspeed up to maintain race or training pace toward the end of the run or race. Finishing sprints should be long efforts over at least a mile, not 200 meter sprints faster than a young dog. Shorten your stride, speed up your leg turnover and stay light on your feet for the entire mile. Use the same tactic running downhill to decrease hamstring damage.

RICE (rest, ice, compression, elevation) and active rest are effective for new strains. You can sit on the ice for the upper hammies; adjust it to hit the right spot. The tendon of origin at the buttock and insertion below the knee can develop a tendonitis. They can take 3 to 6 months to completely heal. Capsaicin cream (e.g. Zostrix) can help to relieve pain and inflammation. Capsaicin interrupts pain signals, but the damage is still there, so do not run. If it hurts, restrict yourself to gentle massage. After the acute phase, cross-fiber massage to help break up scare tissue is suggested for this muscle; set your own pain threshold and get help from an expert. Warm up the muscles with a shower or gentle exercise before messaging. Recondition your muscles gently at first, no speed or hill work until you're back to 75 percent of your usual mileage, and pain free with the injured hamstring just as strong as the uninjured one. Whether running fast or slow, practice good running form.

The hamstrings origin is the ischial tuberosity of the pelvis. The three hammies insert below the knee thus they:
*   Flex the knee and extend the hip;
*   Help to stabilize the knee;
*   Recover the leg for the next stride.
The hamstrings are mainly a recovery muscle. The quads do the work, then as the quads relax and lengthen, the hammies contract to pull the lower leg up and through the stride cycle and set up the upper leg for its next work phase.

Don't stretch beyond your pain reflex. Let your muscle heal while doing gentle stretches; regain hamstring length when the muscle is better.

You'll need an almost locked knee to stretch the lower part of the hammies; bend over your hip joint to stretch the upper part: bend over the hip with a nearly locked knee at the same time to stretch the middle fibers.

The hammies will need two types of exercise to strengthen the entire muscle. Lie on your belly. Keeping the knee on the floor, bend your lower leg up toward your buttock, and then lower it to the floor. Repeat 10-20 times.

Stay on your belly. Keeping your leg straight, raise one foot up 6 to 12 inches and gently let it down for 10-20 reps. After a couple of weeks, add comfortable ankle weights.

Later, strengthen the hamstrings with leg curls in the weight room. Do single leg curls; don't let the weak leg cheat. Don't let the buttocks do the work either. Pool running is an excellent choice to rebuild these hip extensors, as is running backwards. However, running backwards can lead to massive injuries secondary to falling over, hitting posts, walls and people. The safest way to run backwards is not to run at all: use the elliptical trainer with a backward motion.

You can also walk your office chair up the corridor while sat on it. Dig your heels in and gently pull yourself along.

Use ice after all runs, and run 100 meter striders twice a week in addition to your speed sessions. Run speed sessions at appropriate pace, which is rarely faster than 5K pace.

The most relaxing way to stretch the hamstrings is to lay in a doorway with the leg not being stretched through the open door, and the buttock of the leg to be stretched tight against the wall or doorframe. Place the leg to be stretched up the wall or doorframe. Scoot your butt closer to the door, but on the floor and straighten the knee for longer hammies, then switch sides to do the other leg.

GLUTEAL (or Butt) muscles are renowned for aching after distance runners do sprints. A "butt hurt" means you did too many short efforts, too fast, without adequate preparation. Yes, there should be a degree of fatigue, but some runners ask for these muscles to strain by ignoring them most of the year. Don't ignore any muscle group for more than two weeks.

As shown in the downhill running section, the gluts extend the hip in rapid running. Use the stretch from Chapter One plus the hamstring and piriformis advice to keep your butt healthy.

Piriformis Syndrome, or a Butt Pain.

A deeper problem, because the muscle is under the gluteals is piriformis syndrome. Pain in the hip or the center of the butt, with a related pain down the back of the leg can be confused with sciatica. The piriformis muscle goes from your sacrum to the outer part of the hip bone (trochanter of the femur). The piriformis:

* Rotates the hip and leg;
* Maintains your alignment or balance when one foot is off the ground;
* Stabilizes the pelvic region and keeps the thigh bones and knee joints properly aligned over the feet.

Running, which is awfully repetitive, can fatigue the pear shaped piriformis, causing the muscle to tighten, and put stress on the sciatic nerve.

Symptoms include pain at your outer hip. Muscle tightness increases tension between tendon and bone, causing pain or bursitis. It can be a nagging pain in the center of the buttock, a dull ache, or a heavy feeling in your leg.

Piriformis syndrome can also show it self as sciatic neuralgia, that is, pain from the buttocks down to the knees and occasionally into the lower leg. The pain could also radiate up into the lumber region, and can be confused with a herniated disc. Depending on your luck, the sciatic nerve runs under, over, or straight through the belly of the piriformis muscle, and the muscle can inflame your thumb-sized sciatic nerve.

Pain can be aggravated by sitting, doing squats, walking and running. The affected leg is sometimes externally rotated, that is, the toes point out when you relax.

If you drive a long distance with the right foot in external rotation, you can fatigue your piriformis.

Prevention and treatment: Avoid overtraining, ha ha. Let
your muscles recover. Continued running with piriformis syndrome can make it worse and then more difficult to treat. Relax the muscle with ice several times a day and blood will then flow back in to facilitate healing. Massage the area and then stretch to bring in still more nutrients.

The tennis ball trick works nicely. Lie on the floor and put a ball under your butt, a little medial to your hip bone. Ease your weight onto the ball and note the painful areas. You need to work out the trigger points and break up adhesions. Your flexibility will not improve much until you've broken up the adhesions in the fatigued muscle. The ball should actually hurt you a bit. Every 15 to 20 seconds, move the ball toward your midline about an inch at a time along the length of the piriformis.

Icing and massage take patience because the gluteal muscles are on top of the piriformis, so the cold takes a while to reach the target muscle.

Then it will be time to stretch. Lets say your right piriformis hurts. Lie on your back. Cross your right leg over your left knee. You can use the tennis ball again in this position if you wish to get still greater benefits. With your right ankle or the lateral aspect of the foot resting at the front of your left knee or your lower thigh, pull your left knee up toward your chest for 30 seconds, which will push the right foot in front of it and you'll feel the stretch in your right butt before your left gluteals ask you to stop.

The seated hip stretch. Sit on a sturdy bench or surface to help keep your hips aligned. Your right ankle goes on top of your left knee as in the above stretch, but you bend forward at your hips.

You can also do a standing hip stretch using a sturdy table or the back of a sofa. Stand up tall a few inches away from your support and place your right outer ankle on the support. Your hip and your knee will be flexed at 90 degrees, and your knee will be pointing to the right with your right ankle at the same distance from your belly as the knee. The right ankle should be in front of your left shoulder. Toes point away from you and after using your hands to get your leg in this position, you can use them to maintain balance. Keep the left leg straight while bending forward at the hips. Don't role at the waist.

Breathe deeply and relax during all of these stretches and take your time. You'll do both legs of course.

Assuming you cut your mileage in half while treating your problem, once you've got flexibility back and you're pain free, gradually increase training while maintaining a stretching program.

NSAIDs are useful, but don't use them for months while avoiding the syndrome and it's simple treatment. Some people will need physical therapy or ultrasound, and a few will need surgery to release the entrapped nerve.

Orthotics and different running shoes help many people prevent this syndrome. Both will improve your gait. The trouble is, poor posture when sitting for long periods can also cause piriformis syndrome. Get up every hour and take a few minutes walk. When sitting and standing, spread your weight evenly on your buttocks and feet respectively.

<u>Abductors and adductors</u> or inner thigh muscles such as the gracilis which also lifts or flexes the thigh, can be troublesome and masquerade as hamstring injuries. These vital muscles stabilize the hip and knee joints, aid in balance and in running, especially on trails. Have an expert locate the exact spot and you can work out a treatment plan. Include the abductor / adductor machines at the gym and do a set of plies (wide stance with toes pointing out and lower yourself into a one-third squat).

Muscle injuries to the front of the leg are due to overtraining, that is, too many miles before your body has adapted to the load, or too much tempo style hard running. Shin splints were covered earlier, so lets move to the upper leg.

QUADRICEPS STRAINS.

The four-cylinder engine of locomotion. The thigh muscle propels you while stabilizing the knee. Actually, the calf is the main muscle group for moving you forward. The quads cushion the body, set up the calf to do its job, and then devour the ground through the rest of the stride cycle.

The quads are the biggest by volume of the muscle groups, and has multiple functions. If you're not using any other muscle group properly, the first sign can be aching quads. Due partly to their eccentric responsibilities, quads are likely to ache after longer than usual runs, running downhills or if you wear worn out shoes.

Prevention:

* Increase mileage in a steady manner;
* Incorporate hills regularly;
* Practice relaxed downhill running;
* Don't use your quads just to absorb the shock of downhills. Don't fight gravity. Run perpendicular to the ground with a relatively short stride.
* Run downhills on grass if possible;
* Land with a slightly bent knee;
* Build up your calf muscles. Strong calves decrease the quads workload; remember to work the calves by pushing off, especially during the last few miles of each run and the last few reps during speed training;
* Run tall to work your iliosoas muscle group, which helps to lift the thigh.

Do plyometric exercises such as bounding and jumping to improve strength and endurance in the crucial quadriceps.

Work other muscles appropriately so as not to over-stress the quad group. Do your half squats one leg at a time. Single leg squats are another opportunity to work on your balance.

Thighs ache? Cut back mileage by 20 percent or take a couple of days off. Very gentle cross training may be okay. Resume with fewer, less intense miles. Give your athletic body sufficient time to adapt, and then try to increase your mileage again.

Stretch the hip flexors. If you sit for your work, you set up your flexors to shorten. Standing up every hour and walking a few steps is the simplest way to keep the hip flexors loose, while also stopping pressure sores on your butt! Walk to your colleague seven cubicles away or on the next floor instead of e-mailing. Do quad stretches three to four times a day at work, between sets when weight training, and every hour on long runs. The thin sartorius muscle aids in hip flexion; keep your hip joints range of motion intact to keep the sartorius at its optimal length for its work.

Do straight leg raises to reduce the strain on the knees. Also, sit on a table with a weight attached to the ankles. Extend (straighten) the knee and hold in the locked position for 5-10 seconds for 10 repeats. The vastus medialis muscle should be hard. Do both legs.

Leg swings are not just for sprinters and milers, and are superb for strength and balance. Stand on your left foot. Swing your right foot up until your thigh is parallel to the ground with your knee flexed at 90 degrees so that your foot is pointing down. Now swing the right leg behind you until your thigh is at 45 degrees to your left leg. Keep your feet facing the front. Switch legs after a minute. You can use one hand on a support for balance the first few times, then learn to stay upright without assistance from a support.

Abdominal Muscle Strains.

It's tricky to diagnose your own injuries in the mid-section. The pain could be from hip flexors, adductors or abductors. Decrease mileage and see an expert about groin pains. You need to rule out non exercise causes and stress fractures to the hip.

Once you've figured out what the cause of the pain is, strengthen and stretch the area.

Lie on your stomach. Push your shoulders up to make a banana shape which stretches the abdominal muscles. Want to exercises the back muscles? Extend the banana shape by raising the head and shoulders without using your arms, but also raise your feet and legs off the surface.

You can protect the back by keeping the abdominal muscles strong. Do crunches and sit-ups slowly, plus seated knee raises. Sit on the edge of a seat, raise your knees to your chest, and then push the legs out straight. Make the abdominals do some of the work. Seated knee raises also work the Ilio-soas group (Iliacus and Psoas

Major). This pair of muscles help to raise the thigh in fast running
and up hills: they flex the hip. Too much fast running or hill
running for your current fitness level will make these muscles
fatigue or ache and possibly strain.

Crunches only work the upper abdominals. Sit-ups exercise the
other three quarters of the abs! When doing sit-ups on a padded
floor, do a quarter of them right elbow to left knee and a quarter
left elbow to right knee to work the oblique abdominal muscles,
which are some of the seven or so muscle groups which pull the
thorax forward to inflate your lungs. Strong abdominal muscles
help you to run tall and decrease injuries. You're only as strong as
your weakest link: don't let the weak link be a supporting muscle
group.

Don't pull on your head with your hands. Keep your hands
positioned by your ears instead of behind your head. Keep your
head in normal alignment while you do sit-ups and don't do so
many that your form vanishes.

Do your sit-ups slowly enough and you will not need to do sit-
backs. With sit-backs, you start in the up position and keeping your
back straight, you slowly ease back toward the floor. You will feel
the pull on your abdominal muscles as they resist and control the
down movement. Feet getting ready to leave the floor? Hold it
there for a second before returning to the up position. As your
abdominals get stronger, you'll get your back closer to the floor.
Abs real fit? Try it with your arms crossed over your chest!

Prefer to stay on your back while exercising those lower abs.
Do a variation on cycling. One of the best ways to warm up your
huge upper legs muscles before running or stretching is to lie on
your back, then raise your legs up vertically. Hint: hoist your
gluteals off the surface by supporting your butt at the pelvis. Do a
gentle cycling action for a few minutes while taking your hips and
knees through their full range of motion.

Then for your abs, place a hand under your lower back and
press your back into the surface. Suck in your belly. Bring the
knees toward your chest to get your thighs perpendicular to the
surface. Now, lower one leg while straightening at the knee to
touch the surface with your heel, then bring that leg back up.
Switch legs. You can make it harder by keeping both legs in
motion so that one starts the downward motion as the other one
starts the upward motion. You can also negate the heel touch, but

touching the heel confirms that your leg is all the way down. Do keep the entire cycle slow and breath rhythmically, while keeping your tummy tucked in and pressed down.

Side stitch A: Pain below the rib cage due to the diaphragm muscle cramping. It's usually due to improper warmup: Contributing factors are drinking cold fluids just before you run, or gas or food in the stomach.

Low oxygen to the diaphragm causes the stitch, which comes on at fast or slow pace. Regular deep breathing exercises and avoiding the above three errors will decrease the frequency. Do gentle warm ups of ten minutes and ease into your running.

Side stitch B: Stomach ligaments pulling down on the diaphragm secondary to large amounts of cold liquid in the stomach! Sounds just like side stitch A. Decrease this stitch by tightening your abdominal muscles and applying pressure to the painful area. Strengthen the diaphragm with the book on your belly exercise. Lay supine with one hand or a book on your belly. Breathe in and out rhythmically, feeling the air move in and make sure that your abdomen goes up and down, but that your chest barely moves up as you inflate your lungs.

Treat an acute case of stitch with various deep-breathing techniques while either bending over a few degrees, or with your hands on your head. The simplest action, however, is to start again. Walk until you feel relaxed, do some slow deep breathing, then ease back into a slow run. If the diaphragm's blood supply is sufficient, it should not cramp.

Try this stretch to prevent or relieve a cramp. Raise your right arm straight up and bend your trunk gently toward the left. Hold for 30 seconds, release, and then stretch the other side. Do a couple each side before exercising, and any time you get a cramp.

Look at all of your running related injuries objectively and take them as a chance to reassess your training. After finding the cause of each injury, you must correct it and then build up your training again when fully recovered. During prolonged recoveries, do something non-running which you've been meaning to do. Stay healthy, at an appropriate weight and cross-train gently before you return to running.

Chapter Nineteen

CONNECTIVE TISSUES

Soft or connective tissues (tendons and ligaments) can take huge amounts of abuse. Usually, it's stronger than muscle, but push it too far and it will fail. The weakest point will go first; training through the injury can lead to a chronic "itis" such as Achilles Tendonitis. Rehab, using RICE as described in Chapter 18 can be long and slow.

Connective tissue injuries are insidious, creeping up on you week by week. Their stealth makes you change form in little ways, pushing you toward other injuries. As suggested in Chapter 17, it could be your big toe which is causing the knee pain or your hamstring to repeatedly strain. It could be your short right leg that is placing extra strain and work on the structures of your entire left leg.

Most of this chapters problems are overuse or overtraining injuries due to repeating the same stride length thousands of times a day. You can reduce the repetitive stress on muscles and connective tissue by varying your speed, running surface and by using several pairs of running shoes each week.

No matter how softly you land when gliding along the surface, your feet still take a pounding on every stride.

PLANTAR FASCIITIS.

Plantar Fasciitis is caused by an overstretching or inflammation of the plantar fascia, the strong band of tissue making up the arch of the foot. The problem is usually at its attachment to the heel.

Symptoms: Pain at the base of the heel, or under the arch

which may feel like a stone bruise. Pain is worse at the start of the day or run and a bone spur may develop where the fascia has partially torn off the heel. It could also express itself as a pain in the arch of the foot, which radiates toward the toes. Often due to:

* Stress and tension on the fascia from overtraining;
* Tight Achilles;
* A stiff big toe joint;
* A rigid high arched foot;
* Flat feet;
* Overpronation;
* Too thin a heel on running shoes;
* Running on hard surfaces with poor or old cushions (shoes);
* Too much hill or speed training;
* Too many calf stretches over the edge of a stair;
* Too many calf raises.

Should you run through fasciitis? Only if the pain and swelling is mild, or you'll risk a chronic problem. Tape the foot before running, ice after each run, and use the prevention hints below while maintaining fitness with mostly cross training while finding the cause. Pool running is especially good during rehab and while your feet adapt to the increased training of a marathon program. You may need to consider a different marathon 6 months further away.

Prevention: Correct the above. Wear shoes with a higher heel,

good arch support, flexible sole and consider sorbothane insoles. Keep mileage in lightweight racing shoes to a minimum, but sufficient to stay used to running in them. One session each week should suffice. Run on soft surfaces most of the time. Use arch supports or orthotics to prevent the arch from collapsing; use a strip of orthopedic felt under the metatarsal phalangeal joint, (the joint between the toes and the middle of the foot). Stretch and strengthen the calf muscles.

Develop strength under your foot by flexing the toes. Alternate curling the toes as if to pick up a golf ball, then extend the toes up toward the shin.

Also, with the feet flat on the floor, grab a towel and pull it in with the toes. Alternate flexing and relaxing your toes while you're doing calf stretches.

Avoid redamaging the fascia every morning. Gently stretch the fascia by pulling your toes toward you. Don't get out of bed without proper foot support, or you'll rupture the healing spot of your inflamed fascia. Wear support sandals or shoes for that first yet short ambulation. When you're well warmed up, walk in unsupported footwear for part of each day.

Treatment: RICE may help; massage the bottom of the foot using ice made from a disposable cup mold, or a frozen bottle of water. Roll the ice up and back along your entire arch. If this fails, seek specialist advice.

* Ultrasound can help to break up scar tissue;
* Acupuncture is quite successful for plantar fascitis;
* Steroid injections help some people;
* Night splints are a cheap non-invasive option;
* Whirlpools can also give relief.

If the injury is chronic, minor surgery to the toe, or to remove a spur on the heel may be useful. Shock wave therapy is an option to break up the scare tissue, adhesions and to reduce inflammation. On the basis that it has minimal function, some experts recommend cutting the fascia. Better yet: find and address the cause of your problem.

www.deroyal.com/shop or (800) 993-9008 has a kit to help with fasciitis and heel problems.

SUPINATION: under pronation of the foot is not an injury, but supinators are prone to I-T band syndrome, Plantar Fasciitis and Achilles problems so get yourself appropriate shoes so that you run with a neutral gait. Do stretches for all the related muscles. Lightweight slip lasted trainers may help.

METATARSAL INJURIES.
The most important prevention technique is to wear wide, well-padded shoes to allow the foot its natural shape.

Morton's neuroma is an inflammation of the nerve, usually the one which runs between the 3rd and 4th metatarsals and sometimes between the 2nd and 3rd metatarsals. That is where your fiery pain will be during almost any weight bearing activity. Pain in the ball of your foot? Get it checked by a podiatrist. Direct pressure and ultrasound can detect the gristle like nerve.

Neuromas are usually from biomechanical irregularities, including the apparently innocuous bunion and tight shoes, or from repetitive activities. Use pool running and elliptical training instead of 20 percent of your mileage.

Bare foot walking can ease the discomfort, as can ice and NSAIDs. Wear wider shoes in all spheres of life. Metatarsal pads can help, as can orthotics, but cortisone injections may be needed. Surgical removal (going in from the top of the foot) requires only about 6 weeks off from running. Unless your pain is severe, you can run while awaiting surgery.

Stress fracture to the neck of the metatarsal is a subset of March fractures, due to over use and jarring. Signs include swelling, tingling, burning in the ball of the foot or a stone like bruise. Unless you correct the cause, expect the same problem with your other foot.

Requires several weeks of non-impact training e.g. pool running, or rest. The bone may find its best position for you to run, but it may not. Use RICE, wide shoes with cushioning, good insoles, arch supports, and orthotics. Take NSAIDs if appropriate, but not so that you can train through the injury.

Metatarsalgia is pain and inflammation of any of the five metatarsal bones, often associated with a callous secondary to excess weight, high arches and wearing high-heeled shoes. Use the tricks from the last section, and add metatarsal pads at the first sign of pain. Scrunch up a towel with your toes for a few seconds for 5 reps to develop the local muscles and arch strength.

The muscles which propel you forward need to make contact with your fragile feet. The calf muscles' only conduit from the gastrocnemius and soleus to the heel is the Achilles Tendon: It is a runner's second most likely injury site.

Inflamed ACHILLES TENDON or ACHILLES TENDONITIS or TENDINITIS

Symptoms: Dull or sharp pain with dorsiflexion and weight bearing and inflammation of the tendon cord or its sheath. Symptoms range from the back of the heel and ankle, up through the cord and it could extend into the calf muscle. Pain may come on gradually or suddenly; the tendon is especially stiff in the morning. For some runners, the pain disappears after a few miles, giving them several miles of freedom, but with even more pain and inflammation the next day. The Achilles tendon often thickens, sometimes a nodule can be felt, and a cracking sound may be present. Training through the pain can lead to rupture and agony.

Causes: Aging or degeneration of collagen fibers, or inflammation from training at any age (you decide). The tendon tries to compensate for *tight calf muscles*. Stress at footstrike and push-off must be absorbed by the Achilles cord. Damage can be the result of a:

* Gradual mileage increase that catches up with the tendon;
* Sudden introduction of hill work;
* Increased training intensity or sprinting, which stresses and stretches the tendon too much.
* Short, inflexible calf and hamstring muscles, perhaps secondary to increased, slow mileage!
* A lower heel on shoes (running or non-running);
* Running with the weight too far back;
* Hitting the heel heavily on each stride (overstriding);
* High arched rigid foot;
* Overpronation;
* A history of weak feet or Morton's toe (long second toe) predisposes you to this problem.
* The back of running shoes digging into the tendon on every stride is a major culprit.

For some reason, shoe manufacturers insist the tendon needs protecting. Running is a non-contact sport. We need sufficient support for our shoes to stay on, not from being tackled from behind. Shoes with an Achilles dip are just as bad because the top of the dip is often higher than the level at which runners feel pain.

Overpronators are prone to this injury, perhaps because after the tab has slammed into the tendon, it rubs the tendon as the foot rolls inwards; plus the tendon receives an extra twist on every stride.

Prevention: Don't grow older because your tendons become more brittle and less elastic! Wear well fitting and cushioned motion control shoes with heels in good condition: cut the tabs off if necessary, or make two vertical slits where the tendon will go, to allow the now floppy tab to roll gently and almost innocently up and down the tendon. Wear thick socks. Get checked for orthotics. Look for the cause in your case.

Prepare your Achilles for speed and hill sessions with copious stretching of calves; stretch before and after all running. Wear heel lifts and avoid sudden changes in training.

Loose, full length, warm calf muscles will ease the strain on the tendon during all running, not just your quality running. There are many Achilles stretch gismos on the market, but a triangle of wood works just as well.

Treatment: Rest if the Achilles is painful to allow the swelling to decrease. Swelling is part of the healing process. Blood brings in collagen for makeshift repairs, which you will wreck if you run. Apply ice for ten minutes after range of motion exercises and several times a day, and take an anti-inflammatory at the same time: both will help reduce the swelling. Many people find glucosamine supplements of up to 1,500 mgs helpful. When the initial swelling has subsided, ease into a stretching program.

After the initial inflammation has subsided, massage nodules away and do toe raises to build up the calf muscles; do heel drops slowly while standing on a step to stretch the Achilles and calf.

In the acute phase, use heel pads such as sorbothane or orthotics to raise the heel high enough for walking to be pain free. Check your non running shoes because these can also rub the tendon.

Using flat grass areas may help for the first few days back in training. Begin your runs at a shuffle, and then stretch before increasing pace. Grass and dirt reduces the ground impact forces on every stride.

Avoid hills and track speed running until you've stretched the calves for 10 to 20 sessions. Run some of your track miles counter-clockwise.

Cortisone will not help and its use often leads to rupture of the tendon due to continued stress from running on a damaged tendon. A few runners resort to surgery, having scare tissue removed, which eases the tendon's movement within its sheath. Alas, surgery often stimulates more scar tissue and doesn't address the cause.

According to a report presented at the American Orthopedic Society for Sports Medicine, bracing the Achilles was just as successful as surgery for ruptured Achilles Tendons. Think more than twice before having surgery mainly for scare tissue.

A strip of tape applied along the length of the tendon when in the relaxed position will act as a splint, discouraging you from using and stretching the tendon further.

Blood flow to the Achilles is very low. Ultrasound therapy can increase blood flow to the tendon and help to break up scar tissue in tendons and fascia. Unfortunately, ultrasound also blocks nerve activity, which decreases your perception of pain, and can encourage you to train too hard and increase Achilles damage. When treating the Achilles or your I-T band or plantar fascia with several ultrasound treatments, reduce your running significantly for several weeks. Shock wave therapy has decreased pain for some.

Pool run for fitness and find the cause of your problem. It could be that your body needs to catch up with your training. It could be you need to permanently decrease your average weekly mileage by 5 or 10 miles to avoid injury recurrence. If you don't address the short calves, foot control, low heels or inappropriate training, treatment benefits will be short-lived and therefore pointless.

Do calf stretches until you can dorsiflex your foot 10 to 15 degrees, which reduces the stresses on the Achilles.

Here's an exercise suggested by running book author Owen Anderson Ph.D. Stand on a stair or other stable edge which allows you to steady yourself and allows free range of motion for your heel. Raise yourself slowly up onto your toes with both feet. Very slowly lower the heel of one foot to the bottom of its natural range. Put your other foot back on the stair and shift your weight to it. Using that foot, bring both feet together and raise yourself up on your toes again. Do each foot 6 to 10 times. You'll stretch the calves and Achilles when lowering yourself...provided you avoid the stretch reflex by doing it slowly.

Although the Achilles does store significant amounts of elastic energy during every stride while running, your muscles provide 70 percent of the energy which propels you forward.

Should you run: If it does not hurt after a 5 minute warmup, and it does not put extra stress on muscles, run. If you catch the tendonitis early, reduce mileage and slow down. Ice after each run. If the tendonitis is from an unusually long run or tough session, rest it. Tendon swollen? Rest or do non-weight bearing cross training instead of risking a tendon rupture. Don't let it develop into Achilles tendinosis, or a long-term degenerative problem. See an expert if your Achilles ruptures.

SPRAINED OR STRAINED ANKLE.

Ankle ligaments overstretch when you land awkwardly. There may be a popping sound. It takes a couple of months to recover from a true STRAIN. Seek out an expert because x-rays and casting may be needed. Cross train until you can walk without pain. Ice and use NSAIDs in the acute phase.

A SPRAINED ankle has less ligament damage. The main calf muscles are usually strained though, and require nursing back. The big problem is often the smaller stabilizing muscles such as the Peroneous Longus and Tibialis Posterior, plus the flexors and extensors, the everters and inverters of the ankle: they will need to be iced, elevated and rehabbed.

* Grade 1 sprain: The ligaments are stretched but not torn. Pain, swelling and loss of function is minimal.
* Grade 2: A partial ligament tear officially has moderate pain and swelling and some loss of function.
* Grade 3: Complete tear approaches agony, swelling is severe and most function is lost. In England, we would call this a strained ankle.

About 80 percent of runners' ankle sprains are due to rolling the foot inward too far, at 5 to 12 miles per hour. The anterior talofibular ligament is the winner and the calcaneofibular ligament runner up in the most frequently pulled partially apart department. If it hurts you to invert (inwardly turn) your foot after a strain, ice the area which hurts (probably the 4 ligaments round the outer maleoli and up into the muscles on the outer part of the lower leg).

Later, stretch the ankle to its everted position to maintain the ligament's mobility; stretch in the inverted position to regain the
muscles' flexibility. Do your Achilles stretches too.

You'll probably stretch or tear some of your nerves too while
spraining your ankle. The nerves or proprioceptors tell you where
you are in relationship to the ground without your eyes having to
look, and tell your muscles to make the miniscule adjustments
required to keep you upright. Re-teach these nerves how to work
by standing on one foot for 30 seconds and notice the little moves
those lower leg muscles have to make to keep you upright. Do both
legs and advance to closing your eyes. You will also regain muscle
strength with the balancing exercises. Do your shin and ankle
rotations for range of motion and to regain muscle endurance
before strength training.

Lie on your side on your bed with your foot dangling over the
edge. Hang a weight on your foot and lift your toes toward the
ceiling; hold for a few seconds and repeat 10 times. Do your stair
stretch for the Achilles and to help keep the ankle mobile in the
straight up and back mode which you'll need for running. The
wobble board, or standing on a trampoline and other agility
practice will also help. Walking and then jogging a large figure of
8 is useful; as the ankle gets better, make the turns tighter. Check
performbetter.com and fitter1.com for an inflatable disc and
balance board respectively.

<u>Should you run:</u> When you can walk and do toes raises
pain-free, and when you can stay in the skiing stance without pain,
and you can do the 30 second balance exercise, ease into running
with a support such as ace bandage or an air splint. Avoid rough
surfaces for 6 to 8 weeks of running, but then get gently back to
the trails. Be defensive when trail running. Keep the knee slightly
bent on landing and look forward to the minor position changes on
each stride because it builds up the little leg muscles, while the
lower impact on each stride is good for your running longevity.

Reducing the risk of a twisting-type injury:

* Avoid fast running on sections of path with ruts or tree roots,
  for example, in fartlek sessions.
* Don't hold the arms up too high. Run relaxed with a natural
  style. Push the arms straight back to decrease shoulder roll and
  the twisting and strain on your back.

* Wear appropriate shoes for the surface, with sufficient grip. Use studs or dimples, or whatever this year's term for a cross-country sole is. Spikes are great if you do speedwork through mud or on wet grass. Unless you're going sub 16 for 5K, don't use them on the track.
* Beware of excessive cambers and poor road surfaces. Don't run across a hill if the slope is more than a couple of degrees. If a beach is minimally sloped at the low tide bar, or the flat area at high tide, running in both directions will equalize the wear and tear on the ankles, knees and hips.

You need pain-free ankles for successful running. Ankle movement allows you to propel yourself forward powerfully on every stride. Be patient. Regaining full ankle stability can take 6 months.

As mentioned on page 335, beginner runners often get:

SHIN SPLINTS or painful shins. If you have diffuse pain
or tenderness in the lower third of the leg on the inside, or along the entire shin, and if stretching eases the pain, a fracture is unlikely, so you lucky runners can check page 335.

The pain of a Stress fracture is likely to be continuous and restricted to one spot. Do not run.

SHIN STRESS FRACTURE.

If you feel pain when you put pressure on the shin...rest. Stress or hairline fractures don't show up on x-ray until healing is well under way, but they can be confirmed quite early by a bone scan. The dilemma: a fracture requires six to eight weeks non-impact exercise to heal. Use non-running exercise to maintain muscle tone until you've confirmed if you have a fracture. Pool running, elliptical training and cycling are the best exercise options.

When you're ready to resume running, stick to soft surfaces and land softly while giving your bones a final chance to strengthen. Stiffer shoes work for some people, especially for foot fractures because they can reduce the stress on your forefoot; many people with stress fractures higher up the leg prefer a more flexible shoe.

Treadmill running decreases the risk of stress fractures. Increase exercise duration and intensity gradually, and then introduce harder surface running too. Repetitive stress cause these fractures, so vary the stresses with cross training, running on a variety of surfaces, in different shoes and at various training speeds.

The Knee is the most common injury site for entrenched runners, accounting for 25 percent of all injuries, but an even higher percentage of the insidious injuries which runners make themselves suffer. The knee absorbs huge amounts of power, performing twice as much work as the ankle or hip. Heavier runners, and runners who land heavily instead of floating along are at high risk for knee injuries.

Ground impact forces are 2.5 to 3 times your weight. An extra 10 pounds on your frame costs your knees and other joints 25 to 30 additional pounds every time you land on the ground, which is over one thousand times every mile for most people. In addition to increasing injury risk, the extra weight will slow you down by one to two seconds per mile for each pound. Carrying an extra 15 pounds on your thighs, abdomen and elsewhere will cost you 6 to 12 minutes at the marathon.

Another key to knee injury prevention is strong muscles above the joint, especially the vastus medialis or inner quadriceps at the front of the leg. Leg extensions are your first choice, plus half squats, lunges, the straight leg raises and the leg press for whole upper leg strength.

Runners actually suffer from fewer knee injuries than non-exercisers, only one fifth compared to sedentary folk according to the Stanford University Arthritis Center. The moderately training 25-mile per week runner gets fewer injuries than low mileage recreational runners. More running stimulates an increase in the thickness of knee cartilage, which protects you from damage.

You *can* avoid treating the underlying cause of knee injuries by using patellar tendon straps and open patellar neoprene sleeves. These devices may allow you to run longer before you eventually retire from the sport with permanent damage! It's better to find the underlying cause of your knee pain, than to avoid treating it.

Should you run with knee pains: If knee-cap pain eases after warm up exercises, stretching and a few minutes of running, and provided there is no swelling, enjoy lower mileage while addressing the cause.

If the outer thigh pain of I-T band syndrome eases after a few minutes of running, you can also enjoy a lower mileage phase as you find the cause and treat the problem. Now lets expand, because with variations, there are two main knee problems.

CHONDROMALACIA...Runner's Knee or Patellofemoral Syndrome.

This malady moves up on you slowly. It may take considerable time to clear and cure.

Symptoms: Pain or tenderness (often called burning or achy) close to or under the patella (the kneecap); pain at the front or side of the knee. Stiffness of the knee joint. Pain comes on gradually, increases over several weeks, usually in one leg and it's usually your longer leg.

In Chondromalacia, the Patella's cartilage, either directly under the kneecap, or at the side, wears away; it becomes like sandpaper, and often makes a grinding sound as it no longer rides smoothly over the groove of the lower femur. Causes:

* Running on a camber: the slope at the side of the road, or significant mileage across the slope of a hill or beach;
* Long runs; *Tight, weak or fatigued* quadriceps;
* *Tight, overly strong* hamstrings;
* Or (just to confuse us) *weak* hamstrings;
* Going up and down stairs or hills; especially,
* Hyper-extending the knee with downhills;
* Sitting still for long periods;
* Overpronation, which over rotates the knee; the patella gets pulled to the inside of your leg and rubs on the femur;
* Excessive cycling with poor form;
* Stair climbing; Kneeling;
* And sorry people...running too hard, or too much, too early (in the training cycle). Rushed morning or lunchtime runs without a warmup can cause runners knee.

Prevention: Stabilize the foot with well-fitted shoes; use foam, heel and or arch supports to improve fit. Avoid cambers; run on a variety of soft surfaces; try pointing the toe slightly to keep the kneecap in position. Avoid downhills. Reduce the cycling element of your training, or go higher cadence with lower resistance. Keep the knees tracking nicely with no splaying out or in. Before running, do a complete warmup including quadriceps strengthening exercises (leg extensions with the focus on 45 to 10 degrees of flexion at the knee to reduce the strain); don't allow the quads to get more than 50 percent stronger than the hamstrings. Stretch the hamstrings, quads and calves.

Treatment: If you can locate a sore spot, ice can help in the acute phase. Rest for a few weeks, and then do enough running to maintain fitness while allowing the knee to completely heal. Ice after runs. Avoid downhills, cambers and walking downstairs. Swim or pool run if it hurts to run on land.

Experiment with the above to find the cause. Vitamin C may help. Taking aspirin or other NSAIDs several times a day for three months can block cartilage breakdown, but don't risk your intestines and stomach with ulcers unless you're also going to find the cause. Glucosamine, chondroitin or gelatin supplements help some runners.

X-rays and an MRI can check the wear of the joint surfaces. Scraping the surface via arthroscopy may be an option.

Cycle at high cadence to stay fit for life, and when you start running again, build mileage slowly on a variety of soft surfaces.

When swelling is down, strengthen and stretch the quads and hamstrings. The inner quad or vastus medialus oblique is often the weak link. If weak, it allows the outer quad to pull the kneecap out of alignment, placing additional wear and tear on the kneecap. The trusty leg extension machine may not your friend here because it places great strain on the kneecap; stay between 5 and 30 degrees of knee flexion for your repeats.

Use the leg press instead. Do one leg at a time and only drop the weight 30 degrees toward you before pressing it out again. Keep your kneecap aligned with your foot.

Stand on your injured leg and lower yourself slowly to 30 degrees of flexion at the knee. A one-leg squat makes you lift the weight of *your* body. Keep your hips level and face forward with your knees pointed forward. Stand in front of a mirror or window to check form. Do a dozen repeats, and then a set for your good leg, and then a second set for your bad leg. One-legged squats strengthen your upper leg muscles.

Add step-ups and one leg hops on a soft surface, but remember to land softly, and you may avoid knee problems.

Orthotics may help. Choose shoes with good padding and motion-control properties. A rubber sleeve with a hole for the kneecap helps many people: as stated before, don't use this device as an excuse to avoid quad exercises and stretching.

A tight piriformis (one of the butt muscles) can exacerbate runner's knee by rotating the knee. See page 343.

Patellar Tendonitis: or tendenitis! You might feel a sharp pain where the tendon inserts into the shin bone just below the kneecap. Pain is worst at ground impact (of the foot). This is a sub-set of Runner's Knee.

Causes are as for Runner's Knee, but especially downhills, overtraining, landing hard on a straight knee instead of a flexed knee, and overstriding. Hint: your foot should be traveling backwards by the time it touches the ground with the knee flexed at about 15 degrees. Claw the rest of your body forward with your foot.

Use the leg press for your quads, a knee strap but not a neoprene sleeve if you feel like it, and ice for comfort.

ILEOTIBIAL BAND SYNDROME or I-T BAND SYNDROME.

Symptoms: An inflammation or stabbing pain on the outside of the knee or at the hip. Pain usually increases gradually on a run, but the pain may cease afterwards.

Cause: The strong I-T band goes from the outside and front of the pelvis, down the thigh to insert on the upper part of the fibula, just below the knee. The I-T band helps to stabilize the knee. Where it passes by the outside of the knee, small sacs or bursa of fluid should cushion the I-T band from rubbing against the bone. The sacs or the band may become inflamed. The Ileotibial band rubs against the lateral femoral condyle each time you bend your knees, especially when running downhill or on a camber. Friction results in tenderness of the outer knee at the top of the tibia and inflammation. Causes include:

* Running downhills, especially sloped surfaces like the side of the road; usually the curbside leg is affected.
* A sudden change in surface or training;
* Excessive foot movements; Overpronation;
* Poor shoe choice; insufficient lateral support;
* Warn out shoes: outer part of the shoe still looking good? The midsole may already be dead, and the cushioning has gone.
* Worn out body from overtraining, especially long runs;
* Tightness in the I-T band; Bowed legs;
* Weak hip abductors or poor hamstring flexibility;
* Unequal or weak quad strength or leg length differences predispose you to I-T.
* Too many laps of the track in one direction.

Some studies show that women are at higher risk for I-T Band Syndrome due to wider hips (on average).

According to a Stanford University study, weak gluteus medius muscles, the main hip abductors, can cause I-T band syndrome. To correct this, lie on your side and raise your straightened leg up and thus away from your middle. Turn the foot slightly upwards for these leg lifts. Do 15 to 30 reps with a one to two second hold at full abduction and visit the gym for weight training!

Other Preventions: Make training changes slowly. Replace your shoes: think stability. Motion control shoes stop unwanted motions...provided you get the right type for your feet and legs. Walk or warm up properly before moving at fast pace. Avoid hill repeats on a camber; if you must run on a camber or sloped road, keep the injured leg on the higher side; better yet, avoid road running because even a flat road surface is harder than dirt and grass. Avoid tight bends, corners and downhill running on asphalt.

Use the grass or dirt for downhills when possible. Run 300s and 500s in lane 5, instead of 400s in lane one. You'll run more straights and with less leaning over. Do your recoveries on the outside of the track, or on the grass. Change direction for some repeats. Do your I-T stretches (emphasize the hip) and stretch the other major muscles.

According to Dr. Michael Fredericson MD of Stanford University, the most effective I-T stretch is the hip lean. To stretch the Right I-T band, stand on your left leg, take the right foot around the back of the left and place it next to your left foot. Raise your arms and slowly lean away from the right hip to give a high force upon the I-T tissue from hip to knee.

Strengthen the weak quad with straight leg raises, leg extensions (if it does not exacerbate your problem), and the leg press. Exercise your hip abductors during weight training. Stretch these two groups plus the hamstrings and gluts. Do weight training for the hamstrings too. See a podiatrist to check if an orthotic insert for your running and your leisure shoes would help. Avoid hill running if your knees continue to hurt, or run a series of up-hill repeats on a long hill and get a ride back down, or leave a bike at the top and cruise down.

Treatment: Attack the causes; reduce mileage and take anti-inflammatory drugs for about 10 days. Use ice regularly. Massage and trigger point stimulation may help. Cortisone may help relieve the bursa. Surgery is an option - removal of the inflamed area or splitting the I-T band.

The top end of the band can cause problems too. A dull ache along the outer thigh may occur one to two miles into your runs; it often disappears at the end of the run. The bursa or fluid sack over the greater trochanter may become inflamed. Do your I-T stretches.

To decrease both types of knee insult, don't do stair climbing in rehab. Cycling at high cadence and elliptical training are more rhythmic.

Hip or Low back pain. Symptoms: Soreness, tension or
pain in the back, which if it's sciatica:
* May radiate down the buttock and back of the leg; with
* Tingling or numbness in the leg or foot;
* Plus, hamstring tightness; and,
* Secondary muscle spasms in the upper back or shoulders.
Sciatica is due to pressure on the sciatic nerve, the thick nerve which originates in the lower back goes down each buttock and the back of the legs. Sciatica usually affects one leg at a time, and can include shooting pains, or pins and needles. Piriformis syndrome can also cause the pain. Sciatica can come on slowly with a dull ache in the lower back.

Back pain is a common problem for the new runner, due to weakness after years of under use. Causes include:

* Leg length difference;
* Old back strains or vertebral disk problems, (the area of leg pain depends upon the origin of the spinal irritation);
* Weak abdominal muscles (see page 347);
* Failure to warmup properly;
* Leaning back or too far forward when running.

When running up and down hills you're likely to feel back pain after or toward the end of a hill session if you do them with bad form, make a sudden increase in the number of repeats, or try running too fast for your body. As this would make it an acute injury, you'll require active rest. Ten to 14 days later do another hill session, but with fewer reps and run perpendicular to the slope at 5K effort.

Prevention: Avoid being overweight. Whether purely a muscle problem or the sciatic or femoral nerve problem, you need to strengthen the abdominal muscles to improve posture and decrease irritation to the nerves. To reduce the strain on your lumbar spine, work on posture in all phases of your life. Do sit-ups with the legs bent, and the feet tucked in close to the buttocks.

Stretch hamstrings while easing the back through its range of motion. There is a direct correlation between tight hamstrings and bad backs, though it's difficult to say which comes first. Stretch the buttock muscles, I-T band, the piriformis and the calf muscles too of course. Lift (everything) properly by keeping the load close to you. Keep your back straight when lifting, use your leg muscles for the lift and avoid leaning or twisting while doing the lift.

Wear cushioned shoes on soft surfaces. Avoid sitting in one position for long periods.

Treatment: Exercise is better than rest for many back problems, and doubles your chance of being pain free in a year: however, a few non-running days in the acute phase is prudent. Use cross training if running hurts. Otherwise, keep to soft surfaces and avoid hills. Take NSAIDs and use ice alternating with moist heat. Have a massage or manipulation by an expert. Raising the feet should help to relax the initial strain, so use pillows at night. Try sleeping on your side with a pillow between your knees to take tension off of your lower back. Seek medical advice. An MRI is non-invasive. Find the cause or your back pain will come back.

There are medical conditions unrelated to running which can cause back pains, including the referred pain of heart attacks, gallstones, bladder infections and cancers. Initially, the back pain may be your only clue that you have a medical problem. Groin pains are also a clue to infections, especially if you can feel the lymph nodes.

If you repeatedly suffer from connective tissue injuries, or you have chronic injuries to the knee or Achilles, check to see if you need a full-length orthotic. Orthotics can prevent the feet collapsing inward on every stride, and enable you to push evenly off the ball of the foot, and from between the two biggest toes.

Most of the time, your training reaction takes weeks or months to show itself, either as improved performances, or aching limbs and injury, depending on how close to your optimum training you are. If injury occurred, you may need some days or weeks to get over it. Find the cause of your injury and then rebuild slowly.

Recovery, Injuries and Racing.

Aging, or a history of years of hard training and racing decrease your capacity to absorb landing forces (your elasticity), let alone to store that energy for your next stride. Taking one year off from running every 4 or 5 years gives all of your connective tissues a chance to regroup and completely heal from the previous few years of training and racing.

To paraphrase Tim Noakes MD, your Achilles won't rebound energy like a pogo stick forever.

You can still run an easy 40 minutes three days per week during your recovery year, but for the rest of your healthy exercise do non-impact activities such as cycling, swimming, pool running, elliptical training, weights and mobility and strength with yoga and pilates.

The break from racing also gives you a chance to regroup mentally. There comes a point in most races where it is your brain which keeps you going. A year off can bring back your enthusiasm for racing, and give you a better chance to run just as fast on the age-graded system as you did 2 years ago.

Some of you will prefer a modified down year at age 38, 43, 48 etc when you do half your usual mileage, and "jog" your 6 favorite races a minute per mile slower than last year while enjoying the atmosphere. Make sure the races are only one-third of <u>this</u> years weekly mileage.

At age 39, 44, 49 etc, you may do a gradual training build-up to reach peak condition for your new age group at 40, 45, 50 etc.

<u>Need more Injury Advice?</u> Your local running club or coaches probably know of experts. Also:
American Academy of Podiatric Sports Medicine
(800) 438-3355 - aapsm.org

American Chiropractic Association
(800) 986-4636 - amerchiro.org

American College of Sports Medicine
(317) 637-9200 - acsm.org

American Orthopaedic Society for Sports Medicine
(708) 292-4900
American Physical Therapy Association
(800) 999-2782 - apta.org

American Massage Therapy Association
(847) 864-0123 or (888) 843-2682   amtamassage.org
Or National Certification Board for Therapeutic Massage and Bodywork (800) 296-9664 ncbtmb.com
ART (Active Release Techniques) a form of scare tissue release. activerelease.com

Click where it hurts for 100 injuries at sportsinjuryclinic.net
Looking for trails? See trailrunner.com
Yoga for runners? Try bodywisdommedia.com
Pilates your passion? reabnyc.com has 8 classes.
Yoga and pilates CD at yogafit.com
Achilles short or got plantar fasciitis? thesock.com
<u>*www.liquidice.biz*</u> *for an ice wrap*

For detailed Cross Training: See *Best Half-Marathons.*

Appendix I

Health Benefits of Exercise

Do it at the right intensity and there's no pain with exercise. This is a partial list from Best Half Marathons. Decrease risk of:

Heart disease (the leading cause of death in western society)
Stroke or cerebrovascular accident (CVA) which is the third leading cause of death.
Cancer: From lung and breast to colorectal cancer.
Gallbladder surgery.
Decreases surgery complications.
Decreases the severity and the side effects from diabetes.
Lowers total cholesterol while improving your good cholesterol levels (HDL).
Trims your belly and gets rid of excess fat.
Decreases your common cold risk and makes it easier for you to recover from a cold because your immune cells circulate at a higher rate than when not exercising.
Decreases the pain of arthritis.
Reduces Tylenol needs.
Decreases Insomnia.
Reduces Deep Vein Thrombosis (DVTs) or blood clots.
Regular aerobic exercise improves the quality of your sleep and decreases the time that it takes to fall asleep. Makes you more productive and content during your active hours.
Elevates mood, releases tension and reduces anxiety and depression. Increases cognitive function and concentration.
Improves the health of your baby. You'll improve fetoplacental growth rates. Your postpartum recovery will be faster.
Stronger bones & fewer fractures from osteoporosis.

Appendix II

An Internet Question.

Lets see how helping a fellow runner can help all runners. Here is the marathon training of a sub 3-hour guy who is looking to do 2.50. He struggled (was sluggish) almost every time he went out for an hour run five days per week. His sessions in the build up included two interval workouts of 8 times 2 miles at 6:20 pace (goal time) or 2:46 marathon pace.

He fell apart at 20 miles in the marathon, and doesn't know how he managed to finish. He was on a very consistent 2:49 pace through mile 17.

Since that marathon, he decreased the number of days running to increase the quality of training. The last 10 Wednesdays he's included 5 to 6 one-mile repeats at 5:30 pace with a 60 second rest, with the last one at around 5:16 pace. He includes a 3 mile warm up and cool down. His philosophy is 10 out the door, i.e., he runs ten miles or not at all. He only runs 4 days per week, logging 50-52 miles. He also has 7 consecutive Saturday long runs of 20 miles.

Another run is what he calls a tempo when he does 7 of the 10 miles at 7 minute pace. The other day is around 7:30 pace.

Two weeks ago, he ran his interval workout on a Friday and then followed with a 20 in a 35-degree downpour on Saturday.

He recently ran 27:20 for 5 miles.

At age 32, he is trying to come up with researched based training rather than just tempo and intervals for a marathon.

He would like our opinion on how his body might hold up in comparison to his first marathon! What changes would you make to my training? Here was my reply.

You have many good points to your program. As you're making a return to running, you will make progress at the marathon with any training. You'll gradually maintain pace for 20, then 22 and eventually the entire 26.2.

But as you say, a little science will not hurt you: 4 runs per week are probably the best way to use 50-52 miles, (the same as Chapter 14), but do consider these pointers.

Add some variation to your long run...which needs to be at 7:30 per mile or SLOWER for a 2.50 marathon. Alternating 17, 20 and 22s give a challenge once every three weeks. Sneak in a 15 the week that you rest up for short races (one per month), and you'll have a nice 4 week rotation. When your weekend race is more than 10K, don't do a 17 the next day. Instead, run enough miles to reach 20 for the weekend. Example: 10 mile race with a 2 mile warm up and one mile cooldown, cruise 7 at easy pace the next day. The following weekend, start your 17 and longer rotation.

Check Chapter 14s two speed sessions per week schedule. It has only 11 runs of 20 miles in its 38-week schedule and one run of 22. Running a 20 week after week does work for some people, but more than three in a row is probably counterproductive except for 100 miles per week runners.

The midweek long run should also be 12 most weeks, except for once a month when you rest for a weekend race!

Your weekly mile repeats are at 10K to 5K pace based on your 5 mile time. This is an excellent session, at 90 to 95 percent of VO2 max. You're probably better off running them slower and for longer reps. As you've perfected the ability to run mile reps, you should not be doing them every week.

Restrict yourself to 10K pace for most Intervals. Interval training at 10K pace is easier on your body than 5K pace, yet still improves your VO2 Maximum and running economy. Note: Some runners have high VO2 maximum but poor running economy; some have excellent running economy but poor VO2 maximums. You need to perfect both.

Decreasing speed to 10K race pace but running longer repeats stimulate your oxygen uptake ability or your VO2 max system and force you to run more economically (if you think about your running form).

Longer repeats at 10K pace keep you in your training zone for a greater percentage of your training. Use 2K to 2 mile repeats at 10K pace.

You will also need to train at 5K pace though, so why not use mile repeats at 5K pace once every three weeks. Add in some shorter repeats at 3K pace to run at 100 % of VO2 max, or about 98 % of max heartrate. 4 x 500 meters at 3K pace at the end of 4 x one mile at 5K pace works fine. More options in Chapter Six.

I do like the 2-mile repeats at close to half marathon pace to improve your anaerobic threshold. However, 6:20 per mile is actually no-mans land for you. It's faster than you need to run at to stimulate aerobic endurance, mitochondria, blood volume, and red blood cells etc, yet it's slower than anaerobic threshold pace. You should probably run at half marathon to 15K race pace nearly every week to practice economy at modest tempo. 85 to 90 % of max HR is great training and very easy to sustain.

Scientifically speaking, based on that 5 mile race, those two-mile repeats should also be at or under 6 minutes per mile to stimulate your anaerobic threshold. Alas, two sessions are not enough, and 16 miles at 6.20 pace is probably excessive, unless you do it once instead of a half marathon, and after resting up and about 5 to 6 weeks pre-marathon to allow for recovery.

Threshold pace training gives huge rewards from 6-mile sessions, or not much more than 10 percent of your average weekly mileage, but should be done nearly every week.

Strictly speaking, your 7 mile tempo is not tempo pace, which would also be 6 minute miles based on your 5 mile time. Tempo pace is anaerobic threshold or 15K to half marathon race pace. 25 minutes or 4 miles is probably the limit for tempo pace running, after a short rest, another 2 miles would be fine at your mileage.

The goal of any speed session is to be able to run 10 to 20 miles the next day, which you did in the rain recently. Of course, having to bundle up in nasty conditions helps most runners to restrain training pace, so we should look forward to cold days when we wear three layers of clothing.

Match each speed session with a long run for a consistent training program. The long session at half marathon pace would be the exception to the rule, and could be a substitute for a 20.

I see no hills in your training. One out of every 8 sessions should be hill repeats or a very hilly course with surges at 5K intensity. Flatland dwellers can use bridges and treadmills for hill training. Adding a fifth run would increase endurance, but also increases injury risk. Five mile runs can be a joy. You don't have to restrict yourself to 10 or zero.

Adding weight training for 30 minutes, plus 30 minutes of cross training such as biking, elliptical training or running in the pool would be a preferable way to increase training. Because they are less specific, you usually need to spend more time cross training to get the equivalent of a mile of running. A combination of cross training activities can maintain or improve your running fitness.

Avoid long runs after weight training because your biomechanics can suffer due to fatigue in the last few miles, increasing injury risk. Weight training before a short run works well though, especially if you add 20 to 30 minutes of aerobic cross training at the end to give yourself the equivalent of a medium long run. Want to run long and weight train on the same day? Run first. Feed and hydrate, and then do the weight training.

Rest is achieved with your 4-day program, and hopefully you will decrease mileage by 25 % in the penultimate week and do half your usual training in the final week before your next marathon. Both will increase the chances of maintaining pace.

Monitor your carbohydrate and liquid intake every week but especially the last week. See Chapters 8 & 9. Practice taking in 200 calories per hour in your liquids, and replace 50 to 70 percent of the liquid that you sweat. Do the same in your marathon to help you maintain pace or to avoid bonking.

Start your marathon a bit slower. Run 2:51 to 2:52 marathon race pace for the first 10 miles, then increase the pace by 5 seconds per mile (2:49 pace) until the 20 mile point. If you still have the legs, increase by another 2 to 5 seconds a mile for your sub 2:50.

Not prepared to accept 15K pace or 85 to 92 percent of your maximum heartrate as lactate threshold pace? Buy a lactate analyzer and do finger stick blood tests at various intensities e.g. one mile tempo runs at current half marathon pace and at 5 seconds per mile speed increments to find your actual threshold point. Take longer than usual rests during this test because you'll probably do six one mile repeats and finish at close to 10K pace. See fact-canada.com

Record your level for speed and heartrate because your speed at threshold pace will improve as you get stronger, and as your running economy improves, but eventually decrease as you age.

Appendix III

Organizing your Track Night

Tuesday or Wednesday track groups often focus exclusively on running repeats at 5K pace or faster, which works for many runners because long reps at this pace are hard to do on your own. However, many runners miss out on three crucial intensities: 10K and 15K race pace to improve running economy and anaerobic threshold, and hill repeats.

Why not have a 4 week rotation so that everybody knows what the goal is, and can adjust the weekend session to meet his or her needs. If you meet every Tuesday, you could do.

1st Tuesday every month, 15K intensity
2nd Tue   10K effort
3rd Tue   5K speed
4th Tue   3K pace cruising
5th Tuesday when present, fartlek away from the track.

Rotate 3 sessions at each intensity (see chapters 5 to 7) and you'll only do each session 4 times per year with the group.

As mentioned elsewhere in this book, you can train with people who are faster or slower than you are. The month that the group is doing a 25 minute run at 15K intensity, some of the runners can do 2 x 10 minutes at 10K effort, or 3 x 6 minutes at 5K speed. You all get to help each other.

In week three, the slower runners may be at 3K pace, so on week 4 they will need to run slower than the fast guys to avoid running at mile pace. They could take a 10 second head start for each 600 meter rep and have the fast guys run even pace to catch them at the finish. You could also take a head start for mile reps at 5K or 10K effort in weeks 2 and 3 so that everybody is training at the same intensity.

THE AUTHOR

In 1994, David Holt ran 75 minutes for the half-marathon as part of his build-up for a serious marathon. Four weeks later his 2.37 over achieved on the prediction tables, (Slovic and others). His marathon was clearly the result of strength and endurance from a decade of competent and varied training.

Holt did not race marathons until well past his running peak. Slovic and the other prediction options for the marathon would have given Holt's 31.16 for the 10K, 53 minute 10 miles and 71 minutes for the half-marathon in 1987 and 1988 a projected 2:27:34 to 2:33:42 finish but he was too attached to medium distances to race longer than 20 miles.

At age 47, David cross trains copiously with biking, elliptical training, pool running, swimming and weight training.

David Holt's other printed books are:

Running Dialogue,

10K & 5K Running, Training & Racing,

5K Fitness Run and

Best Half-Marathons.

His next printed book will be 5K Fitness Walk, available in 2,005.

Holt has sold articles to Runner's World and Running Times, and writes a coaches corner for the Internet's Transitiontimes.com.

Holt's E-books include:

10K & 5K Running: Jog, Run and Train to Race 5K to 10 Miles is the e-book version of the printed 10K & 5K Running.

301 Balanced Eating & Nutrition Tips: Don't Diet for Exercise & Health.

401 Injury Prevention and Treatment tips to Walk, Jog, Run or Train 6 days a week.

Athletic Cross Training for Runners & Triathletes: Pool run, weight or elliptical train, bike & walk or jog to fitness or the triathlon.

INDEX

Marathon Pacing Chart

The small marathon pacing chart on page 381 shows just 5 miles at 5 seconds per mile slower than even pace at the start. You can make your own pace band with a slower early pace as described in Chapter 10 & 12, giving you steeper negative splits. You can also visit runnersworld.com and go through "marathon training" to find a pace band maker.

Page 381s chart gives only 5 sample time goals because the author is too lazy to make a chart at 2 second per mile intervals. Just kidding friends, you may actually get away with being over ambitious by 5 seconds per mile. As demonstrated by recent marathon performances by the world record breakers Radcliffe, Khannouchi and Tergat, and by United States 2004 Olympic medalists Deena Kastor and Meb Keflezighi, most of us should aim for negative splits.

Even pace marathon tables are extinct, so work out your finish goal time (pages 225-233) and then:

Divide by 26.2 to get your exact pace per mile at even pace. Decide how much slower you will run the first 5 miles and write your split times on your arm with waterproof ink or on waterproof paper to guide you.

Luckily, because of the crowds, most of you will be forced to run your first mile even slower. The 20 seconds or so that you think you've lost in the first mile can easily be made up from mile 15 to 26.2. Don't wind your way madly through the crowds and waste energy. The timing chip tied to your shoe will give the official time that you crossed the start line. Don't just go for the nice numbers shown on page 381.

Kastor's Bronze and Keflezighi's Silver medals at Athens in 2004 broke a 20 year Olympic drought for US marathoners. Their storming second halfs showed the best way to run a fast marathon and the best way to cope with hot conditions.

Stay in control and well hydrated as you ease through the first half of your marathons so as to give your body it's best chances of giving you your *Best Marathon*.

Goal Time or Pace.

	3 hours	8 minute miles	4 hours	4.5 hrs	5 hours
Ave speed	6:52	8:00	9:10	10:18	11:27
First 5 miles					
Each at	6:57	8:05	9:15	10:23	11:32
5 miles in	34:45	40:25	46:15	51:55	57:40
2nd 5 miles	6:52	8:00	9:10	10:18	11:27
5 mile split	34:20	40:00	45:50	51:30	57:15
10 mile time would be	69:05	1:20:25	1:32:05	1:43:25	1:54:55
Repeat the previous 5 miles for a 5 mile split of	34:20	40:00	45:50	51:30	57:15
At 15 miles	1:43:25	2:00:25	2:17:55	2:34:55	2:52:10

Somewhere during the 4th 5 mile section, you'll pick up the pace by 5 seconds per mile, but you only need 5 of your last 11 miles to be this quick. Maybe you'll start from the top of the overpass at mile 16, or it could be 18. Allow the course to decide when it's best to speed up slightly and reap the rewards of your easy start.

The average pace for the last 11.2 miles will only be 2.3 seconds per mile faster than from mile 5 to 15.

Ave speed of last 11.2	6:49.7	7:57.7	9:07.7	10:15.7	11:29.7

Page 240 shows a slightly different way to break up your race based on a 3 hour marathon, and you can adapt it for your own goal time.

5K Fitness Run: Walk, Jog & Train for Fun, Health & to Race the 5K.

220 pages, ISBN 0965889750…$14.95

Jogging and running programs, health tips, motivation, cross training and finding the time to run 12 to 30 miles per week. Includes numerous training programs based on time or mileage for all types of joggers and runners, plus 40 pages on cross training and chapters on stretching and nutrition.

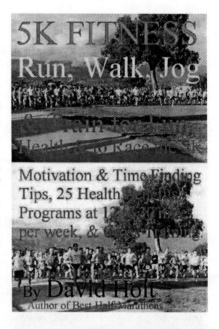

10K & 5K Running, Training & Racing:

ISBN 0965889718 $17.95

The Running Pyramid takes runners to the next level with 5 training phases including mileage base, hill running, anaerobic threshold training and Intervals to improve running economy and VO2 maximum.

Pick your mileage level at 20, 30, 40, 50 and 60 to 80 miles per week, then pick your intensity level and use the program that works for you, and refer to the detailed chapters as needed.

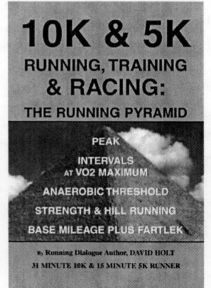

Best Half-Marathons:

marathon.

220 pages, ISBN 0965889769 is $17.95 Order Best Half-Marathons from any bookstore on main street or the Internet, on paper or as an e-book. The half-marathon is a more sensible goal for new runners. Use its 40 pages on cross training, plus running to get fit.

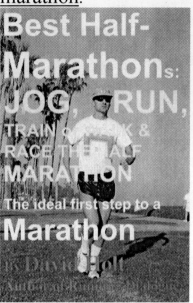

A year or more of half-marathon training, plus racing 3 to 4 half-marathons also lays a great foundation to run well at the...

The book in your hands is <u>Best Marathons</u> ISBN 096588970X. Order from stores on the high street, main street or the Internet for $17.95.

e-book format is also available from Internet retailers like Amazon.com or Barnes and Noble.

Want to buy your non-running friend a book, order <u>Best Half-Marathons</u> (see above) or choose from page 382.

For printed copies of <u>Best Marathons, Running Dialogue, 10K & 5K Running, Training & Racing, Best Half-Marathons</u> or <u>5K Fitness Run</u>, you can also mail your orders to.
    David Holt 3335 Richland Drive #4, Santa Barbara, CA 93105 Payment by check or money order please. $15.00 per book includes shipping. Tell me which books you are ordering!

David's advice also at http://www.runningbook.com

Printed in the United States
67461LVS00004B/110